The Paperless Medical Office Workbook

SECOND EDITION

Using Harris CareTracker

Virginia Ferrari

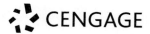
CENGAGE

Australia • Brazil • Mexico • Singapore • United Kingdom • United States

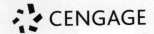

***The Paperless Medical Office Workbook:
Using Harris CareTracker,*** **2nd Edition**

Virginia Ferrari

SVP, GM Skills & Global Product Management:
Jonathan Lau

Product Director: Matthew Seeley

Product Team Manager: Stephen Smith

Senior Director, Development:
Marah Bellegarde

Senior Content Development Manager:
Juliet Steiner

Content Developer: Kaitlin Schlicht

Product Assistant: Mark Turner

Marketing Manager: Jonathan Sheehan

Senior Content Project Manager:
Thomas Heffernan

Art Director: Angela Sheehan

Production Service: SPi Global

Cover Images: VAlex/Shutterstock.com,
Vectorphoto/Shutterstock.com, smartdesign91/
Shutterstock.com, Bryan Solomon/
Shutterstock.com, Blan-K/Shutterstock.com,
Aha-Soft/Shutterstock.com, RedKoala/
Shutterstock.com

For product information and technology assistance, contact us at
Cengage Customer & Sales Support, 1-800-354-9706.

For permission to use material from this text or product,
submit all requests online at **www.cengage.com/permissions**.
Further permissions questions can be emailed to
permissionrequest@cengage.com.

Library of Congress Control Number: 2017957038

ISBN: 978-1-337-61421-4

Cengage
20 Channel Street
Boston, MA 02210
USA

Cengage is a leading provider of customized learning solutions with employees residing in nearly 40 different countries and sales in more than 125 countries around the world. Find your local representative at: **www.cengage.com.**

Cengage products are represented in Canada by Nelson Education, Ltd.

For your course and learning solutions, visit **www.cengage.com.**

Purchase any of our products at your local college store or at our preferred online store **www.cengagebrain.com.**

Printed in the United States of America
Print Number: 01   Print Year: 2017

Contents

List of Activities

Preface

Electronic technology is the major means through which workers communicate in today's health care environment. *The Paperless Medical Office Workbook: Using Harris CareTracker, 2nd Edition* is an electronic health record solution that integrates instructional theory with state-of-the-art Practice Management and Electronic Medical Record (EMR) software.

Harris CareTracker PM and EMR is one of the most advanced cloud-based practice management systems (PMs) and EMRs in the industry. The product is certified through the Certification Commission for Health Information Technology (CCHIT®) and is used by thousands of providers throughout the country. The Harris CareTracker product provides state-of-the-art features and user-friendly software, and is compliant with governmental mandates.

The PM side of Harris CareTracker is a sophisticated practice management system that automates time-consuming administrative tasks such as eligibility checks, scheduling, reminders, patient visit documentation, and claims submission. Its features include:

- Interactive dashboards that prioritize work lists automatically.
- A rules-based, front-end clinical editing tool that scrubs outgoing claims prior to submission.
- An online code lookup software that boosts coding accuracy.

The EMR side of Harris CareTracker monitors and measures all clinical data and prioritizes anything that needs attention. Some of the outstanding features of Harris CareTracker EMR include:

- Automatic refill requests
- Chart management
- Lab management
- Medication history
- Prescription (Rx) writing
- Report management

PURPOSE OF THE TEXT

The Paperless Medical Office Workbook: Using Harris CareTracker, 2nd Edition, was written to fill a void in today's EMR training market. There are many EMR training solutions available but this workbook provides 20–25 hours of step-by-step training activities that simulate typical work flows in ambulatory health organizations. This text takes students through critical information on integrating Electronic Health Record (EHR) software into the medical practice, and then offers step-by-step guidance on how those principles can be applied using the Harris CareTracker PM and EMR software.

Chapter 1 serves as an introduction to the EHR, including its benefits and core functions. Activities in Chapter 1 guide students through how to set up their computers for optimal performance, register their credentials, and create their personal Harris CareTracker training companies. Chapters 2 through 10 contain step-by-step front and back office activities for the students to complete. At the end of each activity, students are asked to print a screenshot or report that captures the work they have completed. Students are encouraged to keep this documentation in an "assignments" folder to be turned in to their instructor. Chapter 11 provides comprehensive case studies without the benefit of step-by-step instructions. Completing the case studies in Chapter 11 affirms proficiency using Harris CareTracker PM and EMR.

ORGANIZATION OF THE WORKBOOK

The Paperless Medical Office Workbook, 2nd Edition, is organized to match the daily flow of a medical office. The first two chapters serve as an introduction to the Harris CareTracker PM and EMR software, and how to navigate it. Beginning with Chapter 3, Patient Demographics and Registration, and continuing throughout the workbook, students follow the logical sequence of what occurs from the time the patient registers and schedules an appointment, through to processing the insurance claim form generated from the patient's visit.

The following breakdown summarizes what is included in each chapter:

Chapter 1: Introduction to the Paperless Medical Office

This chapter briefly discusses the process of converting paper health records to electronic health records and illustrates what occurs in an electronic health network. Students are also instructed on how to update their browser settings to be compatible with the Harris CareTracker software. Students will learn how to set up their computer for optimal performance, register their credentials, and create their Harris CareTracker training company.

Chapter 2: Introduction to Harris CareTracker PM and EMR

Students learn how to log in to Harris CareTracker in this chapter and use the *Help* system. Basic navigation functions of the *Main Menu*, *Home*, and *Dashboard* are presented here as well as the discussion of administrative features available within Harris CareTracker PM. Students will gain a firm understanding of using an electronic messaging system and will demonstrate their knowledge by performing messaging activities.

Chapter 3: Patient Demographics and Registration

In this chapter, students learn the fundamentals of entering patient demographics, registering new patients, and viewing and performing eligibility checks.

Chapter 4: Appointment Scheduling

Scheduling is the central theme of this chapter. Students will learn how to book, reschedule and cancel appointments, add patients to the wait list, and perform activities managing the daily schedule. Users will also learn how to check in patients, create a batch, accept payments, print patient receipts, run a journal, and post the batch.

Chapter 5: Preliminary Duties in the EHR

This chapter is where the EMR side of Harris CareTracker is introduced. Students will learn the significance of Meaningful Use and receive training in how to activate the care management registries. Users will perform basic maintenance functions such as adding a room, adding a custom resource, and managing immunizations. Learning how to navigate through the medical record is a large focus of the chapter.

Chapter 6: Patient Work-Up

In this chapter, students learn the major applications of the *Clinical Today* module—the clinical or EMR side of Harris CareTracker. Students will perform basic check-in duties, and track patients throughout the visit. Learning how to read the tasks menu and complete those tasks is a central focus in this chapter. Tasks may include items such as prescription renewals, electronic *ToDos*, outstanding lab reports or lab reports waiting for a response, and managing open encounters. This chapter emphasizes the importance of time management. In addition to these items, students learn how to record vital signs and chief complaints, view and create flow sheets, create and print growth charts, update the patient on preventative testing and health maintenance items, and create progress notes.

Chapter 7: Completing the Patient Visit

This chapter focuses on what occurs following the patient's examination. Students will learn how to complete requisitions for diagnostic orders for laboratory and radiology orders. Users will also learn how to access the correspondence application, create outgoing and incoming referrals, and complete the visit. Students will resolve open encounters and sign the progress note. In order to generate claims, charges must be captured for the patient's appointment. Students will enter procedure, and diagnostic codes for billing purposes.

Chapter 8: Other Clinical Documentation

In this chapter, users learn how to edit progress notes, add addendums, sign progress notes, and enter results into the patient's medical record. Students learn how to view, customize, graph, and print patient results and record messages. Additionally, users will create and update patient recall letters, and use the clinical export feature to run an immunization report.

Chapter 9: Billing

Students switch back to administrative tasks in this chapter. Once the visit is completed, the financial activities begin. Creating a batch for financial activities, manually entering charges, and editing an unposted charge are just a few of the activities in this chapter. Users will also learn how to generate electronic and paper claims and perform activities related to electronic remittance.

Chapter 10: ClaimsManager and Collections

In this chapter users will learn the functions of the *ClaimsManager* feature in Harris CareTracker and will check the status of unpaid or inactive claims. Generating patient statements and navigating the collections process are also introduced in this chapter.

Chapter 11: Applied Learning for the Paperless Medical Office

This chapter is the finale of the workbook. It includes several case studies that test the users' comprehension of the material presented throughout the text, without providing step-by-step instructions. Students build both competence and confidence from performing activities in this chapter.

NEW TO THIS EDITION

The second edition of this text has been revised to improve student support. Updates include:

- A **Best Practices** guide at the beginning of the book outlines key tips for working in Harris CareTracker PM and EMR.
- A **Student Companion Website** includes some video tutorials and a mapping grid showing chapter activities you can reference for help when completing the Applied Learning Case Studies (Chapter 11).
- To show greater distinction between the different tasks performed in an EMR, the text has been divided into five **modules**: Get Started, Administration Skills, Clinical Skills, Billing Skills, and Apply Your Skills.
- A **Quick Start Guide** begins each module. This Quick Start Guide identifies the prerequisite activities required to advance with the module. Students can review this Quick Start Guide prior to starting a module to ensure that they have not missed any key steps. Students on a wheel curriculum will be able to start the text at four different points (Get Started, Administrative Skills, Clinical Skills, or Billing Skills) by starting with a Quick Start Guide.
- A **Critical Thinking** feature included throughout the chapters helps the student think about and address issues they may face on the job.
- **Required icons** appear next to chapter activities that are required in order to proceed. This helps prevent students from skipping over necessary activities.

As a result of these changes, activities in each chapter have been reorganized and some activities have also been rewritten for greater clarification. In addition to reorganizing the text and updating activities, some content updates have been made. Major content updates include:

- ICD-10 coding with a reference to ICD-9 only for historical information
- Enhanced demographics update
- Notation of required activities

FEATURES

The *Help* system within the Harris CareTracker software includes a plethora of educational materials and training tutorials that provide tips for using Harris CareTracker PM and EMR. In addition to text materials, the Harris CareTracker *Help* system provides training videos that walk users through each function within the system. Because this product is a live program, updated training materials containing the most recent information for Meaningful Use, ICD-10, and HIPAA are available.

The 20–25 hours of hands-on, step-by-step training activities include critical thinking components. Students not only learn how to use the different functions of the Harris CareTracker software but also how to change settings in the software to meet meaningful use goals and to satisfy individual preferences. The *Clinical Today* module within Harris CareTracker PM and EMR assists students in learning how to manage daily, weekly, and monthly tasks, promoting organization, and time management.

Unique features of the text also include:

- **Learning Objectives** state chapter goals and outcomes.
- The **Real-World Connection** feature at the start of each chapter contains information regarding a day-in-the-life of a medical assistant working in a medical practice using electronic health records. The "real world" scenarios are meant to stimulate thought and critical thinking.
- **Professionalism Connection** boxes provide helpful information on how students can best present themselves in a professional manner. This includes showing proficiency in assigned tasks as well as communicating and interacting effectively with patients and staff.
- **Spotlight** boxes highlight important material included throughout the text. It is critical that users of EHR software are familiar with this information.
- **Alert** boxes present critical information to know when completing activities in Harris CareTracker PM and EMR.
- **Required** icons alert students to activities that are required within a chapter in order for them to proceed with that chapter and later activities.
- **Tip** boxes provide helpful hints for using Harris CareTracker PM and EMR.
- **FYI** boxes provide details on functions of Harris CareTracker PM and EMR that are available in real-world settings but are not available in your student version of Harris CareTracker.
- **Step-by-Step Activities** give instructions on how to complete front and back office functions in Harris CareTracker PM and EMR. They feature detailed information on steps to be performed as well as screenshots that illustrate key steps.
- **Case Studies** provide additional opportunity for students to test their ability to complete key chapter activities without the benefit of step-by-step instructions.

DISCLAIMER

Due to the evolving nature and continuous upgrades of real-world EHRs such as this one, as you log in and work in your student version of Harris CareTracker there may be a slightly different look to your live screen from the screenshots provided in the text.

Keep in mind that you will be asked to work in "current dates" when completing activities, so your appointment and encounter dates will not match those used in the workbook screenshots.

When prompted, follow the instructions given in the workbook to complete the activities.

LEARNING PACKAGE FOR THE STUDENT

Student Companion Website

Cengage's Student Companion Website to accompany *The Paperless Medical Office: Using Harris CareTracker, 2nd Edition* is a complementary resource that includes additional support such as a blank Patient Registration Form for additional practice, some video tutorials, and a mapping grid showing which chapter activities you can reference for help when completing the Applied Learning Case Studies (Chapter 11). To access the Student Companion Website from CengageBrain, go to http://www.cengagebrain.com, and key ISBN 9781337614191 in the **Search** window. Locate the *The Paperless Medical Office: Using Harris CareTracker, 2nd Edition* and click on the title. Scroll to the bottom of the page and click on the **Free Materials** tab, then **Save to MyHome**. Once you have added it to "My Home," click on the product under "My Products" for access to the Student Companion Website.

TEACHING PACKAGE FOR THE INSTRUCTOR

Instructor Companion Website

(ISBN 978-1-337-61422-1)

Spend less time planning and more time teaching with Cengage's Instructor Companion Website to accompany *The Paperless Medical Office: Using Harris CareTracker, 2nd Edition*. As an instructor, you will have access to all of your resources online, anywhere and at any time. All instructor resources can be accessed by going to www.cengage.com/login to create a unique user log-in. The password protected instructor resources include the following:

- Answer keys for workbook activities and case studies.
- Mapping of the Applied Learning Case Studies (Chapter 11) to the in-text Activity number for reference.
- Spreadsheet showing which patients appear in which activities as well as what activities are required.
- Blank Patient Registration Form to use for additional assignment/practice.

ABOUT THE AUTHOR

Virginia Ferrari is a former adjunct faculty member at Solano Community College in the Career Technical Education/Business division, where she taught medical front office, medical coding, and small business courses. In addition, she has been a contributing author for other Cengage Learning textbooks, including the Seventh and Eighth Editions of *Medical Assisting: Administrative and Clinical Competencies* and the Second Edition of *Clinical Medical Assisting: A Professional, Field Smart Approach to the Workplace*. Prior to joining Solano Community College, Virginia served as the manager of extended services for one of the fastest-growing physician networks in the San Francisco Bay area. In addition to overseeing the conversion and implementation of electronic medical records, she served on the Best Practice Committee, Customer Satisfaction Committee, Pilot Project for Risk Adjust Coding, and Team Up for Health, a national collaborative for Diabetes Self-Management Education. Virginia holds dual bachelor degrees in sociology and family and consumer studies from Central Washington University and a master's degree in health administration from the University of Phoenix. Virginia also holds certification from the National Healthcareer Association as a Certified Electronic Health Record Specialist (CEHRS), is a previous member of the AAMA Editorial Advisory Committee, and current member of the AAMA Leadership Committee.

System Requirements for Harris CareTracker

MINIMUM REQUIREMENTS

- Intel core or Xeon processor
- Operating System: Windows 7, Windows 8, Windows 10, iPad IOS6
- Windows 7: 8 GB
- Microsoft Internet Explorer 11.
- Acrobat Reader
- Adobe Flash
- Java
- 1024 × 768 resolution

THIRD-PARTY SOFTWARE

Third-party software (such as Yahoo! and Google toolbars, or Norton and McAfee) does not follow the rules setup in Internet options; therefore it tends to block Harris CareTracker functionality with respect to pop-ups. If this does happen, then you need to add training.caretracker.com and rapidrelease.caretracker.com to the allowed or safe sites lists of those programs. Follow the instructions in the next section, Internet Settings (Add as Safe Site).

INTERNET SETTINGS
(Add as Trusted Site)

1. Open Internet Explorer browser window.
2. On the menu bar, click Tools and then select Internet Options from the menu. Internet Explorer displays the Internet Options dialog box.
3. Click the Security tab and then click Trusted Sites.
4. Click Sites. Internet Explorer displays the Trusted Sites dialog box.
5. In the Add this website to the zone box, type: training.caretracker.com
6. Click Add. Internet Explorer adds the address to trusted sites.
7. Repeat steps 5 and 6 for rapidrelease.caretracker.com.
8. Deselect the Require server verification (https:) for all sites in this zone checkbox.
9. Click Close to close the Trusted Sites box.
10. Click OK on the Internet Options box to save your changes.

Compatibility View Settings

1. In Internet Explorer 11, launch the website for which you want to disable Compatibility View (www.cengage.com/caretracker).
2. If the menu bar is not visible, press the **Alt** key to display the browser menu.
3. On the browser menu, click the Tools > Compatibility View Settings. The browser opens the Compatibility View Settings window.
4. In the "Websites you've added to Compatibility View" section, remove caretracker.com if it appears there.

BANDWIDTH RECOMMENDATIONS

If there are multiple workstations utilizing Harris CareTracker, then each will require a minimum of 300 kb of bandwidth per active workstation with a DSL or Cable connection. For a T1 or Dedicated connection, a minimum of 60 kb per workstation is required.

RECOMMENDED SCREEN RESOLUTION

The recommended screen resolution is 1024 × 768.

SUPPORTED BROWSER

Harris CareTracker supports only Internet Explorer 11 for desktop devices. Safari for iPad may also be used. Mozilla Firefox and Google Chrome are not yet supported.

Best Practices for Harris CareTracker

Certain best practices should be followed whenever you are working in Harris CareTracker. A list of these best practices is provided below. Continue reading for more information on these best practices.

- Before beginning work each day, check the News application in CareTracker for updates from Harris CareTracker and Cengage. To do so, click on the Home Module and then click on the News tab.
- Check your browser. Use only Internet Explorer 11 (IE 11) or Safari for iPad.
- Check Compatibility View settings. "Display intranet sites in Compatibility View" and "Use Microsoft compatibility lists" should be unchecked.
- Clear your cache each time you start working in Harris CareTracker.
- If you receive a "Duplicate Session" error message, close your browser window. Then open a new Internet Explorer browser window. In the new window, select File>New Session.
- Prior to completing an activity, read all of the activity directions first, before completing any steps.
- When directed to "print," if a print button is not available in Harris CareTracker, take a screenshot of your work.
- Properly log out when you are finished working.
- For technical support questions, check your student companion website for solutions. If you can't find a solution to your issue, contact Cengage.

Check Your Browser

Harris CareTracker supports only Internet Explorer 11 and Safari for iPad.

To Determine Your Browser

You can determine the basic type of browser you are using by looking at the icon at the bottom of your computer screen, in the Start Menu, on the Desktop, or on your Task Bar. Internet Explorer or Safari for iPad are required for using Harris CareTracker. **Figure 1** shows the Internet Explorer icon. **Figure 2** shows the Safari icon

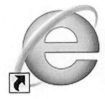

Figure 1
Internet Explorer
Icon

Used with permission from Microsoft

Figure 2
Safari Icon

Used with permission of Apple Inc.

(which is compatible with Harris CareTracker for iPads only). **Figure 3** shows other icons that are *not* compatible with Harris CareTracker (Google Chrome, Microsoft Edge, and Mozilla Firefox).

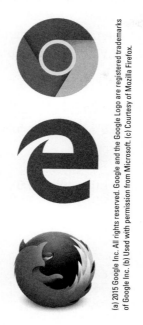

(a) 2015 Google Inc. All rights reserved. Google and the Google Logo are registered trademarks of Google Inc. (b) Used with permission from Microsoft. (c) Courtesy of Mozilla Firefox.

Figure 3 Google Chrome, Microsoft Edge, and Mozilla Firefox Icons

To Determine Your Browser Version

There are multiple versions of Internet Explorer. You must be working in Internet Explorer 11 to use Harris Care-Tracker. To determine which version you have, click on the Internet Explorer icon on your device. In the browser window, click on "Help" to bring up the Help menu (**Figure 4**). Click "About Internet Explorer" and you will see the pop up showing what version of IE you are using (**Figure 5**).

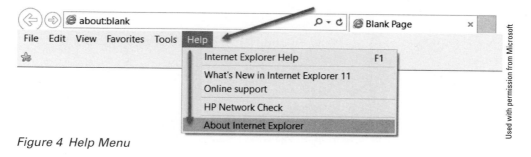

Used with permission from Microsoft

Figure 4 Help Menu

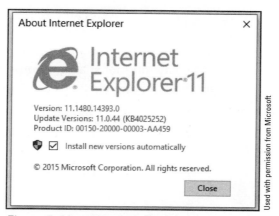

Used with permission from Microsoft

Figure 5 About Internet Explorer

To Locate Internet Explorer in Windows 10

Newer Windows computers may not have Internet Explorer installed and you will need to install prior to working in Harris CareTracker. To locate IE 11 in Windows 10, select the Start button and search for "Internet Explorer." If IE 11 is installed, you will see it pop up at the top of the search results. Search Microsoft's Support page for more help if needed, or to install IE 11 on your Windows computer.

Check Compatibility View Settings

You will need to change your Compatibility View Settings as follows.

1. Open up Internet Explorer 11 (IE 11).
2. Click on the Tools menu tab.
3. Select the Compatibility View settings option (**Figure 6**).

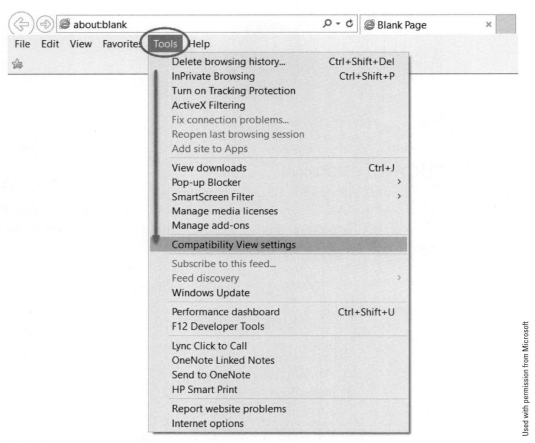

Figure 6 Compatibility View Settings

4. In the resulting popup, uncheck the "Display intranet sites in Compatibility View" option (Figure 7).
5. Uncheck "Use Microsoft compatibility lists" (**Figure 7**).
6. Click Close.

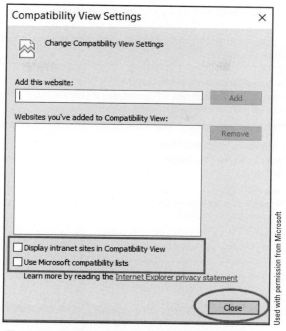

Figure 7 *Change Compatibility View Settings*

Clear Your Cache

You should clear your cache each time you begin working in CareTracker. To clear your cache in Internet Explorer 11:

1. Open an Internet Explorer® browser window.
2. From the *Tools* menu, select *Internet Options*. Windows® displays the *Internet Options* dialog box.
3. On the *General* tab, in the *Browsing history* section, click *Delete...* (**Figure 8**). Windows® displays the *Delete Browsing History* dialog box.

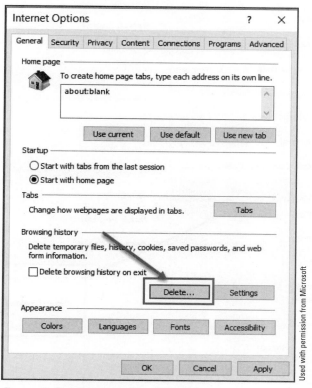

Figure 8 *Delete Browsing History*

4. Deselect the *Preserve Favorites website data* checkbox (**Figure 9**).

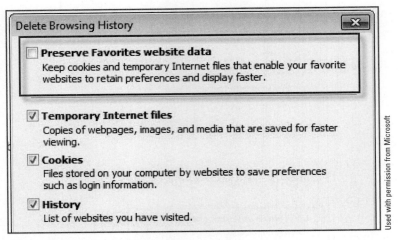

Figure 9 Preserve Favorites

5. Select the *Temporary Internet files, Cookies,* and *History* checkboxes only.
6. Click *Delete*.
7. Click *OK* when finished.

To clear your cache in Safari for iPad:

1. Tap *Settings* from your iPad® home screen.
2. Tap *Safari*® from the *Settings* pane on the left. The *Safari*® *Pane* displays *Clear History, Clear Cache,* and *Clear Cookies* at the bottom (**Figure 10**).

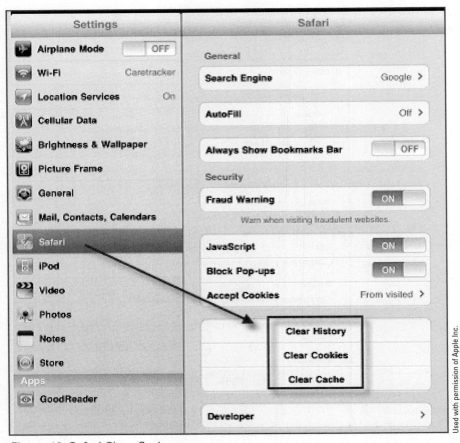

Figure 10 Safari Clear Cache

3. Tap *Clear History*. iPad® displays a confirmation window.
4. Tap *Clear* in the confirmation window.
5. Repeat steps 3 and 4 to clear your cache and cookies (refer to Figure 10).

Resolve a "Duplicate Session" Error Message

If you receive a "Duplicate Session" error message, close your browser window. Open a new Internet Explorer browser window. In the new window, select File > New Session. You should now be able to access Harris CareTracker.

Take a Screenshot

Throughout the text you will be instructed to "print" or in some cases, take a screen shot, of your work to submit to your instructor as confirmation of activity completion. To take a screenshot with your PC:

1. Find the screen you need to print out (this will usually be noted in your "end of activity print instruction").
2. Using your keyboard commands, take a screenshot. Depending on the computer you are using, the way you take a screenshot may vary. Typically, a screenshot can be captured using the Print Screen [PrtSc] key on your computer. Some users may need to press the key [Alt] and [PrtSc] to capture only the active window.
3. Open a Word document.
4. Using the Paste command, paste the image from the screen onto your Word document. This can also be accomplished by either right clicking your mouse and choosing one of the Paste options, or by left clicking anywhere in the Word document and pressing the keys [Ctrl] and [V] to paste the image onto the Word document.
5. Save the Word document and submit the document to your instructor as advised (electronically or paper).

Log Out of Harris CareTracker

It is important to properly log out of CareTracker when you are done with your session. Do not simply close the window, but instead, click on *Log Off* in Harris CareTracker **(Figure 11)**.

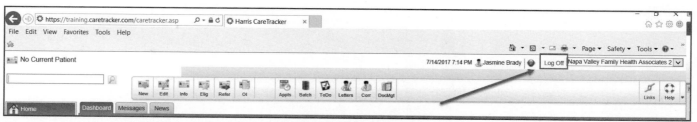

Figure 11 *Properly Log Off Harris CareTracker PM and Physician EMR*

Courtesy of Harris CareTracker PM and Physician EMR

Contact Cengage for Technical Support When Needed

If you have technical support questions while working through the activities in *The Paperless Medical Office*, check your student companion website for help. You can access your student companion website through logging in or creating a free student account at login.cengage.com, clicking on Find Free Study Tools, searching for and adding the ISBN 9781337614191 and then clicking on the product under My Products. If you are unable to resolve your issue through the support posted to the student companion website, then contact Cengage technical support at www.cengage.com/support.

 WARNING!! Do not purchase a "used textbook," as the credentials would have already been registered and cannot be used again. You must have a new textbook with your own credentials in order to be able to create your training company for work in Harris CareTracker.

MODULE 1
Get Started

This module includes:

- Chapter 1: Introduction to the Paperless Medical Office
- Chapter 2: Introduction to Harris CareTracker PM and EMR

In order to complete activities in Harris CareTracker, you must first set up your computer for optimal functionality. You will then register your credentials and create your Harris CareTracker training company.

If you are beginning your work starting with this module, follow along from the beginning and complete all the Required ⚑ activities as you move sequentially through the text.

Introduction to the Paperless Medical Office

Learning Objectives

1. Set up your computer for optimal functionality when using Harris CareTracker PM and EMR.
2. Create a Harris CareTracker training company.
3. Describe core functions, advantages, and disadvantages of the EMR/EHR.
4. Summarize administrative workflows in Harris CareTracker.
5. Identify clinical workflows in Harris CareTracker.

Real-World Connection

Welcome to Napa Valley Family Health Associates (NVFHA), your Harris CareTracker training company! Our practice is located in the beautiful Napa Valley in California. The practice consists of four providers, six medical assistants, one X-ray technician, and a medical lab scientist who oversees our laboratory. As a medical assisting student, you will rotate among our four providers:

- Amir Raman, DO (Specialty—Internal Medicine)
- Anthony Brockton, MD (Specialty—Family Practice)
- Rebecca Ayerick, MD (Specialty—Family Practice/Pediatrics)
- Gabrielle Torres, NP (Specialty—Family Practice)

We are a busy family health center and take care of patients across the lifespan. To be considered for a job in our practice, you must have a caring attitude, have strong administrative and clinical skills, and get along well with people of all ages and all socioeconomic backgrounds.

We are a practice that believes in a proactive approach to health care. We look for ways to improve patient outcomes while driving down health care costs. As a matter of fact, we recently applied for and received NCQA Patient-Centered Medical Home (PCMH) Recognition. The PCMH is a care delivery model whereby patient treatment is coordinated through their primary care provider to ensure the patient receives the necessary care when and where they need it, in a manner they can understand. Becoming a PCMH is a way of organizing primary care that emphasizes care coordination and communication to transform primary care into "what patients want it to be." Medical homes are intended to lead to higher quality care, lower costs, and improved outcomes. We chose Harris CareTracker PM and Physician EMR as our electronic health record system because of its robust functions and reporting capabilities, which are essential to a PCMH model.

This workbook focuses on technical skills, but do not be surprised if you learn a few other skills along the way! Throughout the text, you will be challenged to think critically and perform to the best of your ability. Your first challenge is to carefully read the instructions and implement all of the settings for the activities/features outlined in this first chapter. Failure to implement the recommended settings may result in an inability to perform some activities. Let's get started!

SET UP COMPUTER FOR OPTIMAL FUNCTIONALITY

Learning Objective 1: Set up your computer for optimal functionality when using Harris CareTracker PM and EMR.

In order to complete activities in Harris CareTracker, you must first set up your computer for optimal functionality. You will then register your credentials and create your Harris CareTracker training company. Because it may take up to 24 hours for your student company to be created, you will complete the activities in Learning Objectives 1 and 2 now.

Readiness Requirements

In order to use Harris CareTracker, you must meet the minimum system requirements and update your browser settings. You'll walk through these requirements in the activities in this chapter.

 TIP You will find up-to-date *System Requirements and Recommendations* in the *Help* system of Harris CareTracker at *Help > Contents tab > System Requirements and Recommendations* folder. Chapter 2 will introduce you to *Help* and the various content and training available.

To use Harris CareTracker PM and EMR, your computer must have Internet Explorer® version 11. Other browsing software (outside of Safari® for iPad®) may work differently with the application. See the System Requirements section for further technology requirements. Chrome and Firefox are not currently supported. While iPads are compatible with Harris CareTracker, Macs cannot be used to register an access code, also known as your credentials. In an EHR, credentials are the login information required to access the software, which is the assigned username and password.

Disable Third-Party Toolbars

Remove all third-party toolbars (Google, Yahoo!, Bing, AOL, etc.) from Internet Explorer®. Third-party toolbars cause random performance and functionality issues within Harris CareTracker PM and EMR. Complete Activity 1-1 to disable toolbars.

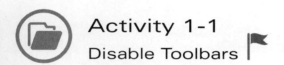

Activity 1-1
Disable Toolbars

1. Open an Internet Explorer® browser window.

2. Right-click on the menu bar. The browser displays a list of toolbars. Active toolbars appear with a check mark to the left of the name (**Figure 1-1**).

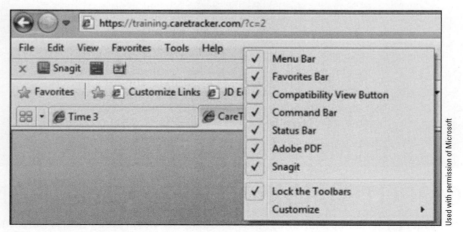

Figure 1-1   Disable Toolbars

3. Uncheck the toolbars you want to disable (Google, Yahoo!, Bing, AOL, etc. if displaying). Internet Explorer® disables the toolbar if that toolbar does not have a check mark next to it.

Setting Up Tabbed Browsing

Tabbed browsing allows you to open multiple websites in a single browser window. It is very important to set this up to access several patient charts at one time in a single browser. This will make switching between patients much easier and enables you to have multiple items open on the task bar. Complete Activity 1-2 to set up tabbed browsing.

Activity 1-2
Set Up Tabbed Browsing

1. Open an Internet Explorer® browser window.

2. Select *Tools > Internet Options* from the browser menu. The *Internet Options* dialog box displays.

3. In the *Tabs* section, click *Tabs*. The *Tabbed Browsing Settings* dialog box displays.

4. Select the following options noted below and in **Figure 1-2**:

    • Warn me when closing multiple tabs

    • Always switch to new tabs when they are created

    • Show previews for individual tabs in the taskbar*

    • Enable Tab Groups*

    • When a new tab is opened, open: Your first home page

    • When a pop-up is encountered: Let Internet Explorer decide on how pop-ups should open

    • Open links from other programs in: A new window

    *Takes effect after you restart your computer

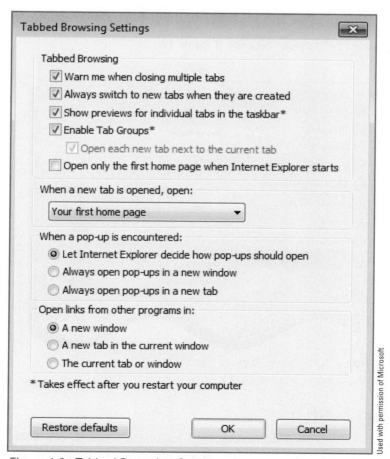

Figure 1-2   Tabbed Browsing Settings

5. Click *OK* to close the *Tabbed Browsing Settings* box.

6. Click *OK* on the *Internet Options* box to save your changes.

Disable Pop-Up Blocker

A pop-up window is a small web browser window that appears on top of the website you are viewing. This allows you to avoid having to navigate away from the current window you are viewing. Harris CareTracker PM and EMR uses the pop-up mechanism, enabling an efficient workflow. Many computers have firewall protectors that alleviate nonsense pop-up ads from displaying as you work on a website. However, you must enable pop-ups to use the functionality within Harris CareTracker PM and EMR. Complete Activity 1-3 to turn off pop-up blocker in Internet Explorer® and Safari®.

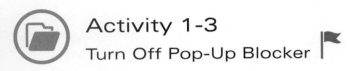

Activity 1-3
Turn Off Pop-Up Blocker

1. To disable pop-up blocker in Internet Explorer, open an Internet Explorer® browser window.

2. Select *Tools* > *Pop-up Blocker* > *Turn Off Pop-up Blocker* from the browser menu.

To disable pop-up blocker in Safari® for iPad®:

1. Tap *Settings* from your iPad® home screen.

2. Tap *Safari®* from the *Settings* panes on the left. The *Safari®* pane displays the browser options.

3. Tap *Block Pop-ups* to turn off pop-up blocker (**Figure 1-3**).

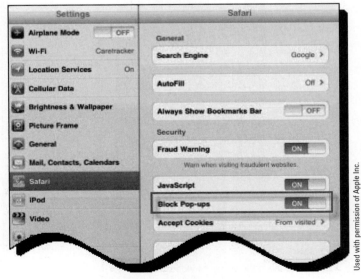

Figure 1-3 Safari® Pop-up Blocker

Change the Page Setup

It is important to change the default margin, header, and footer settings to print letters, forms, and claims in Harris CareTracker PM and EMR. Complete Activity 1-4 to change page setup.

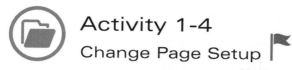

Activity 1-4
Change Page Setup

1. Open an Internet Explorer® browser window (one such as your Harris CareTracker training company). **Note**: You must have an actual website up, not just a blank/new tab.

2. On the browser menu bar, click *File*. Then choose *Page setup* from the menu. Internet Explorer® launches the *Page Setup* dialog box.

3. Delete the values in the *Margins* (*inches*) fields. Leaving these fields blank will automatically set their value to zero.

4. Select *Empty* in each of the *Header* and *Footer* fields. Click *OK*.

Downloading Plug-ins

A plug-in is a program that works with Harris CareTracker PM and EMR to give added functionality. Follow each link to download the required plug-in for free, if you don't have the plug-in already.

- Adobe Reader (*www.adobe.com, search for "Reader"*)
  - *To view, navigate, and print PDF files.*
- Adobe Flash (*www.adobe.com, search for "Flash Player"*)
  - *To view animation and interactive content.*
- Java (*www.java.com*)
  - *To run applications and applets that use Java technology. Java is required to view prerecorded sessions.*

Adding Trusted Sites

Add *training.caretracker.com* and *rapidrelease.caretracker.com* to the trusted site list. Otherwise some functionality may be blocked, such as running ActiveX controls and installing browser plug-ins. Adding trusted sites also allows your computer to distinguish between secured sites and harmful sites. Complete Activity 1-5 to add trusted sites.

Activity 1-5
Add Harris CareTracker to Trusted Sites

1. Open an Internet Explorer® browser window.

2. On the menu bar, click *Tools* and then select *Internet Options* from the menu. Internet Explorer® displays the *Internet Options* dialog box.

3. Click the *Security* tab and then click *Trusted Sites*.

4. Click *Sites*. Internet Explorer® displays the *Trusted sites* dialog box.

5. Deselect the *Require server verification (https:) for all sites in this zone* checkbox.

6. In the *Add this website to the zone* box, type *training.caretracker.com*.

7. Click *Add*. Internet Explorer® adds the address to trusted sites.

8. In the *Add this website to the zone* box, type *rapidrelease.caretracker.com*.

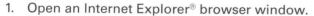

9. Click *Add*. Internet Explorer® adds the address to trusted sites (**Figure 1-4**).

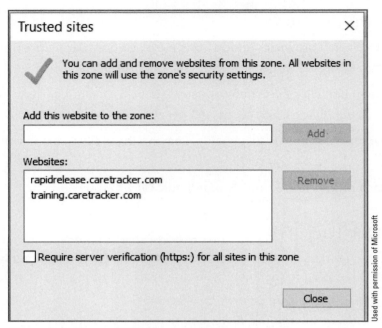

Figure 1-4   Trusted Sites

10. Click *Close* to close the *Trusted Sites* box.

11. Click *OK* on the *Internet Options* box to save your changes.

Clearing the Cache

The cache is a space in your computer's hard drive and random access memory (RAM) where your browser saves copies of recently visited web pages. Typically, these items are stored in the *Temporary Internet Files* folder. It is important to clear your cache on a regular basis and at every release for Harris CareTracker PM and EMR to function more efficiently.

 IMPORTANT!! You must clear your cache prior to logging in to Harris CareTracker PM and EMR. If you are already logged in, log out of Harris CareTracker before clearing your cache.

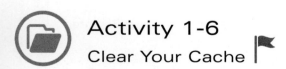

Activity 1-6
Clear Your Cache

To clear your cache in Microsoft Internet Explorer® 11:

1. Open an Internet Explorer® browser window.

2. From the Internet Explorer® 11 *Tools* menu, select *Internet Options*. Windows® displays the *Internet Options* dialog box.

3. On the *General* tab, in the *Browsing history* section, click *Delete...* (**Figure 1-5**). Windows® displays the *Delete Browsing History* dialog box.

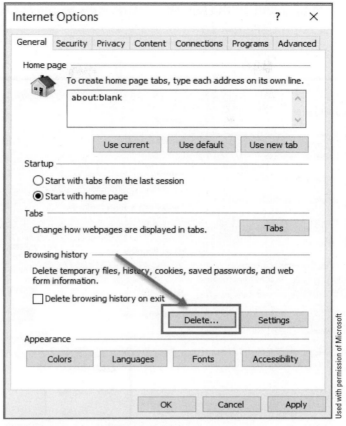

Figure 1-5   Delete Browsing History

4. Deselect the *Preserve Favorites website data* checkbox (**Figure 1-6**).

5. Select the *Temporary Internet files and website files, Cookies and website data*, and *History* checkboxes only.

6. Click *Delete*.

7. Click *OK* when finished.

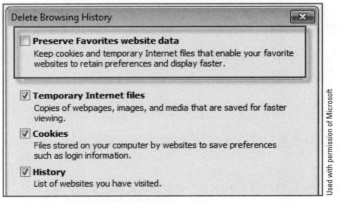

Figure 1-6   Preserve Favorites

To clear your cache in Safari® for iPad®:

1. Tap *Settings* from your iPad® home screen.

2. Tap *Safari®* from the *Settings* pane on the left. The *Safari® Pane* displays *Clear History*, *Clear Cache*, and *Clear Cookies* at the bottom (**Figure 1-7**).

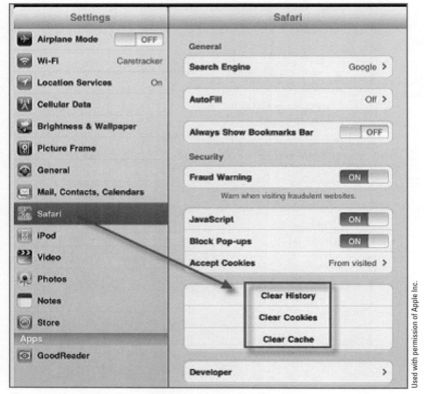

Figure 1-7   Safari Clear Cache

3. Tap *Clear History*. iPad® displays a confirmation window.

4. Tap *Clear* in the confirmation window.

5. Repeat steps 3 and 4 to clear your cache and cookies (refer to **Figure 1-7**).

Setting Your Home Page

Your home page is displayed when Internet Explorer® first opens. You can choose to set Harris CareTracker PM and EMR as your home page if necessary.

Activity 1-7

Setting Harris CareTracker as Home Page

1. Open an Internet Explorer® browser window.

2. Select *Tools > Internet Options* from the browser menu. The *Internet Options* dialog box displays.

3. In the *Address* box of the *Home page* section, type: *http://www.cengage.com/CareTracker* (**Figure 1-8**).

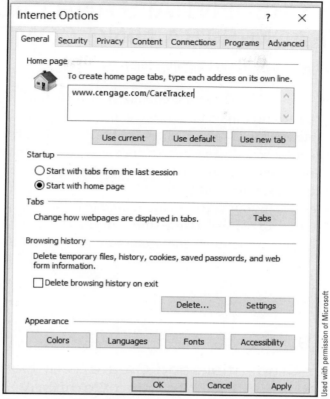

Figure 1-8   Home Page

4. Click *OK*. Harris CareTracker PM and EMR will display as your home page the next time you open Internet Explorer®.

Disable Download Blocking

Complete Activity 1-8 to disable download blocking.

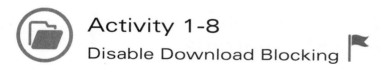

Activity 1-8
Disable Download Blocking

1. Open an Internet Explorer® browser window.

2. Select *Tools > Internet Options* from the browser menu. The browser displays the *Internet Options* dialog box.

3. Click the *Security* tab.

4. Click the *Internet* (globe) link.

5. Click the *Custom level...* button.

6. Scroll down to the *Downloads* section.

7. In the *File Download* section, click *Enable*. Click *OK*.

8. Click *OK* in the *Internet Options* window to close it.

Now that you have set your computer to the required settings to work in Harris CareTracker PM and EMR, you will register your credentials and log in to begin your training.

REGISTER YOUR CREDENTIALS AND CREATE YOUR HARRIS CARETRACKER TRAINING COMPANY

Learning Objective 2: Create a Harris CareTracker training company.

You will be assigned a user name and password (your credentials) to log in to Harris CareTracker PM and EMR. Your preassigned user name and password can be found on the inside front cover of your workbook. Your password must be changed the first time you log in to Harris CareTracker PM and EMR. You will also be prompted to change your password every 90 days for security reasons. The password must consist of at least eight characters with one capital letter and one numeric character. As best practice, write your new password and the date created on the inside cover of your textbook each time you change it.

Before beginning any activities, clear your cache as instructed in Activity 1-6. If you are using a personal computer (PC), only work in Internet Explorer®. Use Safari® for iPad®. Once the cache has been cleared, you may continue by registering your credentials and creating your Harris CareTracker training company (Activity 1-9).

Activity 1-9

Register Your Credentials and Create Your Harris CareTracker PM and EMR Training Company

1. Go to *http://www.cengage.com/CareTracker* (**Figure 1-9**).

2. The "Domain" is set to *Current*. Do not change this setting—leave as is.

3. The *Product* list is set to "Cengage Learning Harris CareTracker Simulation 1.0" by default. Leave as is.

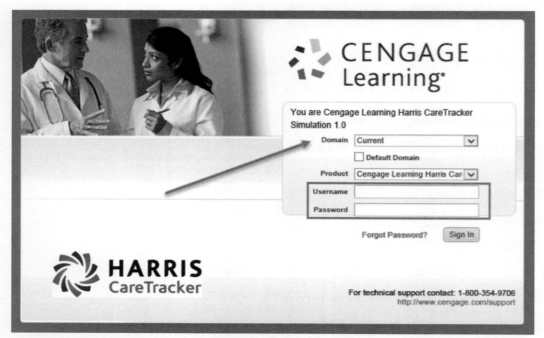

Figure 1-9   Login Screen

4. In the *Username* box, enter the username preassigned to you on the inside front cover of your workbook.

5. In the *Password* box, enter your password. If this is your first time logging in to Harris CareTracker PM and EMR, use the preassigned password located on the inside front cover of your workbook. On your first login, you will be prompted to change your temporary password and complete the *Security Information* and *General Information* fields in the *Operators Settings* dialog box.

TIP Both the username and password are case sensitive.

Your new password:
- Must differ from your old password by at least one character
- Must consist of at least eight characters
- Must contain at least one capital letter and one number; for example: Password5
- Must be reentered in the *Verify Password* field

---

6. Complete the *Security Information* fields by selecting a security question and providing the answer.

7. In the *General Information* fields, enter your *Phone* number (best contact), your *Email* (best contact), and skip the *Direct Email Address* field.

8. Record your new password on the inside cover of your workbook and the date the password was created. This allows for easy reference in case of a lost or expired password.

9. After changing your password and completing the *Security* and *General Information* fields, click *Save*. A message will display indicating that your operator settings have been updated.

10. Close out of the *Success* box. Harris CareTracker will now create your training account and you will receive a notification email when the process is complete. **Figure 1-10** is an example of the notification email you will receive. **Note:** You will not be able to log in to Harris CareTracker until you have received the notification email. It may take up to 24 hours for your Harris CareTracker training company to be created and to receive the notification.

Hello cengage238032,

Your training company has been successfully created. Log in and begin using CareTracker's training environment at training.CareTracker.com

Harris CareTracker has worked with tens of thousands of physicians to create healthier practices and healthier patients. The training environment is a lite version of the complete practice management and EMR solutions we offer to our customers. We look forward to working with you in the future.

Sincerely,
The Harris CareTracker Practice Management and EMR Team

Figure 1-10   Welcome Login Email

Note: On subsequent logins, you will receive a *Message from webpage* that says "There is no Operator Batch Control for this Group." Click "OK" and a dialog box called *Operator Encounter Batch Control* will display when you first sign in. Close out of this box by clicking the *Save* button and then clicking the "X" at the top right of the box (**Figure 1-11**).

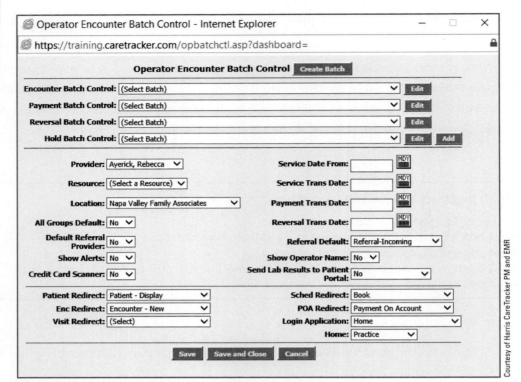

Figure 1-11   Operator Encounter Control Batch Display

CORE FUNCTIONS OF THE EMR/EHR

Learning Objective 3: Describe core functions, advantages, and disadvantages of the EMR/EHR.

The electronic record has many features designed to improve patient care and staff efficiency. The type of software that a medical practice selects will depend on many factors including the type of practice, the goals of the practice, the cost of the software, and individual preferences of the clinicians and staff.

Advantages of Electronic Medical/Health Records

An EMR is an electronic platform that facilitates the needs of a medical practice. An advantage of using a fully integrated practice management and EMR such as Harris CareTracker is that it automates the overall workflow to the greatest extent possible to achieve the maximum amount of practice efficiency. Patient care coordination is improved, and there is a demonstrated reduction in errors, which previously resulted from illegible notes or prescriptions.

Pitfalls of the Electronic Health Record

EHRs have many benefits as described earlier, but there are also a few pitfalls. In the article by the National Center for Biotechnology Information (Menachemi & Collum, 2011), it was noted that despite the growing consensus on benefits of EHR functionalities, there are some potential disadvantages associated with this technology. These include financial issues, changes in workflow, temporary loss of productivity associated with EHR adoption, privacy and security concerns, problems that occur when the system goes down, and other unintended consequences.

Patients and providers express concern over privacy issues related to EHRs and the personal information collected by the federal government. The Affordable Care Act (ACA) mandates the IRS as the collection and enforcement arm for the federal government, which troubles many Americans. In addition, the Department of Health and Human Services (HHS) issues additional rules pertaining to the ACA, there is more intrusion into a patient's medical files, and the patient's privacy is being sacrificed.

The possible repeal and replacement of the ACA is an ongoing debate in Congress, and may result in slight or significant changes to the law. Absent any changes in the law, it is expected that some of the rules and regulations will be changed to fix some of the ACA's obvious shortcomings and deficiencies.

ADMINISTRATIVE WORKFLOWS IN HARRIS CARETRACKER

Learning Objective 4: Summarize administrative workflows in Harris CareTracker.

Workflow is defined as how tasks are performed throughout the office (usually in a specific order), for example, the patient is checked in, insurance cards are scanned, copay is collected, and then the patient is taken to the exam room where vital signs are taken/recorded, and so on. Conducting a comprehensive workflow analysis is a critical step in EHR implementation. **Figure 1-12** is an example of patient flow.

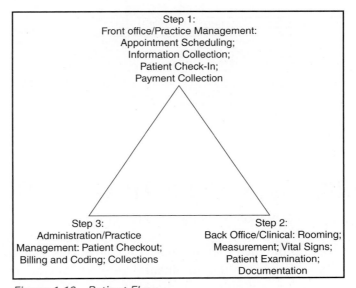

Figure 1-12   Patient Flow

Practice management (PM) software runs the business side of health care, from registering a new patient and scheduling patient visits to coding and billing the patient encounter and generating monthly reports. Harris CareTracker PM software can be customized to user preferences. PM software maximizes provider productivity and meets rigorous scheduling demands. Alert messages, a master index, and insurance profiles help reduce error and administrative expenses during registration and charge entry.

The Harris CareTracker PM task sheet (**Figure 1-13**) provides a quick reference guide to the daily, weekly, and monthly tasks for front office, billing, and administrative duties of the medical assistant.

CareTracker Practice Management Task Sheet					HARRIS CareTracker
DAILY TASKS					
FRONT OFFICE			**BILLING**		**ADMINISTRATIVE**

Before Appointment
[ ] Clear cache
[ ] Log In
[ ] Review NEWS
[ ] Review missing
   information
[ ] Work eligibility work list
[ ] Print encounter forms and
   appointment list
[ ] Confirm appointments
[ ] Review/Reschedule
   wait list appointments
[ ] Print unprinted
   correspondence
Optum Patient Portal
[ ] Accept/deny patient
   demographic updates
[ ] Work appointment
   requests
	Day of
	[ ] Create batch
	[ ] Review/work open
	   To Dos, Faxes and Mail
	[ ] Enter demographics
	[ ] Enter ref/auth/cases
	[ ] Book appointments
	
	Patient Contact
	[ ] Check-in
	[ ] Verify insurance and
	   other patient info
	[ ] Check eligibility (walk-ins,
	   new patients, changes)
	[ ] Post co-payment
	[ ] Print receipt
	[ ] Print encounter form
	[ ] Enter visit (MD or staff)
		End of Day
		[ ] Review visits and
		   charges on hold
		[ ] Run journal and
		   balance deposit
		[ ] Post batch
		[ ] Cancel no shows
		[ ] Review appointment
		   conflicts
			[ ] Clear cache
			[ ] Log In
			[ ] Review NEWS
			[ ] Create batch
			[ ] Work the claims worklist
			[ ] Review electronic
			   reports received
			[ ] Correct errors and rebill
			[ ] Close open electronic
			   claim batches
			[ ] Print paper claims
			   /flag as printed
			[ ] Enter charges or
			   save bulk charges
			[ ] Review and save
			   admissions entered
			[ ] Post payments (manually
			   and electronically)
			[ ] Close electronic remit
			   files/or make inactive
				[ ] Review/work open
				   To Dos, Faxes and Mail
				[ ] Work credit balances by batch
				[ ] Work denials
				[ ] Print journal and
				   balance payments
				[ ] Run verify payments
				[ ] Review/reconcile unapplied cash
				[ ] Save admission visits
				[ ] Post batch
				[ ] Check on new insurances
				[ ] Send To Do(s) to others
				   where help is req
				[ ] Work unpaid/inactive
				   claims
				[ ] Generate claims
					[ ] Clear cashe
					[ ] Log In
					[ ] Review News
					[ ] Review/work open
					   To Dos, Faxes and Mail

WEEKLY TASKS					
FRONT OFFICE		**BILLING**	**ADMINISTRATIVE**		

[ ] Print unprinted correspondence
[ ] Review missing encounters
[ ] Open To Do(s) -- open and
   closed client review
[ ] Recalls -- past due follow up
[ ] Review undeliverable/forwarded
   statements/ letters
		[ ] Electronic claim verification
		[ ] Enter Transactions when you verify
		   claims are on file for major payors
		[ ] Work collection accounts
		[ ] Review unbilled procedure balances
			[ ] Verify users have the
			   correct permissions
			[ ] Review and close
			   To Do(s) out to
			   terminated employees
			[ ] Remove terminated
			   employees from list
			   of operators
			[ ] Reset employee passwords
			   as needed
				[ ] Review Rx refill requests
				[ ] Review lab results
				[ ] Review charts
				[ ] Review notes entered
				[ ] Review new Rx's
				[ ] Check on Rx's
				   that may have failed
				   transmission
				[ ] Review orders
				[ ] Review visits	

MONTHLY TASKS					
FRONT OFFICE		**BILLING**			
[ ] Send recalls		[ ] Run bulk apply unapplieds [ ] Month end close period [ ] Open new fiscal period	[ ] Print month end reports [ ] Review credit balances		
QUARTERLY TASKS					
FRONT OFFICE		**BILLING**	**ADMINISTRATIVE**		
[ ] Read release notes		[ ] Read release notes	[ ] Ensure employees read release notes		
[ ] Attend live or view recorded release training		[ ] Attend live or view recorded release training	[ ] Ensure employees attend live or view recorded release training		
Optum Practice Management TASKS					
[ ] Transmit claims [ ] Software support [ ] Software updates * Only for Full Service Clients					

Courtesy of Harris CareTracker PM and EMR

Figure 1-13   Harris CareTracker PM Task Sheet

CLINICAL WORKFLOWS IN HARRIS CARETRACKER

Learning Objective 5: Identify clinical workflows in Harris CareTracker.

In addition to the administrative and practice management functions, it is vital to have an understanding of clinical duties and definitions. As addressed in the administrative workflow (Learning Objective 4) discussion, it is helpful to follow a workflow assessment guide and checklist. Harris CareTracker *Help* provides an EHR Task Sheet (**Figure 1-14**) outlining clinical workflows.

CRITICAL THINKING   Now that you have completed your Chapter 1 activities, how did the challenge put forth in the Real-World Connection apply? Did you carefully read and implement all of the directions when setting up your computer for the first time? Were you able to successfully create your Harris CareTracker training company? Elaborate on your successes and any challenges you encountered.

HARRIS CareTracker

Harris Caretracker EMR Task Sheet

CLINICAL

Visit	Daily	Weekly and Quarterly
Patient Visit (or Encounter) Activities	**Daily Activities**	**Weekly Activities****
[ ] Review/Update Patient's Clinical Information	[ ] Read Harris CareTracker Mail	[ ] Print Scheduled Charts (every Friday)
[ ] Enter Chief Complaint & Vital Signs	[ ] ToDo(s) Completed(inc.messages from Provider Portal)	[ ] Administrative Review of Quick Tasks
[ ] Review/Update History & Immunization Panes	[ ] Rx Refills Completed Within 48 Hours*	(for all providers)
[ ] Lab/Imaging Results Committed to Chart &	[ ] Review/Submit Saved or Failed Rx(s) New & Renewals	[ ] Order Tracking/Run Overdue Orders Report
Orders are Linked/Completed	[ ] Link Lab/Radiology Results to Open Orders	[ ] Repopulate Registries
[ ] Document Progress Note	[ ] Lab/Radiology Results Committed	[ ] Read Harris CareTracker News
[ ] Review/Resolve Open Activities	[ ] Open Encounter	[ ] Clear Your Cache
[ ] Review/Resolve Pt Care Management Items	[ ] Visits Captured	
[ ] Medications (New/Refills) Completed	[ ] Progress Notes Signed	**Quarterly Activities****
[ ] Lab/Imaging Orders Created	[ ] Incoming Documents	[ ] Ensure employees read release notes
[ ] Patient Education, Referrals, Clinical Letters,	[ ] Scanned or Paper Results Manually Entered	[ ] Ensure employees attend live or
Recalls, & ToDo's Created	[ ] Matched	view recorded release training
[ ] Progress Note Signed	[ ] Signed	
[ ] Communication to Referring Provider &	[ ] Voice Attachments	
Patient as needed (HT&RPP)	[ ] Untranscribed Notes	
[ ] Visit Capture Complete	[ ] Print Scheduled Charts (for next day)	
[ ] Patient Provided Copy of Chart Summary	[ ] Enter Admissions (if applicable)	

*Surescript requirement	Visit Workflow Responsibilities	Which Role?	**Also see Administrative Tasks related to
	Check In		Clinical Oversight on the PM Task Sheet
	Take Back		
	Vital Signs & Chief Complaint (if done prior to PN)		
	Problem List		
	Med List		
	Allergy		
	Update History Pane & Immunizations		
	Open Activity/Patient Care Mgmt Review		
	Complete Orders/Link/Manual Enter Results		
	Progress Note/ Data Entered & Signed		
	ePrescriptions/printed scripts		
	Clinical Orders (Labs/Referrals/Immunizations)		
	Clinical Letters		
	Recall Creation or ToDo for Next Appt		
	Patient Education Handouts		
	Visit Capture		
	Check Out Including ToDos		

Figure 1-14   Clinical Workflows—Task Sheet

SUMMARY

Chapter 1 has introduced you to the paperless medical office and provided you with the background and steps to set up your computer for optimum functionality and to complete the registration of your Harris CareTracker training company credentials.

You will be introduced to the specific features and functionalities of the Harris CareTracker PM and EMR program in Chapter 2.

Introduction to Harris CareTracker PM and EMR

2

Learning Objectives

1. Log in to Harris CareTracker to complete activities.
2. Use the *Help* system to become familiar with key features of Harris CareTracker PM and EMR and to access step-by-step instructions on using each aspect of the system to quickly and successfully complete required tasks.
3. Explain the purpose and location of the *Main Menu, Navigation, Home,* and *Dashboard.*
4. Identify *Administration* features and functions for *Practice Management* and Electronic Medical Records.
5. Use the *Message Center* components for appropriate EHR tasks.

 ## Real-World Connection

Prior to using the EHR software in our practice, medical assistants at NVFHA are required to become certified as "Super Users" of Harris CareTracker PM and EMR, a widely recognized and utilized EHR. The training that employees receive to obtain this status is similar to the training you will receive throughout this workbook. This chapter introduces you to the *Help* system, which features a variety of video links and written training materials that elaborate on the training outlined in each workbook chapter. Employees who utilize these materials typically perform at a higher level than those who do not. Your challenge is to use the *Help* content to enhance the training process and expand your knowledge.

ALERT! Due to the evolving nature and continuous upgrades of real-world EMRs such as this one, as you log in and work in your student version of Harris CareTracker, there may be a slightly different look to your live screen from the screenshots provided in this text.

When prompted, follow the instructions given in the text to complete the activities.

Before you begin the activities in this chapter, review the Best Practices list on page xiv of this textbook. These Best Practices are provided to help you complete work quickly and accurately in Harris CareTracker PM and EMR. Review these Best Practices periodically so that they become second nature.

LOG IN TO HARRIS CARETRACKER

Learning Objective 1: Log in to Harris CareTracker to complete activities.

Activity 2-1
Log in to Harris CareTracker PM and EMR

There are system readiness requirements that must be met before logging in to Harris CareTracker. These instructions are found in Chapter 1, Activities 1-1 through 1-8 and must be completed prior to working in Harris CareTracker. You must "clear your cache" (Activity 1-6) before logging in for each session.

In Chapter 1, Activity 1-9, you registered your credentials and created your Harris CareTracker PM and EMR training company using your preassigned user name located on the inside front cover of your book and the password you created when setting up your training company. Before beginning the activities, clear your cache. If you are using a personal computer (PC), only work in Internet Explorer 11®. Use Safari® for iPad®. Once the cache has been cleared, you may continue by logging in to your student version of Harris CareTracker (Activity 2-1).

1. Go to http://www.cengage.com/CareTracker.

2. The domain is set to "Current" by default (**Figure 2-1**). Leave as is.

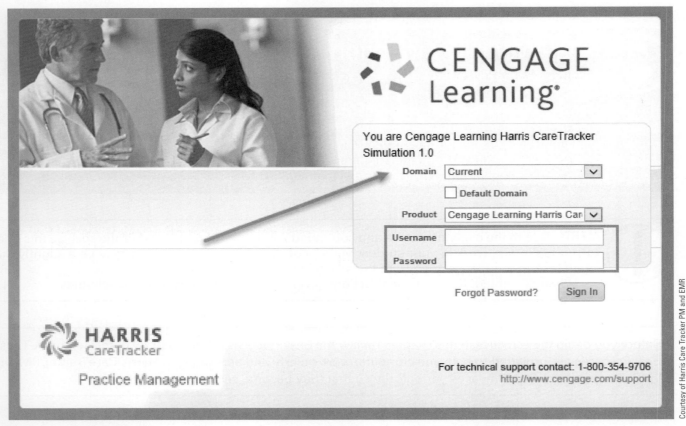

Figure 2-1 Login Screen

3. The product list is set to "Cengage Learning Harris CareTracker Simulation 1.0" by default. Leave as is.

4. In the *Username* box, enter the username preassigned to you. **Note:** Both the username and password are case sensitive.

5. In the *Password* box, enter your password you created in Chapter 1, Activity 1-9. **Note:** As noted in Chapter 1, on each subsequent login, a dialog box called *Operator Encounter Batch Control* will display when you first sign in. Close out of this box by clicking the *Save* button and then clicking the "X" at the top right of the box (refer to **Figure 1-11**).

HELP SYSTEM

Learning Objective 2: Use the *Help* system to become familiar with key features of Harris CareTracker PM and EMR and to access step-by-step instructions on using each aspect of the system to quickly and successfully complete required tasks.

Activity 2-2
Recorded Training—General Navigation and Help

Harris CareTracker PM and EMR *Online Help* ⊙ integrates product help, recorded training sessions, live webinars, support documentation, and quick reference tools to help you learn about and use Harris CareTracker PM and EMR. The Harris CareTracker PM and EMR *Help* system offers an invaluable one-stop resource for both novice and advanced users. It is designed to familiarize the user with key features of Harris CareTracker PM and EMR, and it provides step-by-step instructions on using each aspect of the system to quickly and successfully complete required tasks.

As with all live programs, there are continual updates. The same is true for Harris CareTracker. While Harris CareTracker strives to have the most current information available in *Help*, there are instances where you may notice an update in the program that has not been updated in *Help*. This may include a reference to "Optum" PM & Physician EMR and "Ingenix." The content is the same, regardless of the title reference.

To learn more about Harris CareTracker and the *Help* features provided, click on the *General Navigation and Help System* training under the *Practice Management Recorded Training* header and view the video. The most current versions of documents are always available in *Help* for easy reference. Refer back to the recorded trainings throughout your studies as needed.

1. Click on *Help* ⊙, located at the far right of the screen in the *Name Bar*.

2. At the top of the screen, click on the *Training* button. (**Note:** The *Training* button is to the left of the *Support* button.)

3. Click on "Learn More" under *Recorded Training*.

4. Scroll down to *Practice Management*.

5. Click on the *General Navigation and Help System* topic (**Figure 2-2**) under the *Getting Started* header.

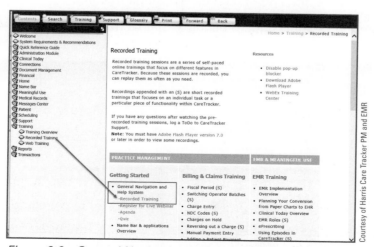

Figure 2-2   General Navigation Help Video

6. Click on the *Recorded Training* link to watch the video.

 Print a screenshot taken during your viewing of the Recorded Training, label it "Activity 2-2," and place it in your assignment folder.

7. After you finish viewing the *Recorded Training*, click on the "X" in the upper-right corner of the *Recorded Training* box. Do not close out of Harris CareTracker.

Activity 2-3
Snipit (S) Fiscal Period

A "Snipit" is a short recorded training that focuses on an individual task or a particular piece of functionality within Harris CareTracker PM and EMR. Snipits are identified with an (S) following the topic header. If you have any questions after watching a Snipit (S) video, you can watch one of the longer recorded training sessions that include the topic. You will view a Snipit (S) in this activity by clicking on *Learn More* under *Recorded Training* (Figure 2-3).

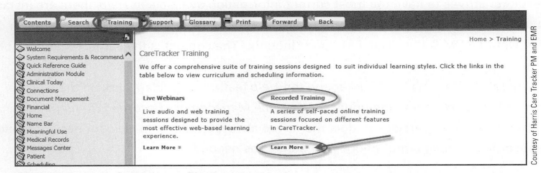

Figure 2-3   Help Snipit Learn More

1. Click on *Help* ⊙.
2. Click on the *Training* button on the toolbar.
3. Click on "Learn More" under *Recorded Training*.
4. Scroll down to the *Practice Management* section. The recorded trainings are grouped by topic area. Any training with an "(S)" at the end of the title is a Snipit training.
5. Click on the *Fiscal Period (S)* topic under "Billing & Claims Training" (**Figure 2-4**).

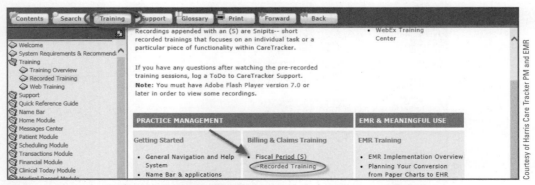

Figure 2-4   Help—Snipit Fiscal Period

6. Click on the *Recorded Training* link to watch the video.

- You must have Adobe Flash Player version 7.0 or later to view a *Snipit (S)* recording. The first time you view a recorded training you may be prompted to download and install the Adobe Flash Player if you do not already have it installed.
- If you find that the *Recording Training* or *Snipits (S)* are running slow or freezing, you may need to log out, clear your cache, and log back in to begin your activities.

Print the Snipit Fiscal Period screen, label it "Activity 2-3," and place it in your assignment folder.

MAIN MENU AND NAVIGATION

Learning Objective 3: Explain the purpose and location of the Main Menu, Navigation, Home, and Dashboard.

There are three applications contained in the *Home* module: *Dashboard, Messages,* and *News* (**Figure 2-5**). There are also three tabs: *Practice, Management,* and *Meaningful Use.* Your Harris CareTracker PM and EMR role determines which applications you can access. Your *Home* screen is set to default to the *Home > Dashboard > Practice* screen.

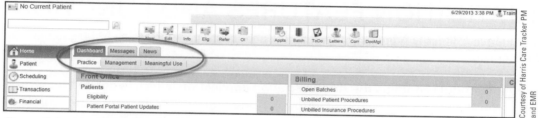

Figure 2-5   Home Application Tabs

Home Overview

In Harris CareTracker PM and EMR, the *Dashboard* is where you find your quick links to front office, billing, and clinical functions and features. The *Messages* application is a communication tool used to manage *ToDo*s, mail messages, and faxes. The *News* application provides the ability to post messages to patients and employees, ensuring that important information is made available in a timely manner. In your student version of Harris CareTracker, you can visit the *News* application for important messages from Cengage and Harris CareTracker, but you will not be able to post messages yourself (**Figure 2-6**).

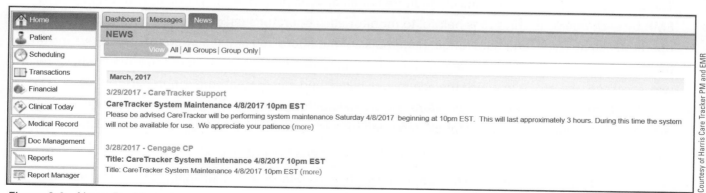

Figure 2-6   News Dashboard

Dashboard Overview

In Harris CareTracker PM and EMR, the *Dashboard* is considered "information central." At a quick glance, you can see a summary of what activity has taken place in your practice, and you can also see what key indicators need to be addressed, such as inactive claims. The *Dashboard* is divided into three tabs: *Practice, Management,* and *Meaningful Use* (**Figure 2-7**).

1. *Practice.* The *Practice* tab contains *Front Office, Billing,* and *Clinical* application summaries.

2. *Management.* The *Management* tab includes the practice's financial and management functions.

3. *Meaningful Use.* The *Meaningful Use* tab measures and tracks a provider's progress toward meeting each of the Meaningful Use requirements and to qualify for the Medicaid and Medicare EHR incentive programs.

Courtesy of Harris Care Tracker PM and EMR

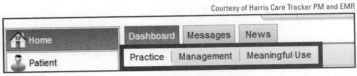

Figure 2-7   Dashboard Tabs

ADMINISTRATION FEATURES AND FUNCTIONS

Learning Objective 4: Identify Administration features and functions for Practice Management and Electronic Medical Records.

The *Administration* module contains the *Administration* application, which is divided into three tabs: *Practice, Clinical,* and *Setup.* Each tab is organized into sections containing links to other applications in Harris CareTracker PM.

Practice–Daily Administration

Although there are numerous features in the *Administration* module, we will focus on the applications you will use during the course of your training relative to practice management.

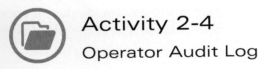

Activity 2-4
Operator Audit Log

The *Operator Audit Log* maintains an audit trail of all actions performed in Harris CareTracker PM and EMR by each operator. This log is helpful to monitor each operator's usage. You can customize the log by operator, activity type, and date range. Regardless of the filters you set, the operator log always includes the date, time, operator's log-in identification (ID), operator's name, the name of the patient whose record was accessed, the group in which the action was taken, and a comment (the action performed).

    The *Operator Audit Log* and *Operators Log* are helpful for your knowledge and understanding regarding privacy issues and the "digital footprint" recorded for each and every action you take in the EHR.

1. Click the *Administration* module. The application opens the *Practice* tab.

2. Click the *Operator Audit Log* link under *Security Logs* (**Figure 2-8**). The application launches the *Operator Audit Log.* **Note:** This may take a few moments to populate.

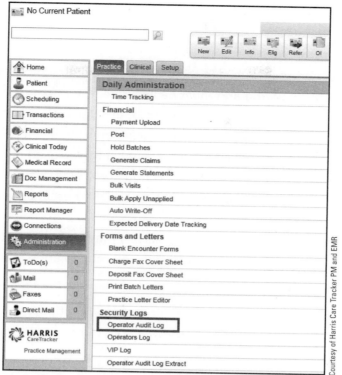

Figure 2-8   Operator Audit Log Link

3. From the *Type* list, select the type of activity for which you want to view a log. Leave as "-Select-" to view a log of all activities. (**Note**: View the drop-down to see the various "Type(s)" of logs available to create.)

4. From the *Operator* list, select the operator for whom you want to generate an audit log (Current Operator). To see a log of all operator activities, you would leave the field as "-Select-."

5. In the *Date* boxes, enter the dates to include in the audit log. (Leave the dates as they are set to run a report for the past seven days.)

6. Click *Show Log*. Harris CareTracker PM displays the log in the bottom half of the screen (**Figure 2-9**). **Note**: This may take a few moments to populate.

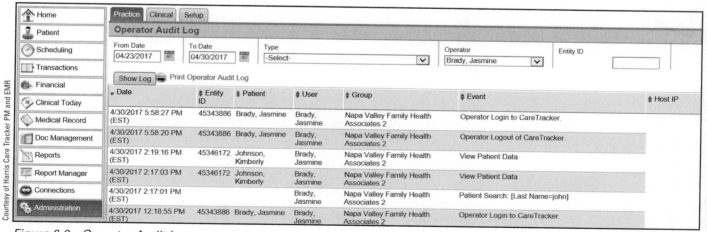

Figure 2-9   Operator Audit Log

To print the log, right-click your mouse on the log and then select Print from the shortcut menu. Label the Operators Audit Log "Activity 2-4" and place it in your assignment folder.

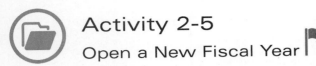

Activity 2-5
Open a New Fiscal Year

Working in the correct fiscal period is crucial in the electronic health record. Transactions and entries are permanently linked to a fiscal period and must be accurate. You must define the fiscal periods for your practice before any charges or payments are entered into Harris CareTracker PM and EMR. You can manage the practice's financials by opening each fiscal period. You can post financials to multiple open periods, but you cannot post financials or create a batch for a closed period. The fiscal period and year you are working in displays in all financial transaction applications, such as *Charge*, *Bulk Charges*, and *Payments on Account*. All reports are linked to the established fiscal periods, not the periods of the calendar year.

Depending on when you begin using this textbook, you may be required to change the fiscal year in addition to opening fiscal periods. This activity instructs you how to open a new fiscal year.

1. Click the *Administration* module. Harris CareTracker PM displays the *Practice* tab.

2. Under the *System Administration* column, in the *Financial* section, click the *Open/Close Period* link (**Figure 2-10**). Harris CareTracker PM displays all of your fiscal periods for the current fiscal year.

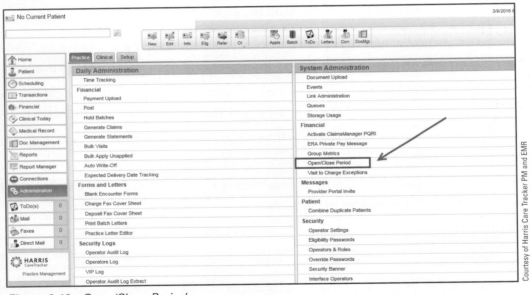

Figure 2-10   Open/Close Period

3. Enter the year in the *Fiscal Year* field. **Note:** If the *Fiscal Year* already displays for the current year you are working, move on to the next step. If you need to change the fiscal year, enter the current year and click *Go*.

4. To open a fiscal year for all groups within your company, select *Y* from the *All Groups* list and then click *Go* (**Figure 2-11**).

5. By default, the beginning and end date of each period is set to the first and last day of the month. Leave as is.

6. Click *Save*.

7. Continue with Activity 2-6 to open a new fiscal period.

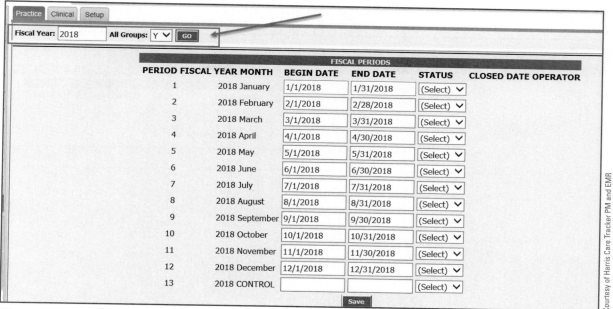

Figure 2-11   Open/Close Fiscal Year

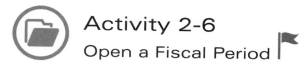 **Print the Open Fiscal Period screen, label it "Activity 2-5," and place it in your assignment folder.**

 # Activity 2-6
Open a Fiscal Period 🚩

On the first day of a new period, the practice administrator must change the status of the period to *Open* to begin posting financials to that period. You can also open a period prior to the first day of the period. It is typical for a practice to have multiple periods open.

You will have to open periods while working throughout the text to reflect the current date(s) of the activities you are working in.

> **(!) ALERT!** Do *not* close a fiscal period unless instructed to do so.

1. Continue from Activity 2-5. If you had already logged out:

   a. Click the *Administration* module. Harris CareTracker PM displays the *Practice* tab.

   b. Under *System Administration/Financial*, click the *Open/Close Period* link. Harris CareTracker PM displays all of your fiscal periods for the current fiscal year.

   c. For multigroup companies, select *Y* from the *All Groups* list and then click *Go* to open a fiscal period for all groups in the company.

2. From the list in the *Status* column, use the drop down and select "OPEN" for the period you want to open. Open the period (month/year) you are currently working in (for example, if the day you complete this activity is January 20, 2018, you would open fiscal period January 2018). **Note**: As you continue your work/activities in Harris CareTracker, you may need to open additional fiscal periods as well. Refer to this activity throughout the text when you need to open additional fiscal periods.

3. Click *Save.* You can now create batches and post financials for this period (**Figure 2-12**).

		PERIOD	FISCAL YEAR	MONTH	BEGIN DATE	END DATE	STATUS	CLOSED DATE	OPERATOR
		1	2017	January	1/1/2017	1/31/2017	(Select)		
		2	2017	February	2/1/2017	2/28/2017	(Select)		
		3	2017	March	3/1/2017	3/31/2017	(Select)		
EXISTS		4	2017	April	4/1/2017	4/30/2017	OPEN		Jasmine Brady
		5	2017	May	5/1/2017	5/31/2017	(Select)		
		6	2017	June	6/1/2017	6/30/2017	(Select)		
		7	2017	July	7/1/2017	7/31/2017	(Select)		
		8	2017	August	8/1/2017	8/31/2017	(Select)		
		9	2017	September	9/1/2017	9/30/2017	(Select)		
		10	2017	October	10/1/2017	10/31/2017	(Select)		
		11	2017	November	11/1/2017	11/30/2017	(Select)		
		12	2017	December	12/1/2017	12/31/2017	(Select)		
		13	2017	CONTROL			(Select)		

Fiscal Year: 2017   All Groups: Y   GO

FISCAL PERIODS

Save

Practice | Clinical | Setup

Courtesy of Harris Care Tracker PM and EMR

Figure 2-12   *Fiscal Period Open*

 Print the Open Fiscal Period screen, label it "Activity 2-6," and place it in your assignment folder.

 ## Activity 2-7
Change Your Password

Every operator must have a user name and a password to log into Harris CareTracker PM and EMR. You are required to change your password every 90 days. Harris CareTracker PM and EMR reminds users seven days before their password expires and gives you the option of changing the password at that time. If your password expires, you can reset it without having to log a *ToDo* to *Support.* You can also use *Operator Settings* to change your password at any time after you begin using Harris CareTracker PM and EMR, even prior to being required to by the system.

> **TIP** It is important that you keep the *General Information* section of the operator settings updated with your current phone number and email address. The application will prompt the operator for an email address if a valid address is not already saved for the operator.

1. Click the *Administration* module. The application displays the *Practice* tab.

2. Under the *System Administration* column, in the *Security* section, click the *Operator Settings* link (**Figure 2-13**). Harris CareTracker PM and EMR launches the *Operator Settings* application.

3. In the *Old Password* box, enter your current password (the one you created in Activity 1-9).

4. In the *New Password* field, enter your new password (enter a personal password you will remember). Record your user ID and new password for future reference:

   a. User Name: _____

   b. New Password: _____

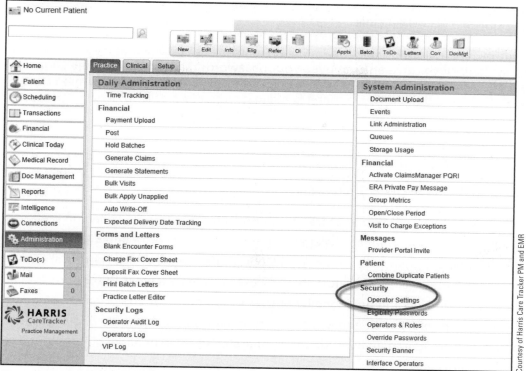

Figure 2-13   Operator Settings

The new password must meet the following criteria:

- The new password must differ from your old password by at least one character.
- The new password must consist of at least eight characters.
- At least one of the eight characters must be a capital letter and at least one must be a number. For example: "Password5."

5. In the *Verify Password* box, reenter your new password.

6. From the *Question* list, select a security question.

7. In the *Answer* box, enter the answer to the security question.

8. In the *Phone* and *Email* fields, enter your phone number and email address. It is important to keep this contact information up to date because it is used by *Support* to follow up on support issues or *ToDos*. (See **Figure 2-14**.)

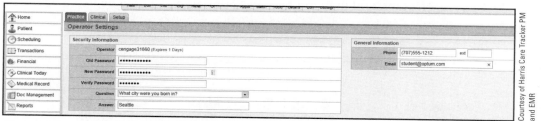

Figure 2-14   Change Password Screen

9. Click *Save*, and you will receive a *Success* pop-up box. Click *Close* on the pop-up box.

📁 **Print the Change Your Password screen, label it "Activity 2-7," and place it in your assignment folder.**

PROFESSIONALISM CONNECTION

The Harris CareTracker PM and EMR software allows management to track where you have been in the system. Never give an employee your password! If an employee uses your sign-in to view a patient's record, there is no way to prove that it was not you. If an employee asks for your password, remind the employee that it is against company policy to give out passwords.

Activity 2-8
Add Your Name as Operator

All Harris CareTracker PM and EMR operators are set up with a user profile based on their responsibilities and duties in a practice. An operator's privileges in Harris CareTracker PM and EMR are determined by the *Role(s)* and *Override(s)* assigned to his or her profile. Roles determine which Harris CareTracker PM and EMR modules and applications an operator can access. Overrides are used either to restrict an operator's access to a certain application and functionality or to grant an operator additional privileges that may not be included in his or her role. For example, if an operator needs access to only one application within the *Financial* module, you could add an override to the operator's profile to allow him or her to access just a particular financial application.

In order to provide a customized user experience, you will now add your name as operator. This also helps easily identify your "training company" operator name as user.

1. Click the *Administration* module. The application displays the *Practice* tab.

2. Under the *Security* header, click the *Operators & Roles* link. The application displays the *Group Operators* list.

3. Click on your operator name. The information will display below your operator name.

4. In the *Name* section:

    a. Skip the *Title* box (not used for operators).

    b. In the *First Name* box, enter your first name.

    c. Skip the *Middle* name box (not used for operators).

    d. In the *Last Name* box, enter your last name.

5. Click *Save*. The application updates your operator name.

6. Log out of Harris CareTracker, and then log back in. Your name will now be listed as the operator (**Figure 2-15**).

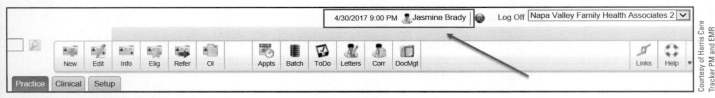

Figure 2-15 Add Your Name as Operator

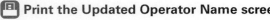
Print the Updated Operator Name screen, label it "Activity 2-8," and place it in your assignment folder.

SPOTLIGHT   The maximum idle time in Harris CareTracker PM is 180 minutes. For security reasons, it is best practice to keep the idle time short, such as 5–10 minutes. The time zone defaults to Eastern Standard Time (EST) if no time zone is set for the operator. Refer to *Help* for instructions to adjust your idle time and time zone.

Activity 2-9
Add Item(s) to a Quick Picks List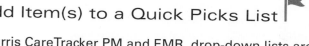

Throughout Harris CareTracker PM and EMR, drop-down lists are available from which you can select field-specific data to help create a more efficient work flow, known as *Quick Picks*. Options available in a drop-down list are built for each practice and are group specific. Your practice can build drop-down options for locations, employers, insurance companies, and financial transactions.

In order for certain data fields to be available as you work in Harris CareTracker PM and EMR, they need to be added to your "quick picks" list. You can add or remove options from a drop-down list in the *Quick Picks Setup* application.

1. Click the *Administration* module and then click the *Setup* tab.

2. Under the *Financial* header, click the *Quick Picks* link (**Figure 2-16**). Harris CareTracker PM and EMR launches the *Quick Picks* application.

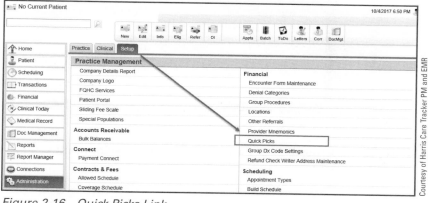

Figure 2-16   Quick Picks Link

3. From the *Screen Type* drop-down list, select the quick picks list to which you want to add an item (select "Form Letters"). The application displays the "quick picks list."

4. Verify that the item you want to add (New Referral) is not already included in the current "quick picks" list.

5. Enter the item you want to add in the *Search* box (enter "New") and then click the *Search* icon. The application displays a search window containing a list of possible matches (**Figure 2-17**). Click on the desired result to select it (select "New Referral"). The application closes the search window and adds the data as an option in the list (**Figure 2-18**).

6. Click on "X" or "Close" to close out of the "Success" dialog box.

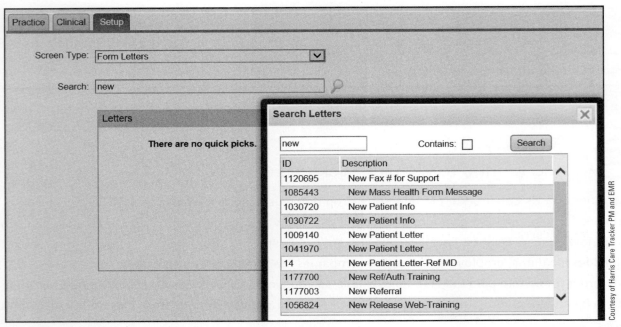

Figure 2-17   New Referral Form Letter

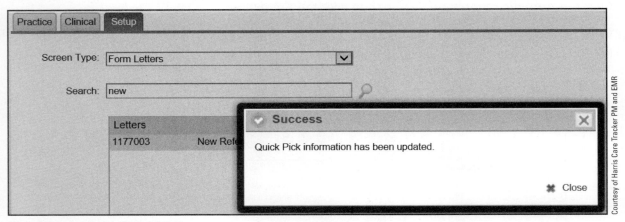

Figure 2-18   Quick Pick Added

💾 **Print the Quick Picks screen, label it "Activity 2-9," and place it in your assignment folder.**

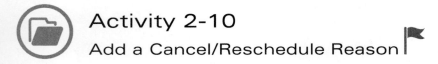

Activity 2-10
Add a Cancel/Reschedule Reason 🚩

The schedule for Napa Valley Family Health Associates has been built into your student version of Harris CareTracker. The practice is responsible for maintaining the schedule template, making changes, and opening future availability, which may be an activity you perform. Refer to *Help* (*Administration Module > Setup > Scheduling*) for steps to make changes in scheduling.

The *Cancel/Reschedule Reasons* application enables you to create company- or group-specific cancellation and reschedule reasons. Once a reason is added and made active, it is available when cancelling or rescheduling appointments via the *Scheduling* module.

1. Click the *Administration* module and then click the *Setup* tab.

2. Under the *Scheduling* section, click the *Cancel/Reschedule Reasons* link.

3. Select the group to which you want to add the reason from the *Group* list. If a specific group is not selected, the reason will be added to all groups in the company (select "Napa Valley Family Health Associates 2").

4. Select the type of reason to add from the *Reason Type* list. There are three options (listed next). For this activity, select "Cancel":

   • (All), which includes both Cancel and Reschedule.

   • Cancel: Makes the reason available when cancelling an appointment via the *Scheduling* module.

   • Reschedule: Makes the reason available when rescheduling an appointment via the *Scheduling* module.

5. Click *Add Reason*.

6. Enter a description of the reason in the *Reason Name* box (enter "Pt went to emergency room").

7. Enter an abbreviated name for the reason in the *Short Name* box (enter "ER").

8. From the *Active* list, select *Yes* to make the reason available for use (**Figure 2-19**).

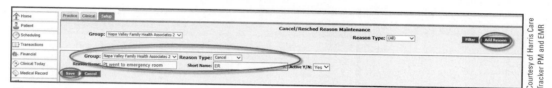

Figure 2-19   Add Cancel Reason

9. Click *Save*.

10. Click on *Filter* and view your cancel reason added (**Figure 2-20**).

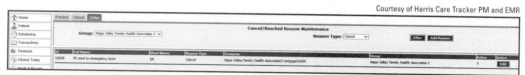

Figure 2-20   Cancel Reason Added

 Print the Cancel Reason screen, label it "Activity 2-10," and place it in your assignment folder.

Activity 2-11
Add a Chief Complaint

The *Chief Complaint Maintenance* application allows you to create a favorite list of MEDCIN-based chief complaints that are available to select from when booking appointments.

1. Click the *Administration* module and then click the *Setup* tab.

2. Under the *Scheduling* section, click the *Chief Complaint Maintenance* link. The application launches the *Chief Complaint Maintenance* feature.

3. Click the *+ New Complaint* link. The application displays the *Add New Complaint* dialog box.

4. From the *Group* list, select the group for which you want to add a chief complaint (select "Napa Valley Family Health Associates 2").

5. In the *Chief Complaint* field, click the *Search* icon. The application displays the *Complaint* search window. **Note:** If the name of the complaint is known, enter the full or partial name of the complaint in the *Search* box. For this step just click on the *Search* icon. The application returns the available results.

6. Scroll down and click on the complaint you want to add (select "New Patient (1000248)," **Figure 2-21**). The application populates the *Chief Complaint* box with the selected complaint. **Note:** This may take a few moments to populate. Wait until *New Patient* is added to the *Chief Complaint* box before moving on.

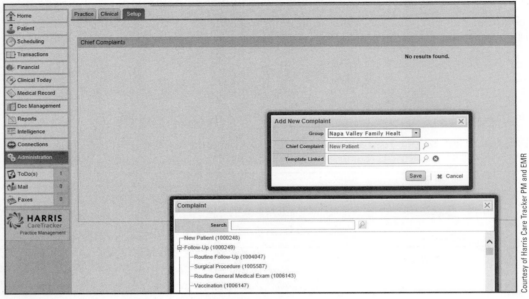

Figure 2-21   Chief Complaint Maintenance

7. In the *Template Linked* field, click the *Search* icon. The application displays the *Template* search window. Scroll down and click the "+" sign next to "Internal Medicine." Scroll down and select "IM OV Option 4 (v4) w/A&P."

8. Click *Save*. The new complaint is now added to the *Chief Complaint Maintenance* screen (**Figure 2-22**). Note again, this may take a few moments to populate. Do not click on *Save* more than once or you may receive an error message.

Courtesy of Harris Care Tracker PM and EMR

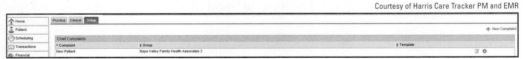

Figure 2-22   New Complaint Saved

 Print the New Patient Chief Complaint screen, label it "Activity 2-11," and place it in your assignment folder.

Activity 2-12
Add a Custom Resource

The *Custom Resources* application of the *Administration* module is where you can add, define options, and assign classes for resources. Resources can be people, places, or things. Providers are always considered a resource, but an exam room or a piece of equipment can also be considered a resource. Something that requires a schedule is considered a resource because it has specific availability with the days and times it can provide certain services. If the resource does not need a set schedule, then it is not considered a "resource" in Harris CareTracker PM and EMR.

1. Click the *Administration* module and then click the *Setup* tab.

2. In the *Scheduling* section, click the *Custom Resources* link. Harris CareTracker PM displays the *Resource* page. All providers in the practice are listed as *Available Resources*.

3. (FYI) If you are adding the custom resource for a particular provider in your group, select the provider from the *Provider* list and then click the left arrow button.

4. Click *New* next to the *Available Resources* list. Harris CareTracker PM displays a dialog box, prompting you to enter a name for the resource.

5. In the dialog box, enter a name for the resource you are creating. Enter "Obstetric 2-D Ultrasound Machine" (**Figure 2-23**).

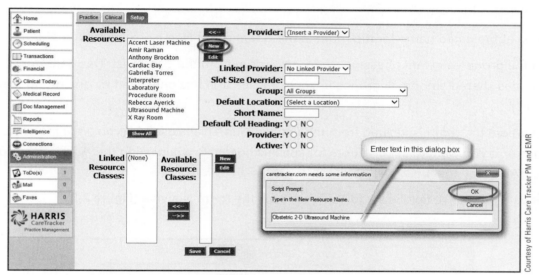

Figure 2-23   Add a Resource

6. Click *OK.* The application adds the resource to the *Available Resources* list (**Figure 2-24**).

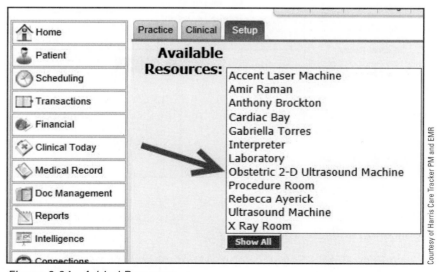

Figure 2-24   Added Resource

📇 **Print the Added Resource screen, label it "Activity 2-12," and place it in your assignment folder.**

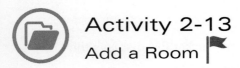

Activity 2-13
Add a Room

It is important to have an efficient appointment workflow to better serve patients. The *Room Maintenance* feature helps you set up rooms to keep track of where the patients are during their visit by updating their location throughout their appointment (e.g., exam room one, nursing station).

1. Click the *Administration* module and then click the *Setup* tab.

2. In the *Scheduling* section, click the *Room Maintenance* link.

3. Click *Add*.

4. Enter the name you want to assign to the room in the *Room Name* box (enter "Exam Room # 2").

5. Enter an abbreviated name for the room in the *Room Short Name* box (enter "Ex 2").

6. Select the group you want to assign to the new room from the *Group* list. This determines whether the room is shared among all groups in your practice or if it is only used by one group (select "All Groups").

7. Select where the room is located from the *Location* list. This is useful if you are a multilocation practice or if you want to set up floors for specific hospitals when using the *Admissions* application (select "All Locations").

8. By default, the *Active* field is set to *Y*. This means the room is active (**Figure 2-25**).

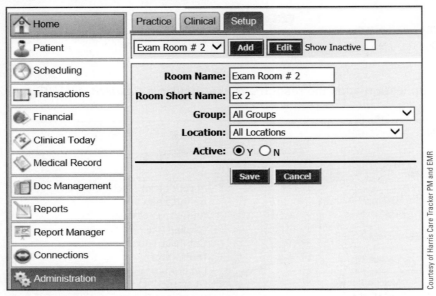

Figure 2-25   Add a Room

9. Click *Save*. The application adds the room.

10. Click back on the *Administration > Setup > Room Maintenance* link to view the newly added "Exam Room # 2" in the drop-down list (**Figure 2-26**).

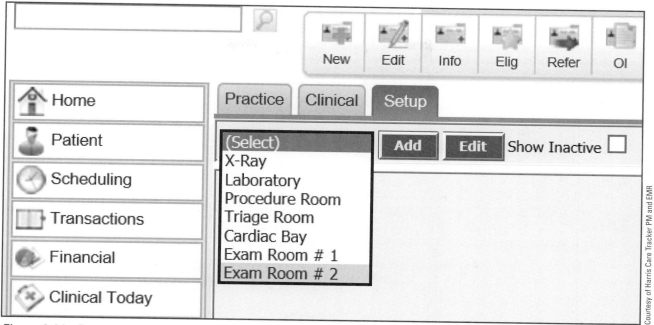

Figure 2-26   Rooms

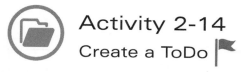 Print the Add a Room screen, label it "Activity 2-13," and place it in your assignment folder.

MESSAGE CENTER

Learning Objective 5: Use the Message Center components for appropriate EHR tasks.

The *Message* application is a communication tool that allows you to manage customer, staff, and patient communications. The *Message* application is a combination of the following features:

- *ToDos. ToDos* are Harris CareTracker PM and EMR's internal messaging system that serve two primary functions: assigning a coworker a task and communicating with the Harris CareTracker PM and EMR Support team.

- *Mail.* The *Mail* application is similar to any standard email application and allows you to send, receive, organize, and reply to internal email messages.

- *Queues. Queues* allow you to send *ToDos* to a group of people instead of an individual person.

- *Fax.* The *Fax* feature provides the ability to send and receive electronic faxes through Harris CareTracker PM and EMR.

Activity 2-14
Create a ToDo 🚩

The *ToDo* application is Harris CareTracker PM and EMR's internal messaging system that allows you to assign administrative and patient-related tasks within your practice as well as communicate with the Harris CareTracker PM and EMR support team. You will know you have an open *ToDo* if a number appears next to the *ToDo* link in the left navigation pane. In the *ToDo* application, you can review each *ToDo* that has been sent to you, reply to a *ToDo*, transfer a *ToDo*, take ownership of a *ToDo*, or close a *ToDo*. The application is updated in real time.

1. Click the *Home* module and then click the *Messages* tab. The *Messages* application displays all of your open *ToDo*(s).

2. Click on the *ToDo* icon on the *Name Bar*. The application displays the *New ToDo* window (**Figure 2-27**).

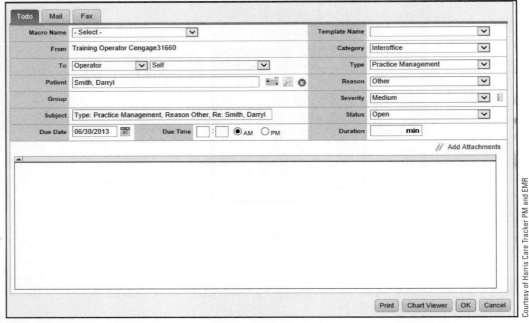

Figure 2-27   ToDo Dialog Box

3. Leave the *Macro Name* blank.

4. By default, the *From* list displays your name.

5. In the *To* list, click the required options. The *To* list includes the categories described in **Figure 2-28**. Select "Operator" in the first field and "Self" in the second field.

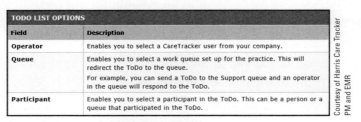

Figure 2-28   List Options for ToDo

6. If you are sending a *ToDo* to a patient, enter his or her full or partial last name in the *Patient* box (enter "Smith") and then click the *Search* icon. When the search window opens, click on the name of the patient in the search results (select "Smith, Darryl").

> **TIP**   If the *ToDo* is not patient related, you would click the *Delete* icon ⊗ to remove the name from the *Patient* field. You can click the *Info* icon to view the patient's contact information in the "At a Glance" patient information window.

7. By default, the *Subject* box displays information based on the selection in the *Type* and *Reason* lists in the right-hand column. However, you can change the subject if necessary. Leave as "Practice Management, Reason Other."

8. The *Due Date* automatically defaults to today's date and *Due Time* box defaults blank. Depending on the *ToDo*, enter the date and time by which the *ToDo* should be completed. This is important to track overdue items. For this activity, leave *Due Date* as today's date and leave the *Due Time* blank.

9. Leave the *Template Name* field blank.

10. From the *Category* list, select the *ToDo* category (leave as "Interoffice").

11. In the *Type* list, click/confirm the type of the *ToDo* (leave as "Practice Management").

12. In the *Reason* list, click/confirm the reason for the *ToDo* (leave as "Other").

13. In the *Severity* list, select the priority level of the *ToDo* (leave as "Medium").

14. The *Status* list is set to "Open" by default. Leave as is.

15. In the *Duration* box, enter the total time spent working on the *ToDo* (enter "5").

16. In the content box, type in "Test ToDo."

17. Click *OK*. The *ToDo* will disappear and show in your *Messages Dashboard* (**Figure 2-29**).

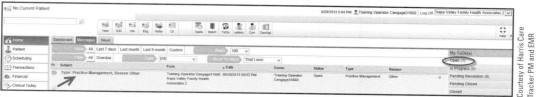

Figure 2-29   Student-Created ToDo

Print the Messages dashboard with the completed ToDo, label it "Activity 2-14," and place it in your assignment folder.

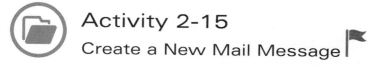

Activity 2-15
Create a New Mail Message

The *Mail* application allows you to communicate electronically with staff members, providers in your *Provider Portal,* and patients activated in the *Patient Portal.* The mail feature works the same as other email applications, enabling you to open, view, create, send and receive, and delete messages. In addition, you can link attachments such as patient encounter notes, documents, results, referrals and authorization forms, set priorities, and more.

You can use templates to create preformatted content for mail messages. For example, you can create a standard mail message used for outgoing referrals. Any time that template is selected the mail message is automatically populated with the text in the template. Templates are created in the *Event Manager* application in the *Administration* module.

1. Click the *Home* module and then click the *Messages* tab. The *Messages Center* opens and displays all of your open *ToDos*.

2. Click *Send Mail*, located on the bottom right of the page (**Figure 2-30**). The application displays the *Message* dialog box.

3. Leave the *Macro Name* as is (-Select-).

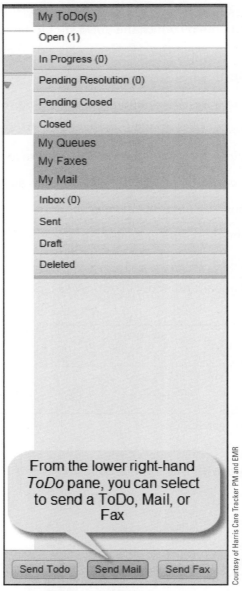

Figure 2-30 Send Mail

4. The *From* list defaults to the operator creating the mail message and cannot be edited.

5. In the *To* field, click the *Search* icon. Harris CareTracker PM and EMR opens the *Select Operators* dialog box.

6. Place a check mark in the box by *your* login name (see example in **Figure 2-31**).

7. Click *Select*. The application closes the *Select Operators* dialog box.

8. If a patient is in context, the patient name displays in the *Patient* box. However, you can also send a mail message about a different patient by clicking the *Search* icon. For this activity, you will leave the patient field blank. If a patient is in context, click the red "x" at the end of the patient name field to remove the patient from context.

9. In the *Subject* box, enter the subject of the mail message (enter "Test Mail Message").

10. Leave the *Template Name* field blank.

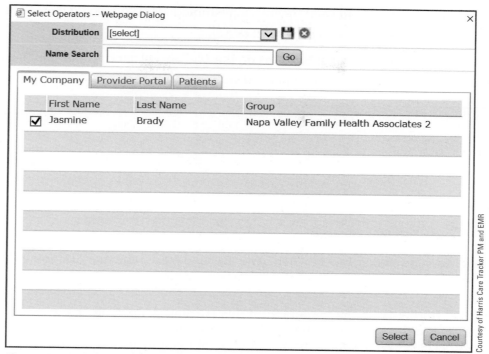

Figure 2-31   Select Operators Dialog Box

11. By default, the *Severity* list displays "Medium." However, you can change the priority of the mail message if necessary. Leave as is.

12. (FYI only) To link patient data or to add attachments, refer to the instructions in *Help*. Do not link or add any data.

13. In the message dialog box, enter the message and format the information if necessary. Enter "Test Mail Message" (**Figure 2-32**).

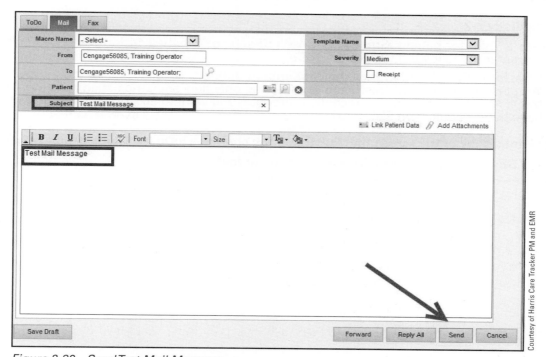

Figure 2-32   Send Test Mail Message

14. Click *Send*. If you did not want to send the message immediately you would click *Save Draft* to save the message and send later. For this activity, click *Send*.

15. To view your sent message, click the *Sent* link on the *My ToDo(s)* pane on the right side of the screen (**Figure 2-33**) or the *Mail* link on the left-hand side of your screen.

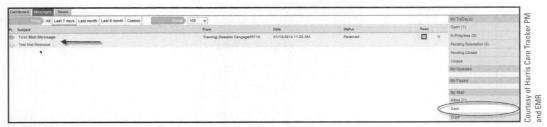

Figure 2-33   Sent Mail Message

 Print the Sent Message screen, label it "Activity 2-15," and place it in your assignment folder.

CRITICAL THINKING   In the beginning of this chapter, your challenge was to utilize the *Help* materials to enhance the training process and expand your knowledge. Which features in *Help* did you access? What topics did you find most helpful? If you experienced any challenges completing the activities, did you log in to *Help* to look for support? If not, why not?

CASE STUDIES

Case Study 2-1

Add "Paul T. Endo" to the "Refer Provider To" quick picks list. (Refer to Activity 2-9 for guidance.)

 Print a copy of the screens that illustrate your added quick pick. Label the *Paul T. Endo* screenshot as "Case Study 2-1." Place in your assignment folder.

Case Study 2-2

Create a *ToDo* for patient Kimberly Johnson. (Refer to Activity 2-14 for guidance.) For this case study, enter the following text for the *ToDo*:

"Test ToDo (CS 2-2): Dr. Ayerick, patient Kimberly Johnson called to establish as a New Patient. Your practice is currently restricted to accepting only new pediatric patient. She was referred by Dr. Alfred Peretti who has recently retired. Do you want to accept her as a new patient, or have her schedule with Gabriella?"

 Print a copy of the screen that illustrates you created a ToDo for Kimberly Johnson, label it "Case Study 2-2," and place it in your assignment folder.

MODULE 2
Administrative Skills

This module includes:

- Chapter 3: Patient Demographics and Registration
- Chapter 4: Appointment Scheduling

As a health care professional you may use Harris CareTracker PM and EMR to search for patients in the database, edit a patient's demographics, register a new patient, perform eligibility checks, and schedule appointments. These tasks are performed first in the practice workflow, before the patient sees the provider. A patient must be registered in the database in order to perform any administrative, clinical, or financial tasks. All the activities you will complete in this module mimic a real-world setting using the administrative features of electronic health records.

QUICK START

Because Harris CareTracker is a live EMR, you will need to complete several tasks to optimize your computer for using the EMR software. **If you have been following along in this book from the beginning and have completed all Required ⚑ activities as you've moved sequentially through the text, then you have already completed the activities below and can move forward. If you are beginning with this module, then you will need to complete the activities below before you can complete any other activities in this Module**.

Be sure you are working in a supported browser (Internet Explorer 11 or Safari for iPad) before you begin. Other browsers (such as Chrome and Firefox) are not supported. Review Best Practices, included on page xiv of this text.

- ❑ Activity 1-1: Disable Toolbars
- ❑ Activity 1-2: Set Up Tabbed Browsing
- ❑ Activity 1-3: Turn Off Pop-Up Blocker
- ❑ Activity 1-4: Change Page Setup
- ❑ Activity 1-5: Add Harris CareTracker to Trusted Sites
- ❑ Activity 1-6: Clear Your Cache
  - *Note: Remember that you should clear your cache each time before you begin working in CareTracker.*
- ❑ Activity 1-8: Disable Download Blocking
  - *Note: Once you have completed the system set-up requirements (Activities 1-1, 1-2, 1-3, 1-4, 1-5, and 1-8), you will not need to repeat these activities unless you change the device you are using or the settings automatically default back to prior settings.*

❑ Activity 1-9: Register Your Credentials and Create Your Harris CareTracker PM and EMR Training Company
  • *Note: It will take up to 24 hours for your CareTracker "Student Company" to be created. Plan accordingly.*
❑ Activity 2-1: Log in to Harris CareTracker PM and EMR
  • *Note: Be sure to write down your new password inside the front cover of your book for easy reference.*
❑ Activity 2-5: Open a New Fiscal Year
  • *Note: Every January 1st, you will need to open a new fiscal year.*
❑ Activity 2-6: Open a Fiscal Period
  • *Note: Every first of the month, you will need to open a new fiscal period.*

Patient Demographics and Registration

Learning Objectives

1. Identify components of the Name Bar.
2. Describe the Patient Module and Demographics features in Harris CareTracker.
3. Search for a patient within Harris CareTracker PM.
4. Register a new patient in Harris CareTracker.
5. Edit patient information in Harris CareTracker.
6. View and perform eligibility checks.

Real-World Connection

Here at NVFHA, we conduct reference checks on all job applicants who make it to a second interview. Our goal is to hire applicants who have a high capacity for "attention to detail." When entering patient demographic information in the electronic health record, it is critical to pay attention to detail because this information impacts so many departments within our practice. If you misspell a patient's name, or put in incorrect address information, it creates havoc for the clinical team searching for the patient's chart, the billing team that has to send out a second billing statement due to incorrect address information, and even the insurance company that reviews a claim for the second time due to demographic discrepancies with the first claim. These types of errors are costly to the practice because they increase employee hours needed to correct the errors and delay reimbursement for service that affect the revenue cycle.

As you go through the activities in this chapter, pay particular attention to your ability to enter information correctly. If you struggle in this area, you may want to slow down a bit and make certain that you're reading the instructions carefully and thoroughly, and are entering the correct information the first time around. Keep this information in mind as you begin your activities. At the end of the chapter, you will be asked to summarize your experience. Are you up for the challenge? Let's get started!

Before you begin the activities in this chapter, refresh your memory on working with Harris CareTracker by referring back to the Best Practices list on page xiv of this textbook. Following best practices will help you complete work quickly and accurately.

NAME BAR

Learning Objective 1: Identify components of the Name Bar.

The *Name Bar*, located across the top of the Harris CareTracker window, provides quick access to the most frequently used Harris CareTracker applications (**Figure 3-1**). A quick reference guide to the various applications launched from the *Name Bar* illustrates each button and a description of the function (**Figure 3-2**). The *Name Bar* allows you to pull a patient into context to perform specific tasks. A patient is "in context" when his or her information appears in the *Name* list and *ID* box, as illustrated on the *Name Bar* picture. To pull a patient into context, you will type in either the patient account number or the first letters of the patient's last name and click *Enter*. Alternatively, you can click on the search patient icon (**Figure 3-3**) 🔍. When the pop-up screen appears, you will enter the first three letters of the last name and first one to three letters of the first name and click on the *Search* button (see **Figure 3-4**) to search. Click on the patient, and he or she will be pulled into context. If no patient is found in the search, you will proceed to creating a new account by registering the new patient.

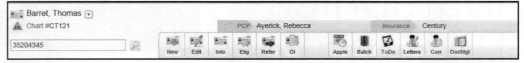

Figure 3-1   Name Bar

NAME BAR	
Button	**Description**
Search	Pulls patients into context by Harris CareTracker PM and EMR ID number, chart number, claim ID, or last name. Enter the patient's first name, last name, or at least three letters of each name to display the Advanced Search dialog box that enables you to select a patient.
Alert	Displays the Patient Alerts window. The Patient Alerts window notifies the operator when key information is missing from a patient's demographics or if any problems exist with the patient's account.
Edit	Launches the Demographics application in edit mode for the patient in context.
New	Launches the Demographics application, enabling you to register a new patient in Harris CareTracker PM and EMR.
Info	Displays a read only summary of the patient's information, including address, contact information, family members, balance information, insurance, etc.
Elig	Displays a history of eligibility checks and enables you to perform an individual electronic eligibility check to ensure that the patient is covered by the insurance company listed as the primary insurance.
Refer	Launches the Referral/Authorization application.
Appts	Displays a list of upcoming patient appointments. In addition, you can view and confirm an appointment, check in/check out a patient, print the encounter form, and perform various other tasks pertaining to the appointment.
OI	Displays information pertaining to dates of service. For example, you can obtain information such as associated procedures, financial transactions and claim activity, and make financial transactions such as payments, adjustments, refunds, and more.
Batch	Launches the Batch application, allowing you to create a new batch to enter charges and post payments and adjustments. In addition, you can also set up personal settings when using Harris CareTracker PM and EMR. For example, the main application to launch when logged on to Harris CareTracker PM and EMR.
ToDo	Launches the Harris CareTracker PM and EMR messaging tool, allowing you to communicate with other staff and the Harris CareTracker PM and EMR Support Department.
Letters	Generated and prints letters to send a patient.
Corr	Displays a queue of letters generated and enables you to print the letters to send to patients.

Figure 3-2   Description of Name Bar Applications

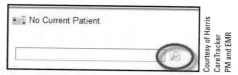

Figure 3-3   Search Patient

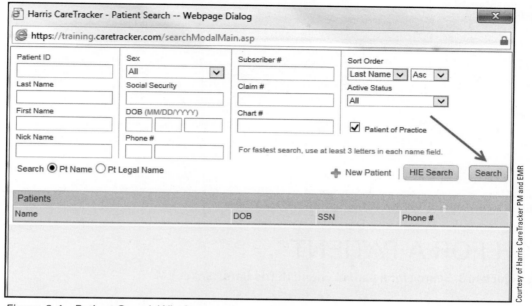

Figure 3-4   Patient Search Window

To access a patient previously in context, click the arrow next to the patient's name (**Figure 3-5**). To remove the patient from context, select *None*.

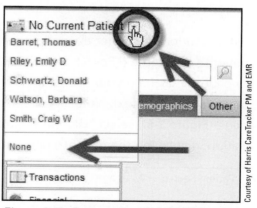

Figure 3-5   Patients Previously in Context

DEMOGRAPHICS

Learning Objective 2: Describe the Patient Module and Demographics features in Harris CareTracker.

The *Demographics* application in the *Patient* module is where new patients are registered and added into the Harris CareTracker PM and EMR system. A patient's record will contain basic identifying information and is where pertinent health insurance information is captured. You will record a patient's personal information such as his or her name, address, phone number, date of birth (DOB), Social Security number, marital status, sex, insurance, and employment information necessary to create a patient registration and electronic chart. Demographics in the medical field can be described as defining or descriptive information on the patient (e.g., name, address, phone number[s], sex, insurance information, DOB [age], ethnicity) (**Figure 3-6**).

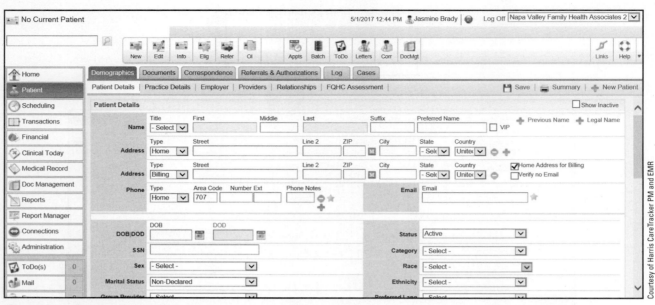

Figure 3-6   Demographics Screen

SEARCH FOR A PATIENT

Learning Objective 3: Search for a patient within Harris CareTracker PM.

Activity 3-1

Search for a Patient by Name *(currently in the database)*

PATIENT: Frank Powell

1. In the *ID* search box on the *Name Bar* located under the patient name (or No Current Patient) enter the first three letters of the patient's last name ("Pow"), and hit [Enter] (see Figures 3-1 and 3-2 for help). The pop-up will list any patient matching your search criteria (**Figure 3-7**). Click on patient Frank Powell and the patient will be pulled into context. **Note:** If you receive a pop-up asking if you want to navigate away from this page (**Figure 3-8**), select "OK" and Harris CareTracker PM will launch the *Patient Demographics* application, displaying the patient's demographics screen.

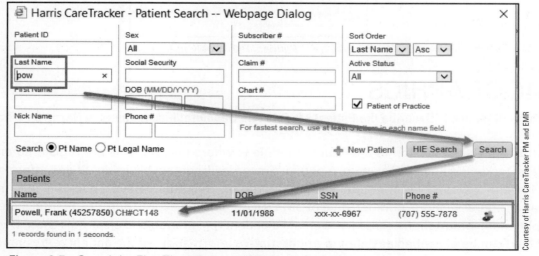

Figure 3-7   Search by First Three Letters of Patient's Last Name

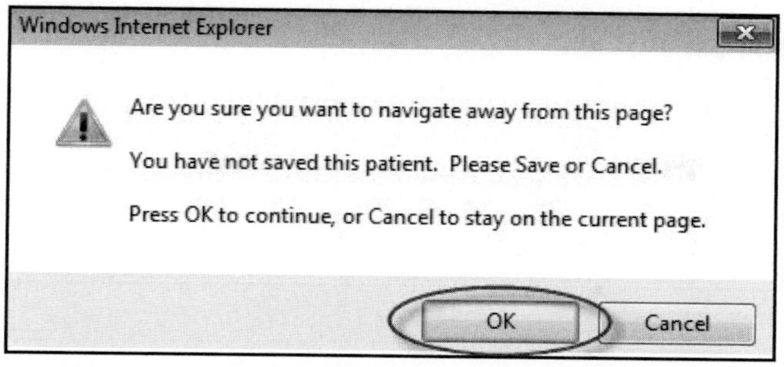

Windows Internet Explorer   [x]

⚠ Are you sure you want to navigate away from this page?

You have not saved this patient. Please Save or Cancel.

Press OK to continue, or Cancel to stay on the current page.

(OK)   Cancel

Figure 3-8   Leave This Page Pop-up Message

Courtesy of Harris CareTracker PM and EMR

✓ **TIP** An alternate method to search for existing patients is:

1. Remove a patient in context by clicking on the drop-down list at the end of the patient's name (**Figure 3-9**) and select "None." The name in the patient field will be removed and "No current patient" will display.

Courtesy of Harris CareTracker PM and EMR

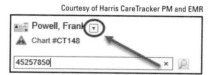

     Powell, Frank [▼]

     ⚠ Chart #CT148

     45257850   [×] [🔍]

Figure 3-9   Remove Patient from Context Drop-Down

2. With "no current patient" in the ID search box, click on the *Search* icon 🔍, which will bring up the *Patient Search* box.

3. In the *Patient Search* box, enter at least three letters of the patient's last ("Pow") and first name ("Fra"). A previous name such as a maiden name or an alias cannot be used to search for a patient.

4. Click the *Search* button. The *Patient Search* box displays a list of patients that match the information entered (see Figure 3-7), along with the patient ID and chart number.

5. Click the *Family* icon 👥 to view the patient's family members registered in Harris CareTracker PM and EMR (if applicable).

6. Verify the "second identifier" such as DOB or last four numbers of the Social Security number, and then click the specific name to launch the patient into context (see Figure 3-7).

---

2. Record the patient's ID number, chart number, and Social Security number for additional activities related to searching for a patient. _____

🖨 **Print the Patient Demographic screen displayed, label it "Activity 3-1A," and place it in your assignment folder.**

3. Repeat Activity 3-1 by searching for four additional established patients by name. Record their ID number, chart number, and Social Security number for future searches.

    a. Kevin Johnson _____

    b. Jane Morgan _____

    c. Kirk Johnson _____

    d. Abby Zuffante _____

🖨 **Print the Search Results screen for each patient, label it "Activity 3-1B," and place it in your assignment folder.**

PROFESSIONALISM CONNECTION

Registration is often the first encounter patients experience during the initial office visit. The medical assistant responsible for this task sets the tone for the remainder of the visit. If the medical assistant is curt and unfriendly, the patient may feel uneasy and tempted to leave; however, if the medical assistant is friendly and courteous, the patient will likely feel more at ease and comfortable proceeding with the remainder of the visit.

PROFESSIONALISM CONNECTION

Start every conversation with a patient whether over the phone or in person by asking for a minimum of two identifiers. Most offices have the patient state their first and last name followed by their birth date or phone number. This helps to confirm that you are in the correct chart and reduces the risk of documenting in the wrong chart.

REGISTER NEW PATIENTS

Learning Objective 4: Register a new patient in Harris CareTracker.

Activity 3-2
Register a New Patient

For this activity, you will register a new patient, one who is not in the current database (**Figures 3-10 and 3-11**). It is important to register all patients in the Harris CareTracker PM and EMR system with their demographics information such as name, contact information, date of birth, insurance and employer information, and more. This information is required to ensure proper treatment as well as to facilitate billing. Prior to registering a new patient, always search the database to be certain that the patient has never been registered. Use two patient identifiers when searching to avoid creating a duplicate account.

TIP Navigate through each field in demographics by pressing the [Tab] key and Harris CareTracker PM and EMR will automatically format the entry, regardless of the way it is entered. For example, by tabbing through the *First Name* and *Last Name* boxes, Harris CareTracker PM and EMR automatically applies title case to the name, meaning the first letter of each name is capitalized. To navigate back to a field, press [SHIFT+TAB].

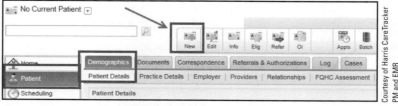

Figure 3-10   New Patient Link

Courtesy of Harris CareTracker PM and EMR

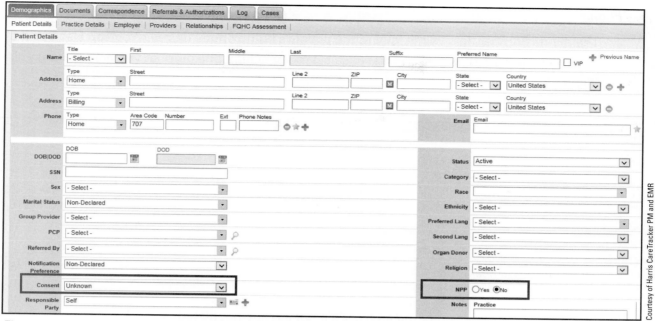

Figure 3-11   New Patient Demographic Screen with Consent Fields Highlighted

To register new patient Jordyn Lyndsey, refer to Source Document 3-1 (Patient Registration Form) and Source Document 3-2 (NPP) found at the end of this activity (pages 59–60). First, search the existing database to confirm the patient (Jordyn Lyndsey) has never been registered. After confirming she is not in the system, click *New* on the *Name Bar.* Harris CareTracker PM displays the *Patient Details* window. Register "New Patient" Jordyn Lyndsey's demographic information, responsible party, insurance, and employer information from her patient registration form. When finished, click *Save.*

1. *Name:* Enter the patient's full legal name. Include a nickname if used, for example, Jordy for Jordyn in the *Preferred Name* box/field.

2. Ms. Lyndsey is considered a "VIP." Place a check mark next to the *VIP* box at the end of the *Name* line.

3. *Address:*

   a. In the *Line 1* box, enter the patient's street address (house number + street name).

   b. In the *Line 2* box, enter the patient's apartment or condominium number, if applicable.

   c. In the *Zip* box, enter the patient's zip code (**Figure 3-12**).

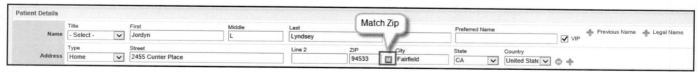

Figure 3-12   Patient Address Fields   Courtesy of Harris CareTracker PM and EMR

   d. Press the [Enter] key. Harris CareTracker PM automatically populates the *City, State,* and *Country* fields based on the zip code. **Note:** Unless a separate billing address is entered, the patient's home address becomes the billing address by default.

   e. Confirm that a check mark is in the "Home Address for Billing" box. If not, click on the box.

   f. If needed, click the + icon to add additional address fields.

4. *Phone*:

    a. The phone number field will default to the patient's home phone number. You can also use the drop-down feature from the *Type* list to select the type of phone number you are entering (**Figure 3-13**).

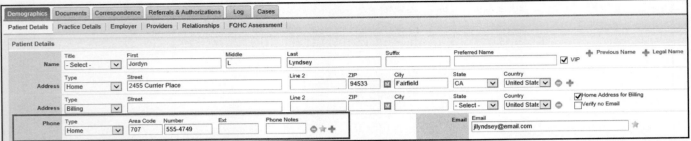

Figure 3-13   *Patient Phone Number Fields*

Courtesy of Harris CareTracker PM and EMR

    b. In the *Area Code* field, enter the area code if not already populated.

    c. In the *Number* field, enter the phone number. You do not need to enter a hyphen (it will automatically be added as you enter the phone number).

    d. (FYI) If the phone number entered requires an extension, enter the extension in the *Ext* field.

    e. In the *Phone Notes* field, enter any notes related to the patient's contact information, for example, "OK to leave message, do not call after 8 P.M." and so on. (Enter whether okay to leave detailed message as noted in Source Document 3-1 here.)

    f. Click on the *Set as Preferred Contact* ☆ icon at the end of the line.

TIP   Steps to deactivate or activate a phone number

- If a patient's phone number is no longer active, click the *Deactivate* icon at the end of the phone number line to make it inactive (**Figure 3-14**). By clicking on the *Deactivate* icon, the phone number will be deactivated but will remain in the patient's record. Harris CareTracker PM and EMR grays out deactivated phone numbers as a visual reminder.
- Click the *Activate* icon to reactivate a phone number.

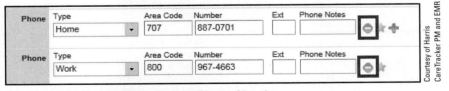

Courtesy of Harris CareTracker PM and EMR

Figure 3-14   *Deactivate a Patient Phone Number*

---

    g. In the *Email* field, enter the patient's email address on the same line as the patient's home phone number. Enter the email address exactly as you would if you were sending an email. Harris CareTracker PM will validate the email address format when the record is saved. **Note:** If a patient does not have an email address, place a check mark in the "Verify no Email" box. When checked, the *Email* field will be grayed out.

5. *Date of Birth* (DOB) (Age): Enter the date of birth in MM/DD/YYYY (or mm/dd/yy—six-digit) format, or click on the *Calendar* icon 🗓 to select a DOB.

6. *SSN* (Social Security Number): Enter the patient's Social Security number. Do not include dashes. This field must contain the nine digits or be left blank. Once you save your edits, the first five digits will be encrypted and only the last four digits display.

7. *Sex*: Enter the patient's sex. If no sex is entered, a claim cannot be sent.

8. *Marital Status*: Enter the patient's marital status, if known or declared. Choose the status from the drop-down list.

9. *Group Provider*: Select from the drop-down list the provider listed on the patient registration form.

10. *PCP* (Primary Care Provider): Select the PCP for the patient noted on the registration form from the drop-down list. (**Note:** If you were searching for a provider who is not on the list, you would click the Search icon 🔍 to the right of the field, type in as much information as you have [minimally last name and state], and search for providers (**Figure 3-15**). You would normally select the provider listed on the patient registration form.

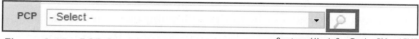

Figure 3-15   PCP Search Icon   Courtesy of Harris CareTracker PM and EMR

11. *Referred By*: This field is referring to what physician, if any, referred the patient to the practice. From the drop-down list, select the most appropriate. If you do not find the referring physician in the drop-down list, you can search the National Provider Identifier (NPI) database. For this activity, the referring providers are in your quick-pick drop-down list.

12. *Notification Preference*: From the drop-down list, select the preferred method of communication noted in Source Document 3-1.

13. *Consent*: From the drop-down box, select from the options: Unknown, Yes, No, or Revoked. Review Source Documents 3-1 and 3-2 and determine if *Consent* and *NPP* have been given. Enter the appropriate response in each field.

14. *Advance Directive*: The *Yes* and *No* fields are grayed out and cannot be changed in your student environment. Using the drop-down in the -Select- field, select "Patient Refusal" for this activity. **Note**: In a live environment, you would have to add the Advance Directive document to the system before the *Yes* can be checked by clicking the plus sign to the right and add the document. Then, *No* will change to *Yes* once the document is saved.

15. *Responsible Party*: Enter the responsible party information from the patient registration form and insurance card. The only option available from the drop-down list is "Self." Leave as "Self" for new patient Jordyn Lyndsey. **Note**: If you click on the + icon to the right of the field, the *Add Responsible Party* dialog box will pop up (**Figure 3-16**), and you can add a responsible party if it is other than "Self." Using the *Search* icon 🔍 in the *Add Responsible Party* box allows you to search the practice's database. There is also a *Relationship* field, and from the *Relationship* list you can select the patient

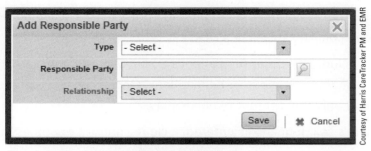

Figure 3-16   Add New Responsible Party

whose demographic information is being completed. When a relationship is selected, the patient's name is displayed in the *Responsible Party* field.

16. *Status*: This field is used to note the patient's status. Choose "Active" for new patients. (Other choices from the drop-down list would be used as appropriate, for example, Deceased, Discharged, Followed by Another M.D., Inactive, Moved Out of Area, or Not a Patient of Practice.)

17. *Category*: From the drop-down list, select the most appropriate category (if any). Leave *Category* as "-Select-" when registering a new patient. Categories available are Bad address, Collections, and High deductible. (**Note**: Additional categories can be added through the *Administration* module if the practice chooses to do so.)

18. *Race*: In the drop-down menu, select from the following options: American Indian or Alaskan Native, Asian, Black or African American, Native Hawaiian or other Pacific Islander, Patient Refusal, or White.

19. *Ethnicity*: In the drop-down menu, select from the following options: Hispanic or Latino, Not Hispanic or Latino, or Patient Refusal.

20. *Preferred Lang*: Select the preferred language of the patient from the drop-down menu.

21. *Second Lang*: Select the patient's second language from the drop-down menu, if applicable.

22. *Organ Donor*: Identify whether the patient is an organ donor (if noted on the patient registration form).

23. *Religion*: Select the patient's religion from the drop-down menu (if noted on the patient registration form).

24. *NPP* (Notice of Privacy Practices): Referring to the Patient Registration packet, select the radio dial button "Yes" or "No" indicating whether the NPP has been signed/recorded. Always confirm if the *Consent* and *NPP* were signed by the patient, and check "Yes" on the demographics screen. Harris CareTracker will automatically "date stamp" when the *NPP* and *Consent* information were entered.

25. *Notes* (*Practice* or *Clinical*): Enter any notes that you want to include for this patient. In the lower-right-hand corner of the demographics screen, check the box *Trigger Patient Flash Note*. That will activate the notes to flash when you pull the patient into context. For example, "requires electric exam table."

26. *Insurance Plan(s)*: Complete the fields with information from the patient registration form (Source Document 3-1).

   a. A subscriber (policy holder) is an individual who is a member of a benefits plan. For example, in the case of family coverage, one adult is ordinarily the subscriber. A spouse and children would ordinarily be dependents. The *Subscriber* field defaults to "Self." Leave this selection if the patient is the subscriber. (Jordyn Lyndsey is the subscriber, so leave as "Self.") If an individual other than the patient or the responsible party is the subscriber, click on the + icon at the end of the *Subscriber* field.

TIP To Add a New Subscriber

In this activity, you do <u>not</u> need to add a new subscriber, but you may need to add a new subscriber in future activities and certainly in the real-world setting. To add a new subscriber:

1. Click the + icon next to the *Subscriber* field (**Figure 3-17**). Harris CareTracker PM displays the *Add Subscriber* dialog box.

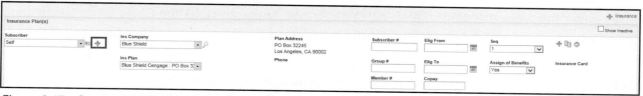

Figure 3-17   *Search Icon in the Subscriber Field*   Courtesy of Harris CareTracker PM and EMR

2. In the *Add Subscriber* dialog box, you will select the appropriate *Type, Subscriber,* and *Relationship.*

3. To search for the *Subscriber,* click on the *Search* icon. (**Note:** Only search the database if the subscriber was ever a patient of the practice.) If the subscriber is not found in the database, close the *Search Patients* window and click the *Copy* icon in the *Add Subscriber* dialog box. Harris CareTracker PM displays demographic fields for the new subscriber information.

4. Complete the demographic information for the subscriber in the fields provided. You must enter the subscriber's *Name, SSN, DOB, Sex,* and *Insurance* information at a minimum.

b. In the *Ins Company* field, select the subscriber's insurance company from the drop-down list (**Figure 3-18**). Verify that you have the correct insurance plan by double-checking the address displayed next to the insurance plan name. The insurance plan will populate with the name and address if you select a plan from the drop-down list. If the plan name is not in the list, search the Harris CareTracker PM database.

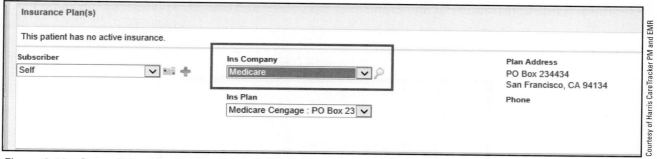

Figure 3-18   *Select Subscriber's Insurance Plan*

c. In the *Subscriber* # field, enter the subscriber number listed. The subscriber number refers to the insurance policy number.

d. (If applicable) Enter the group number in the *Group* # field. The group number typically identifies the employer. The use of group numbers varies among insurance carriers, so be sure to enter the numbers in accordance with each carrier's numbering policy.

   e. (If applicable) Enter the member number in the *Member #* field. (There is no member number for this patient.) The member number is typically assigned to individual family members on the policy.

   f. In the *Elig From* and *Elig To* fields, enter the subscriber's effective dates of coverage with a particular insurance carrier. Often the date entered in the *Elig From* field will match the patient's employment start date if the patient is covered through that employer. The *Elig To* field remains blank until the patient changes insurance plans. To complete the eligibility fields, you can either enter the dates manually in MM/DD/YYYY format, or you can click the *Calendar* icon and select a date. In the case of Jordyn Lyndsey, the *Elig From* date would have been her 65th birthday, since she is a Medicare patient.

   g. If the subscriber is required to pay a copayment, enter the copayment amount in the *Copay* field. Do not use dollar signs. When charges are entered for the patient, Harris CareTracker PM will automatically calculate and carve-out the copayment amount for private pay (the amount for which the patient is responsible). The carve-out occurs only if the copay amount is entered in the *Copay* field.

   h. The *Sequence* field indicates whether the insurance plan entered for the patient is the primary (first in order), secondary (second in order), or tertiary (third in order) insurance. The number of insurance plans entered on a patient's demographic determines the numbers that display on the *Sequence* list. Select "1" for the primary insurance, select "2" for the secondary insurance, and so on. For example, if the secondary insurance plan saved on a patient's demographic becomes the primary insurance, you would then change the plan's sequence to "1" instead of "2." (Select "1.")

   i. Confirm that the patient has signed the Assignment of Benefits/Financial Agreement, and select "Yes" from the *Assignment of Benefits* drop-down menu (other options from the drop-down list are "No" or "Patient Refused"). It is imperative that patients sign the Assignment of Benefits authorization so the practice may bill the insurance company for reimbursement.

27. The last field in the *Patient Details* tab is where photos are added. This feature is not active in your student environment. Skip over this field.

28. Prior to navigating to another tab or application, be sure to scroll down and click *Save* to save your entries. Harris CareTracker PM and EMR saves the patient and assigns a unique identification number. The newly registered patient is also pulled into context. After completing the new patient registration activity, you may receive a pop-up alert advising you of missing information (**Figure 3-19**).

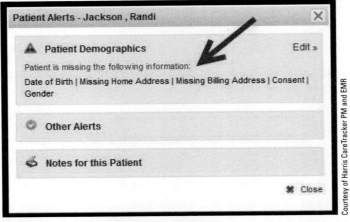

Figure 3-19   Patient Alerts Pop-up Box

29. To make further entries to patient demographics, click Edit in the Name Bar. Then, at the top of the *Demographics* screen, click on the *Employer* tab, to the right of the *Patient Details* tab.

30. Click on the + *New Employer* link on the left side of the screen and complete the fields with information from the patient registration form (Source Document 3-1).

    a. A list of the practice's most common patient employers is available from the *Employer* field drop-down list. Select the appropriate employer choice from the drop-down list. When an employer is selected from the list, the employer's work address information will be populated in the *Address* fields.

TIP To Search for an Employer

In this activity, you won't need to search for an employer, but you may need to do so in future activities. To search for an employer:

    1. If the patient's employer is not an option in the *Employer* drop-down list, search Harris CareTracker PM's employer database. This can be done by clicking the *Search* icon next to the *Employer* field (**Figure 3-20**). This will open the *Search Employers* window. If the employer is not listed, you can click the + *New Employer* link and add the employer information.

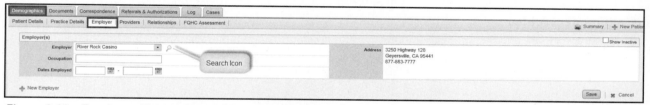

Figure 3-20   Employer Field in Patient Demographics Screen   Courtesy of Harris CareTracker PM and EMR

    2. Enter the name of the employer in the *Employer Name* field. In addition, you can narrow the search by entering the employer's city and state. Click on the *Search* button to display a list of the employers that match the information entered.

    3. By clicking on the appropriate selection, the employer's name, address, phone number, and fax number are entered into the respective fields.

    b. The patient's occupation should be entered in the *Occupation* field, for example, "P/T Bookkeeper."

    c. Enter the start and end dates in the *Dates Employed* fields as noted on the Patient Registration form (Source Document 3-1) (if any). If the patient is presently an employee, no ending date is entered. A date can be entered into either of the fields manually |in MM/DD/YYYY format, or by clicking on the *Calendar* icon and selecting the appropriate date.

    d. Click *Save*.

31. Now update the emergency contact information with the following steps:

    a. Click on the *Relationships* tab.

    b. Click the drop-down next to "Add Relationship."

    c. Select *Emergency Contact* and the "Add Emergency Contact" dialog box will appear.

    d. Leave the drop-down in the *Patient* field as "-Select Patient-."

    e. In the *Non-Patient field*, enter the name of the *Emergency Contact* (Janet Jones).

    f. Use the drop-down next to "Relationship" and select the appropriate relationship as noted on the patient registration form (Child).

    g. In the "Phone" field, enter the information as noted on the patient registration form (use *Mobile* for the *Phone Type* and enter the phone number listed in the Registration Form).

    h. Click "Yes" as "Preferred."

    i. Then click *Save*.

32. If necessary, click *Edit* and continue the full registration process for any missing information. It is important to know that all fields should be completed, although they are not required. The pop-up will also alert you to missing information such as primary location (should be "Napa Valley Family Associates [NVFA]"), preferred language, secondary language, ethnicity, race, organ donor status, religion, and more. Click *Save* to save any changes made.

33. (FYI) There are additional tabs in the *Demographics* application that may or may not be used by the practice.

Print the completed *Patient Details* and *Employer* screens, label them "Activity 3-2," and place them in your assignment folder.

Source Document 3-1

Patient Registration Form

NVFHA

Patient's Last Name	First (legal name)	First (Preferred name)	Middle Name
Lyndsey	Jordyn		L

Address (Number, Street, Apt #)	City	State	Zip Code
2455 Currier Place	Fairfield	CA	94533

Mail will be sent to the address listed above, unless patient indicates a different address (leave blank if same as above)

Send mail to Address (Number, Street, Apt #)	City	State	Zip Code

Phone Options	Phone Number	Okay to leave detailed message	Call this number (circle one)
Home	(707) 555 - 4749	Yes _X_ No _____	(1st) 2nd 3rd choice
Cell	( ) -	Yes ____ No _____	1st 2nd 3rd choice
Work	( ) -	Yes ____ No _____	1st 2nd 3rd choice

Would you like to communicate by Email	Yes _X_ No __	Email Address	jllyndsey@email.com

Date of Birth	Sex	Social Security Number
1/17/1952	Female _X_ Male ____	000-00-9118

Marital Status (*circle one*)	What is your preferred language / secondary language
Single / Married / Divorced / (Widowed) /Partner	English

Race (*circle one*)

African American (Black) / Asian / Bi-Multi-racial / Pacific Islander-Hawaiian / Caucasian–White / Native American Eskimo Aleut / Decline to state / Other

Ethnicity (*circle one*)

Hispanic-Latino / (Non-Hispanic-Latino) / Other

Religion	Baptist		Organ Donor	Yes _____ X _____	No _____

Are you new to our practice	Who referred you to our practice	Who is your Primary Care Physician
Yes __X__ No _____	Amir Raman	Amir Raman

Additional Notes

Emergency Contact

Emergency Contact's Name	Relationship to patient	Phone
Janet Jones	Daughter	(510) 555 - 2246

On-Line Patient Portal Communication via Email

On-Line communication is used for non-urgent message/requests only. NVFHA uses secure technology to protect the privacy and confidentiality of your personal information. Only you, your physician, and authorized staff can read your message.

What is your preferred method of communication?	Phone _X_ Letter _____ Patient Portal _____ Email _____

Insurance Information

Subscriber (Insurance Holder) Name	Date of Birth	Relationship to patient	Subscriber Phone Number
Self	/ /		( )

Health Plan Information	Primary Health Plan	Secondary Health Plan
Health Plan Name	Medicare Cengage	
Health Plan Address	PO Box 234434, San Francisco, CA, 94134	
Group Number	CARE 1357	
Subscriber Number	CARE 1357	

Elig Date From	1/17/2017	Copay	N/A

Patient Employer Information

Employer Name & Address (Number, Street, Apt #, City, State, Zip Code)	Employer Phone Number
Carneros Inn	( )

Occupation	P/T bookkeeper	Start Date	6/19/2014

Assignment of Benefits • Financial Agreement

I hereby give lifetime authorization for payment of insurance benefits to be made directly to **Napa Valley Family Health Assoc.,** and any assisting physicians, for services rendered. I understand that I am financially responsible for all charges whether or not they are covered by insurance. In the event of default, I agree to pay all costs of collection, and reasonable attorney's fees. I hereby authorize this healthcare provider to release all information necessary to secure the payment of benefits.

I further agree that a photocopy of this agreement shall be as valid as the original.

Date: **XX/XX/20XX** _____ Your Signature: *Jordyn Lyndsey*

Method of Payment: ☐ Cash ☐ Check ☐ Credit Card

Source Document 3-2

NVFHA

NOTICE OF PRIVACY PRACTICES (NOPP)

ACKNOWLEDGEMENT OF RECEIPT

Patient Name: Jordyn L. Lyndsey

(Please Print)

By signing this form, you acknowledge receipt of the Notice of Privacy Practices of NAPA VALLEY FAMILY HEALTH ASSOCIATES. Our Notice of Privacy Practices provides information about how we may use and disclose your protected health information (PHI). We encourage you to read it in full.

Our Notice of Privacy Practices is subjected to change. If we change our notice, we will provide you with the revised notice or you may obtain a copy of the revised notice by accessing our website at http://www.nvfha.org or contacting our organization's customer service department at (707) 555-1212.

If you have any questions about our Notice of Privacy Practices, please contact the Privacy Officials at the medical practice you visit or the Quality Improvement Department at (707) 555-1212.

- -

I acknowledge receipt of the Notice of Privacy Practices of NAPA VALLEY FAMILY HEALTH ASSOCIATES.

Date: **XX/XX/20XX**

Name: Jordyn L. Lyndsey

(Please Print)

If legal representative give relationship:

Inability to Obtain Signature	Date:

Why:

Provider Representative: _____ Provider Rep Signature: _____

(Print)

Activity 3-3

Print the Patient Demographics Summary

Medical practices may find it useful to print a patient's demographic report for a variety of reasons. Some practices will give a copy of the printed report to a patient at check-in to verify information and to make any necessary corrections/updates. Following this workflow will help identify inconsistencies between the patient information and information stored in your practice management software.

1. Pull a patient into context (New Patient—Jordyn Lyndsey).

2. Click the *Patient* module. Harris CareTracker PM and EMR displays the *Demographics* tab.

3. Click the *Print* 🖫 icon to the left of the *Summary* link in the upper-right corner of the *Demographics* application. Harris CareTracker PM displays your printing options, along with a *Patient Summary Printout* screen (**Figure 3-21**). (**Note:** It may take a little time to generate the report.)

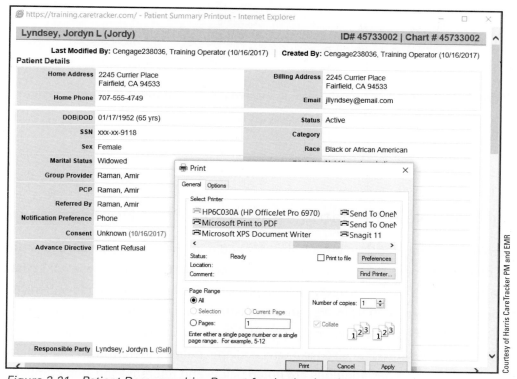

Figure 3-21   *Patient Demographics Report for Jordyn Lyndsey*

4. Choose a printer listed in the *Print* dialog box to print the patient demographics summary (**Figure 3-22**). (Alternatively, you can close the print prompt box and take a screenshot of the report, or right click on the report and select *Print*.)

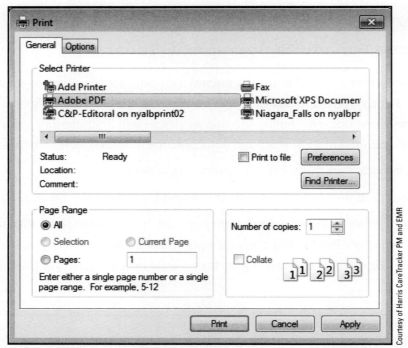

Figure 3-22   Print Prompt Screen

 Print the *Patient Demographics* report, label it "Activity 3-3," and place it in your assignment folder.

Activity 3-4
Register a New Pediatric Patient and Print Demographics

Register new pediatric patient Francisco Powell Jimenez and print his demographics. Search the existing database to confirm the patient has never been registered. After confirming he is not in the system, click *New* on the *Name Bar.* Harris CareTracker PM displays the *Patient Details* window. Register Francisco Jimenez's demographic information from his patient registration form using the information in Source Document 3-3 (Registration Form), located at the end of this activity. When finished, click *Save* and then print the demographics report. Because Francisco is a new pediatric patient, there will be slight changes in the registration process. Those changes/additions are noted below and reference the step number in Activity 3-2.

1. *Name*: Enter the patient's name.

2. *Address*:

   a. In the *Line 1* box, enter the patient's street address (house number + street name).

   b. In the *Line 2* box, enter the patient's apartment or condominium number, if applicable.

   c. In the *Zip* box, enter the patient's zip code (**Figure 3-23**). Click on the [Match] icon. Harris CareTracker PM automatically populates the *City*, *State*, and *Country* fields based on the zip code.

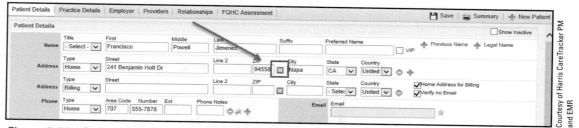

Figure 3-23   Patient Address Fields

d. Leave the check mark in the "Home Address for Billing" box.

3. *Phone*:

a. The phone number field will default to the patient's home phone number. Enter the patient's phone number from his Patient Registration form (**Figure 3-24**).

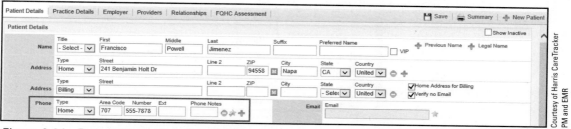

Figure 3-24   Patient Phone Number Fields

b. In the *Area Code* field, enter the area code if not already populated.

c. In the *Number* field, enter the phone number.

d. In the *Phone Notes* field, enter any notes related to the patient's contact information as noted in Source Document 3-3. For example, "Do not leave detailed messages."

e. Click on the *Set as Preferred Contact* ⭐ icon at the end of the line.

f. Leave the *Email* field blank. Place a check mark in the "Verify no Email" box to the above and right of the email field.

4. *Date of Birth* (DOB) (Age): Enter the date of birth in 08/31/YYYY format (use last year for the year in this field).

5. *SSN* (Social Security Number): Enter the patient's Social Security number. Do not include dashes.

6. *Sex*: Enter the patient's sex.

7. *Marital Status*: *Marital Status* defaults to "non-declared." Choose the status from the drop-down list.

8. *Group Provider*: Select from the drop-down list the provider listed on the patient registration form.

9. *PCP* (Primary Care Provider): Select the PCP for the patient noted on the registration form from the drop-down list.

10. *Referred By*: From the drop-down list, select the most appropriate. Leave as "-Select-" if no referring provider is noted (do not enter a non-provider in this field for this activity).

11. *Notification Preference*: From the drop-down list, select "phone."

12. *Consent:* From the drop-down box, select from the options: Unknown, Yes, No, or Revoked. Because Francisco is a pediatric patient, select "Unknown."

13. *Advance Directive*: The advance directive field defaults to "No." Because Francisco is a pediatric patient, leave as is.

14. *Responsible Party*: Enter the responsible party information from the patient registration form and insurance card. The only option available from the drop-down list is "Self." Because new patient Francisco is not the Responsible Party, you will follow step 15.

15. Click on the + icon to the right of the field, the *Add Responsible Party* dialog box will pop up (see **Figure 3-25**), and add the responsible party noted on the patient registration form.

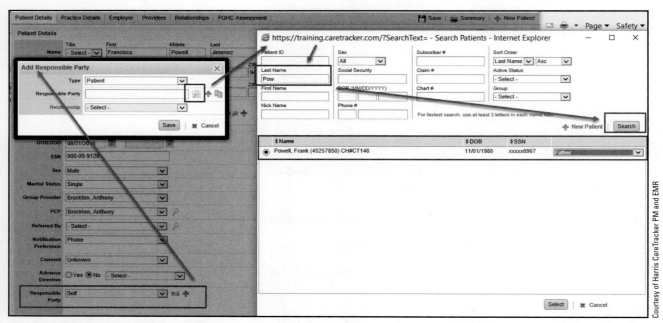

Figure 3-25   Add New Responsible Party

16. Click on the *Search* icon in the *Add Responsible Party* box that allows you to search the practice's database. Because Francisco's father, Frank Powell, is the *Responsible Party*, enter his name in the *Search Patients* box and click Search.

17. When Frank Powell's name appears, click on the radio dial button to select him, and use the drop-down to the right of the SSN field and select "Father."

18. Click *Select* and the *Search Patients* dialog box disappears.

19. In the *Add Responsible Party* box, the *Relationship* field now contains "Father."

20. Click *Save* and the *Relationship* is saved.

21. *Status*: This field is used to note the patient's status. Choose "Active" for new patients.

22. *Category*: From the drop-down list, select the most appropriate category (if any). Leave Category as "-Select-" when registering a new patient.

23. *Race*: In the drop-down menu, select the race indicated on his patient registration form.

24. *Ethnicity*: In the drop-down menu, select the ethnicity indicated on his patient registration form. If there is no entry, select "Patient Refusal."

25. *Preferred Lang*: Select the preferred language of the patient from the drop-down menu. If no entry is on the patient registration form, leave this field as "-Select-."

26. *Second Lang*: Select the patient's second language from the drop-down menu, if applicable.

27. *Organ Donor*: Identify whether the patient is an organ donor (if noted on the patient registration form). If there is no entry, leave as "-Select-."

28. *Religion*: Select the patient's religion from the drop-down menu. If there is no entry, leave as "-Select-."

29. *NPP* (Notice of Privacy Practices): Select the radio dial button "No" because Francisco is a pediatric patient.

30. *Notes* (*Practice* or *Clinical*): Enter any notes that you want to include for this patient. For example, enter in the *Practice Notes* "Direct any communications to Mr. Frank Powell, Francisco's father."

31. *Insurance Plan(s)*: Use the scroll feature on the right-hand side of the *Patient Details* window to display the entire *Plan(s)* field.

   a. The Subscriber field defaults to "Self."

   b. Click on the + at the end of the *Subscriber* field to add a new Subscriber (patient's father, Frank Powell).

   c. Harris CareTracker PM displays the *Add Subscriber* window (**Figure 3-26**).

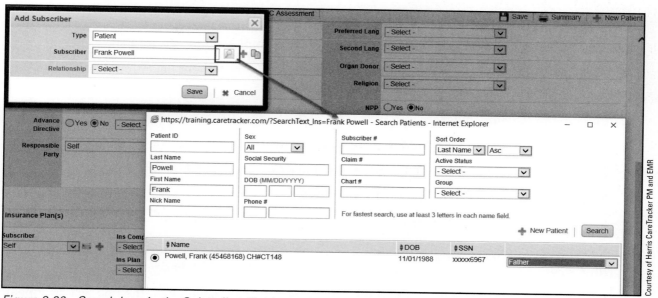

Figure 3-26   *Search Icon in the Subscriber Field*

   d. In the *Add Subscriber* dialog box, you will select the appropriate *Type* (Patient); Enter *Subscriber* (Frank Powell) and, click on the *Search* 🔍 icon. Select "Frank Powell" (by clicking the radio dial button) and then selecting "Father" from the drop-down next to the Social Security number in the *Search Patients* dialog box (see Figure 3-25).

   e. Click the *Select* button at the lower right of the *Search Patient* dialog box. The box will disappear.

f. In the *Add Subscriber* dialog box, you will see Frank Powell as the *Subscriber* and "Father" as the *Relationship*. Click on *Save* and Frank Powell is pulled into the *Subscriber* field in the *Insurance Plan(s)* section.

g. *Ins Company* field: Refer back to the patient registration form and using the drop-down, select the insurance information. Once selected the *Ins Plan* will automatically populate.

h. In the *Subscriber #* field, enter the subscriber number listed.

i. (If applicable) Enter the group number in the *Group #* field.

j. (If applicable) Enter the member number in the *Member #* field. (There is no member number for this patient.)

k. In the *Elig From* and *Elig To* fields, enter the patient's birth date (08/31/XX—use last year). The *Elig To* field remains blank until the patient changes insurance plans.

l. Enter the copayment amount in the *Copay* field. Do not use dollar signs.

m. Leave the *Sequence* field as "1."

n. Confirm that the patient has signed the Assignment of Benefits/Financial Agreement, and select "Yes" from the *Assignment of Benefits* drop-down menu (patient's father, Frank Powell, signed the patient registration form, which includes the Assignment of Benefits/Financial Agreement).

32. The last field in the *Patient Details* tab is where photos are added. Skip this section as this feature is not active in your student environment.

33. Click *Save* to save your entries. **Note**: Once you have hit *Save*, to make further entries in the *Patient Details* screen, you will have to first click *Edit*.

34. Because Francisco is a pediatric patient, you will skip the *Employer* tab information.

35. Now update the emergency contact information contained in the Patient Registration form with the following steps:

a. Click on the *Relationships* tab.

b. Click the drop-down next to "Add Relationship."

c. Select *Emergency Contact* and the *Add Emergency Contact* dialog box will appear.

d. Next to the *Patient* field, click on the looking glass.

e. In the *Search Patients* dialog box, enter "Frank Powell" and click *Search*.

f. Select "Frank Powell" (by clicking on the radio dial button), and then select "Father" from the drop-down next to the Social Security number (SSN) in the *Search Patients* dialog box.

g. Click the *Select* button at the lower right of the *Search Patient* dialog box. The box will disappear.

h. The drop-down next to the "Relationship" field will auto-populate with "Father." The "Phone" fields will also auto-populate with the information in the database for Frank Powell. Leave these fields as is.

i. Click "Yes" as "Preferred."

j. Click *Save*.

36. (If applicable) Click *Edit* (**Figure 3-27**) and continue the full registration process for any missing information.

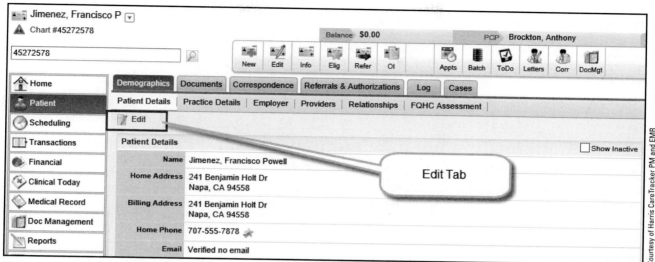

Figure 3-27   Edit Patient Demographics

37. Click the *Print* icon to the left of the *Summary* link in the upper-right corner of the *Demographics* application. Harris CareTracker PM displays your printing options, along with a *Patient Summary Printout* screen (**Figure 3-28**). (**Note:** It may take a few moments to generate the report.)

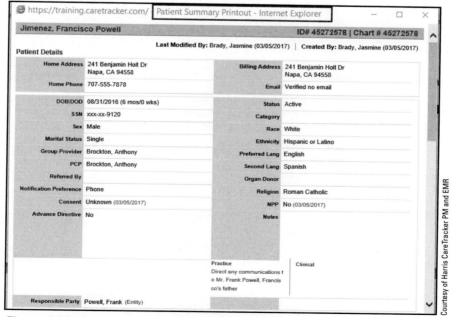

Figure 3-28   Patient Demographics Report for Francisco Powell Jimenez

38. Choose a printer listed in the *Print* dialog box to print the patient demographics summary (see Figure 3-22). (Alternatively, you can close the print prompt box and take a screenshot of the report, or right click on the report and select *Print.*)

📠 Print the *Patient Demographics* report, label it "Activity 3-4," and place it in your assignment folder.

Source Document 3-3

NVFHA

Patient Registration Form

Patient's Last Name	First (legal name)	First (Preferred name)	Middle Name
Jimenez	Francisco		Powell

Address (Number, Street, Apt #)	City		State	Zip Code
241 Benjamin Holt Drive	Napa		CA	94558

Mail will be sent to the address listed above, unless patient indicates a different address (leave blank if same as above)

Send mail to Address (Number, Street, Apt #)	City		State	Zip Code

Phone Options	Phone Number	Okay to leave detailed message	Call this number (circle one)
Home	(707) 555 - 7878	Yes ____ No __X__	(1st) 2nd 3rd choice
Cell	( ) -	Yes ____ No _____	1st 2nd 3rd choice
Work	( ) -	Yes ____ No _____	1st 2nd 3rd choice

Would you like to communicate by Email   Yes ___ No _X_   Email Address _____

Date of Birth	Sex	Social Security Number
8/31/20XX	Female ____ Male _X_	000-00-9120

What is your preferred language / secondary language

Marital Status (*circle one*)

(Single)/ Married / Divorced / Widow /Partner

Race (*circle one*)

African American-Black / Asian / Bi-Multi-racial / Pacific Islander-Hawaiian / (Caucasian–White)/ Native American Eskimo Aleut / Decline to state / Other

Ethnicity (*circle one*)

(Hispanic-Latino)/ Non-Hispanic-Latino / Other

Religion	Catholic	Organ Donor	Yes _____ No _____

Are you new to our practice	Who referred you to our practice	Who is your Primary Care Physician
Yes _X_ No _____	Frank Powell	Anthony Brockton

Additional Notes

Emergency Contact

Emergency Contact's Name	Relationship to patient	Phone
Frank Powell	Father	(510) 555 - 7878

On-Line Patient Portal Communication via Email

On-Line communication is used for non-urgent message/requests only. NVFHA uses secure technology to protect the privacy and confidentiality of your personal information. Only you, your physician, and authorized staff can read your message.

What is your preferred method of communication   Phone _X_   Letter _____   Patient Portal _____   Email _____

Insurance Information

Subscriber (Insurance Holder) Name	Date of Birth	Relationship to patient	Subscriber Phone Number
Frank Powell	11/1/1988	Father	(707) 555 - 7878

Health Plan Information	Primary Health Plan	Secondary Health Plan
Health Plan Name	Century Medical PPO	
Health Plan Address	PO Box 87542, San Jose, CA, 95101	
Group Number		
Subscriber Number	CMED 2478	
Elig Date From		Copay $ 35.00

Patient Employer Information

Employer Name & Address (Number, Street, Apt #, City, State, Zip Code)	Employer Phone Number
Frank Powell - Trinchero Family Estates	(707) 257 - 0200
Occupation Production Supervisor	Start Date 05/01/2011

Assignment of Benefits • Financial Agreement

I hereby give lifetime authorization for payment of insurance benefits to be made directly to **Napa Valley Family Health Assoc.,** and any assisting physicians, for services rendered. I understand that I am financially responsible for all charges whether or not they are covered by insurance. In the event of default, I agree to pay all costs of collection, and reasonable attorney's fees. I hereby authorize this healthcare provider to release all information necessary to secure the payment of benefits.

I further agree that a photocopy of this agreement shall be as valid as the original.

Date: __XX/XX/20XX__   Your Signature: *Frank Powell* _____

Method of Payment: ☐ Cash   ☐ Check   ☐ Credit Card

EDIT PATIENT INFORMATION

Learning Objective 5: Edit patient information in Harris CareTracker.

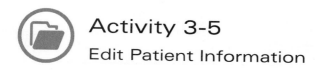

Activity 3-5
Edit Patient Information

It is important to verify accuracy and update (edit) information when a patient schedules an appointment or checks in for an appointment. This makes the treatment process faster and avoids unnecessary complications in billing due to outdated information (**Figure 3-29**).

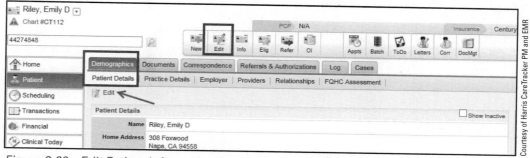

Figure 3-29   *Edit Patient Information Tab*

1. Pull patient Emily Riley into context and click *Edit* on the *Name Bar*.

2. Harris CareTracker PM displays the *Patient Details* window.

3. Click on the *Employer* tab at the top of the screen.

4. Click the *Edit* link at the top left of the screen.

5. Deactivate Ms. Riley's current employer (Napa State Hospital) by clicking on the *Deactivate Employer* icon.

6. Then, click on the + *New Employer* link at the bottom left of the screen. (**Note:** You may receive a pop-up window asking if you want to leave the page. Click on "Leave this page.")

7. You can select a new employer from the *Employer* drop-down menu. Ms. Riley's current employer, Silverado Resort and Spa in Napa, CA, is not listed in the drop-down menu. Instead, click on the *Search* icon, which will open the *Search Employers* window. Enter "Silverado Resort and Spa" in the *Employer Name* field and click *Search*. Click on the appropriate result. The new employer information, including address, will populate in the *Employer* window.

8. Update the *Employer* window with *Occupation* ("Massage Therapist") and *Dates Employed* (use today's date as the start date, and leave the ending date blank) (see **Figure 3-30**).

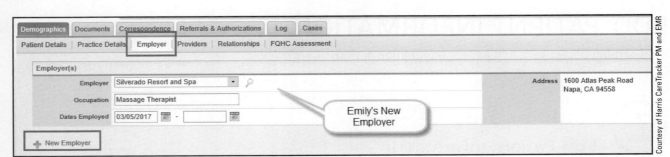

Figure 3-30   *Edited Patient Employer Field*

9. Click *Save*.

10. Click back on the *Patient Details* (Demographics) tab, click *Edit*, change the work address to her new employer just entered and the work phone number to (707)257-0200.

11. Click *Save*.

 Print the updated *Demographics/Employer* screen, label it "Activity 3-5," and place it in your assignment folder.

ELIGIBILITY CHECKS

Learning Objective 6: View and perform eligibility checks.

🔗 **PROFESSIONALISM CONNECTION**

Patients may become frustrated when they are asked if there have been any changes since the last office visit. Some individuals may even become aggravated when you ask to see their insurance card. This is particularly true when the patient just had a recent visit. Your choice of words and tone of voice can make the process less cumbersome. The following statement is an example of a positive directive: "Mr. Timmons, I know you were just in last week, but I just need to make certain that nothing has changed since your last visit, such as your insurance information, telephone number, etc."

 ## Activity 3-6
View and Perform Eligibility Check

The *Eligibility* application enables you to view a history of eligibility checks. It also enables you to electronically check eligibility with the primary insurance as well as the secondary insurance saved in *Patient Demographics*. Harris CareTracker PM and EMR automatically performs eligibility checks every evening for all patients scheduled for appointments for the next five days. Automated batch eligibility checks are performed for a patient once every 30 days regardless of the number of appointments scheduled for the patient during that month. However, it is sometimes necessary to perform individual eligibility checks periodically throughout the treatment and payment cycle or for any walk-in patients. The eligibility check helps to identify potential payer sources, reducing the number of denied claims or bad debt write-offs, and decrease staff hours required for performing manual eligibility checks.

Your student version of Harris CareTracker PM does not have the electronic eligibility feature active. To perform the simulated workflow of an eligibility check, you would click the *Elig* button on the dashboard, and then access payer website or call the insurance company to verify eligibility when electronic access is not available (**Figure 3-31**).

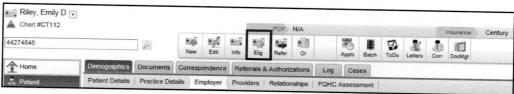

Figure 3-31   *Patient Eligibility Icon*   Courtesy of Harris CareTracker PM and EMR

SPOTLIGHT   If a patient's primary insurance is a non-participating payer and your practice has not signed up to check eligibility for the payers, the *Elig* button is disabled, preventing you from performing electronic checks. This feature is not available on your student version of Harris CareTracker PM.

---

1. Pull patient Emily Riley into context and then click *Elig* on the *Name Bar*. Harris CareTracker PM displays the *Eligibility History* dialog box. In the live version of Harris CareTracker, this box would contain a list of eligibility checks performed for the patient and additional details about the most recent eligibility check. In your student version of Harris CareTracker, you will receive a message stating "No Eligibility History available for this patient."

2. In a live environment, you would click the *Check Eligibility* button in the top right corner to check eligibility. For this activity, you will have to manually simulate checking for patient eligibility. To do this, click the 🗒 + *Add Notes* icon to the left of the *Check Eligibility* button. This will open the *Manual Eligibility* box.

3. Enter information into the *Manual Eligibility* box as shown in **Figure 3-32A**.

    a. *Status*: Select "Eligible."

    b. *Verification*: Enter today's date.

    c. *Mark Reviewed*: Select "No."

    d. *Note*: Enter "Patient is eligible."

    e. Click *Save*.

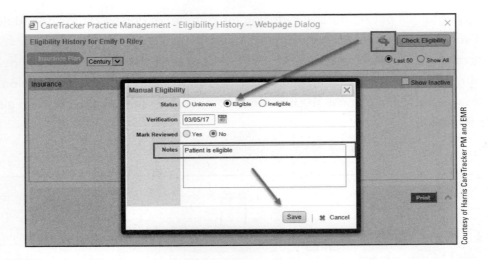

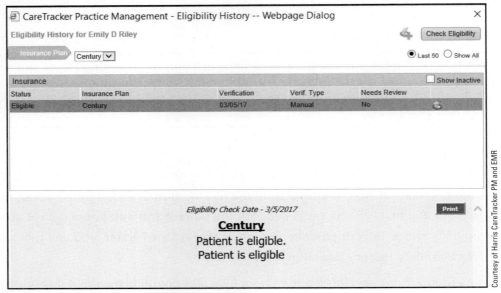

Figures 3-32A and 3-32B   Eligibility Check

4. The manual eligibility check will now show in the *Eligibility History* window (**Figure 3-32B**).

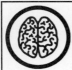 **Print the *Eligibility History* screen, label it "Activity 3-6," and place it in your assignment folder.**

5. Click "X" in the top right corner of the *Eligibility History* window to close out of it.

> **CRITICAL THINKING** Now that you have completed your Chapter 3 activities, how did the challenge put forth in the Real-World Connection apply to you? Did you read each activity in its entirety before you started to enter data? Were you accurate in your entries? Did you struggle with any of the activities or steps? If so, which ones? What measures did you take to correct any errors and move forward with the activity, if any?

CASE STUDIES

Please note, throughout the workbook, end-of-chapter Case Studies related to new patient James Smith will build upon previously completed case studies. If you do not complete Case Study 3-1, later chapter case studies regarding James Smith will not function. There are other Case Studies provided that do not require completion of prior chapter case studies.

Case Study 3-1

Register new patient James M. Smith. Refer to Source Document 3-4 (Patient Registration Form, provided on page 74) in order to complete this case study. Assume that NPP forms have been signed and requisite consent has been given. Mr. Smith is considered a "VIP." Be sure to note that when entering his demographics. Refer to Activity 3-2 for help.

After you register new patient James Smith, print the Patient Demographics report. Refer to Activity 3-3 for help.

Print the Patient Demographics report, label it "Case Study 3-1," and place it in your assignment folder.

Case Study 3-2

Update patient demographics for the following three patients with the date of death (DOD) as indicated. Note that the *Date of Death* (DOD) field is only enabled when the *Status* field has been changed to "Deceased." Refer to Activity 3-5 for help.

A. Francine Quigley—DOD 11/17/2017

B. Cosima Smith—DOD 1/5/2018

C. Bruce Thomas—DOD 1/17/2018

Print the Patient Demographics report for each patient, label them "Case Study 3-2a, b, and c," and place them in your assignment folder.

Source Document 3-4

NVFHA

Patient Registration Form

Patient's Last Name	First (legal name)	First (Preferred name)	Middle Name
SMITH	JAMES	JIM	M

Address (Number, Street, Apt #)	City		State	Zip Code
2455 E. Front, Apt. 205	Napa		CA	94558

Mail will be sent to the address listed above, unless patient indicates a different address (leave blank if same as above)

Send mail to Address (Number, Street, Apt #)	City		State	Zip Code

Phone Options	Phone Number	Okay to leave detailed message	Call this number (circle one)
Home	(707) 221 - 4040	Yes __×__ No _____	(1st) 2nd 3rd choice
Cell	( ) -	Yes ____ No ____	1st 2nd 3rd choice
Work	(877) 833 - 7777	Yes ____ No __×__	1st (2nd) 3rd choice

Would you like to communicate by Email	Yes __×__ No __	Email Address	Jmsmith@email.com

Date of Birth	Sex	Social Security Number
2/23/1965	Female ____ Male __×__	000-00-9009

What is your preferred language / secondary language

English

Marital Status (*circle one*)

(Single) / Married / Divorced / Widow / Partner

Race (*circle one*)

African American-Black / Asian / Bi-Multi-racial / Pacific Islander-Hawaiian /
(Caucasian–White) / Native American Eskimo Aleut / Decline to state / Other

Ethnicity (*circle one*)

Hispanic-Latino /
Non-Hispanic-Latino / Other

Religion	Organ Donor	Yes _____	No _____

Are you new to our practice	Who referred you to our practice	Who is your Primary Care Physician
Yes __×__ No _____	David Dodgin	Rebecca Ayerick

Additional Notes	No call after 8 pm

Emergency Contact

Emergency Contact's Name	Relationship to patient	Phone
Joan Smith	Mother	(510) 478 - 5151

On-Line Patient Portal Communication via Email

On-Line communication is used for non-urgent message/requests only. NVFHA uses secure technology to protect the privacy and confidentiality of your personal information. Only you, your physician, and authorized staff can read your message.

What is your preferred method of communication	Phone __×__	Letter _____	Patient Portal _____	Email _____

Insurance Information

Subscriber (Insurance Holder) Name	Date of Birth	Relationship to patient	Subscriber Phone Number
James M. Smith	2/23/1965	Self	(707) 221 - 4040

Health Plan Information	Primary Health Plan	Secondary Health Plan
Health Plan Name	Blue Shield Cengage	
Health Plan Address	PO Box 32245, Los Angeles, CA, 90002	
Group Number	BCBS987	
Subscriber Number	BCBS987	

Elig Date From	1/1/2010	Copay	$ 25.00

Patient Employer Information

Employer Name & Address (Number, Street, Apt #, City, State, Zip Code)	Employer Phone Number
River Rock Casino, 3250 Highway 128, Geyserville, CA 95441	(877) 833 - 7777

Occupation	IT Support	Start Date	8/25/2009

Assignment of Benefits • Financial Agreement

I hereby give lifetime authorization for payment of insurance benefits to be made directly to **Napa Valley Family Health Assoc.**, and any assisting physicians, for services rendered. I understand that I am financially responsible for all charges whether or not they are covered by insurance. In the event of default, I agree to pay all costs of collection, and reasonable attorney's fees. I hereby authorize this healthcare provider to release all information necessary to secure the payment of benefits.

I further agree that a photocopy of this agreement shall be as valid as the original.

Date: __XX/XX/20XX__ Your Signature: _____ James M. Smith _____

Method of Payment: ☐ Cash ☐ Check ☐ Credit Card

Appointment Scheduling

Learning Objectives

1. Book, reschedule, and cancel appointments.
2. Schedule non-patient appointments.
3. Add a patient to the *Wait List*.
4. Check in patients.
5. Set operator preferences, create a batch, accept payments, print patient receipts, run a journal, and post the batch.

Real-World Connection

Answering the phones and scheduling appointments are two of the most challenging tasks in the medical office. These tasks require an individual who is highly organized, can multitask, and has great communication skills.

Imagine holding the key to your provider's home and controlling which guests have the authority to enter the home and at what times. In some respects, this is similar to what you do when scheduling appointments. Instead of holding the key to the provider's house, you hold the key to the provider's workplace. However, this is only half of the scenario; you must also be cognizant of the severity of the patient's symptoms and the time constraints that prevent the patient from taking the "next available" appointment.

You must ask yourself: Do you have the key attributes of a scheduler? Can you handle the fast pace and keep providers on task, all while accommodating your patients? Consider the desired characteristics of a scheduler as you practice scheduling patients using Harris CareTracker PM. The first step to being a good scheduler is becoming familiar with the software! At the end of the chapter, you will be asked to evaluate your experience scheduling patients. Let's begin!

Before you begin the activities in this chapter, refresh your memory on working with Harris CareTracker by referring back to the Best Practices list on page xiv of this workbook. Following best practices will help you complete work quickly and accurately.

BOOK APPOINTMENTS

Learning Objective 1: Book, reschedule, and cancel appointments.

Building upon activities in Chapter 3, you will now learn how to book (schedule) appointments.

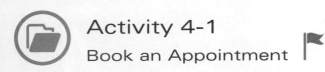

Activity 4-1
Book an Appointment

Booking appointments in Harris CareTracker PM and EMR takes place in the *Book* application of the *Scheduling* module. Both patient and non-patient appointments (e.g., meetings) are booked in this application. You must have a patient in context in the *Name Bar* to book a patient appointment. Three methods are used to book appointments (**Figure 4-1**):

- Schedule directly in *Book*: This allows you to book patient and non-patient appointments by manually moving the schedule to a specific day and clicking on a specific time. You can use the *Book* filters to view the schedule for a specific time, day, location, and provider. Scheduling appointments directly from *Book* gives you the advantage of seeing appointment times that can be double-booked.

- Using *Find*: This allows you to search for the next available appointment time based on specific appointment criteria you set. When searching appointment availability, you can filter your search by provider, location, appointment type, date, day, and time.

- Using *Force*: This allows you to double-book appointments and to book an appointment during a different appointment-type time slot. Forced appointments appear outlined in blue on the schedule.

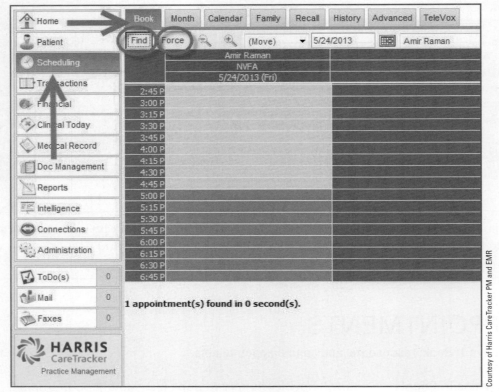

Figure 4-1   Screenshot of Book, Find, and Force

Using established patients in your database as well as building upon your previously registered new patients (from Chapter 3), schedule an appointment for each of the patients in **Table 4-1** by following the directions in Activity 4-1.

ALERT!   Certain scheduling activities will not function in a past date, and billing activities will not function in a future date. It is important to keep this in mind as you schedule patient appointments. Avoid booking too far in the future because that would affect future patient visits and billing activities.

Table 4-1   Patient Appointments to Be Scheduled

PATIENT NAME *PROVIDER*	CHIEF COMPLAINT	TYPE OF APPOINTMENT: RECORD DATE/TIME SELECTED
Jane Morgan *Dr. Raman*	Urinary symptoms	1st available next week/Est. Pt. Sick Date: 2/5/19 Time: 9:30 AM
Ellen Ristino *Dr. Brockton*	Sore throat and nasal congestion	1st available next week/Est. Pt. Sick Date: _____ Time: _____
Craig X. Smith *Dr. Raman*	Wheezing	1st available next week/Est. Pt. Sick Date: _____ Time: _____
Adam Thompson *Dr. Brockton*	Productive cough	1st available next week/Est. Pt. Sick Date: 2/8/19 Time: 8:45 AM
Francisco Powell Jimenez* *Dr. Brockton* (*Registered in Activity 3-4)	New Patient (CPE). In *Notes* field, enter "New Pediatric Patient"	1st available next week/New Patient CPE Date: 2/14/19 Time: 9:00 AM
Edith Robinson *Dr. Raman*	Back pain, six weeks, discuss possible MRI and referral to orthopedist	1st available next week/Est. Pt. Sick Date: 2/15/19 Time: 12:45 PM

To Book an Appointment:

Using the instructions below and the patient data in **Table 4-1**, schedule an appointment for each patient.

1. Pull the patient for whom you are booking an appointment into context on the *Name Bar*.

2. Click the *Scheduling* module. Harris CareTracker PM and EMR opens the *Book* application by default.

3. Display the desired date using one of the following options:

    a. Select an option from the *Move* list to display the schedule for specific time increments such as Next Day, Next Week, 2 Months, and so on.

    b. Manually enter a date in MM/DD/YYYY format or click the *Calendar* ▦ icon to display the schedule for a specific date.

4. Select the provider, location, and the number of days to display, and then click *Go* (**Figure 4-2**).

5. Click on the *time slot* for which you are booking the appointment. (If the schedule is displayed for multiple providers and locations, be sure to click the *time slot* in the appropriate column.) The application displays the *Book Appointment* window.

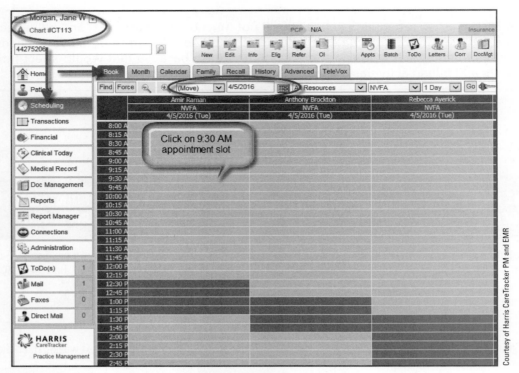

Figure 4-2   Book Appointment for Jane Morgan

TIP If the patient has existing appointments scheduled, the application displays the *Existing Appointments* window. Click *Book Appointment* at the bottom of the window to book a new appointment.

6.   From the *Appointment Type* list, select the appointment type. When you select an appointment type, Harris CareTracker PM and EMR automatically populates the *Task* and *Duration* fields (**Figure 4-3**).

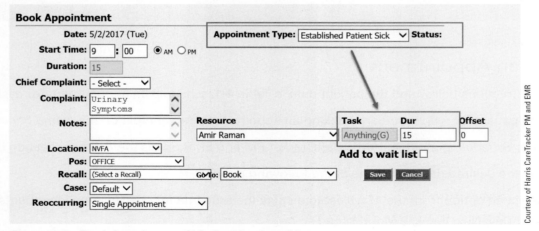

Figure 4-3   Book Appointment Window for Jane Morgan

7.   From the *Resource* list, select the resource (i.e., provider) needed for the appointment.

8.   There are two options for entering a *Chief Complaint* (you can only use option [a]):

   a.   Free text the chief complaint (as noted in **Table 4-1**) in the *Complaint* box (see **Figure 4-3**). For example, enter "Urinary Symptoms" for patient Jane Morgan. (The application will display the complaint in brackets [ ] next to the patient's name on the schedule.)

b. (FYI) From the *Chief Complaint* list, select a chief complaint from the drop-down list. This list is populated with the favorite complaints selected in the *Chief Complaint Maintenance* application in the *Administration* module. (This is not available in your student version. You will use the "free text" option.)

9. In the *Notes* box, enter any notes about the appointment. (Only Francisco Powell Jimenez will need a note entered, as indicated in **Table 4-1**. Notes appear in parentheses next to the patient's name on the schedule and also appear when you move your mouse over the appointment on the schedule.)

 TIP Do not use any symbols when entering appointment notes or patient complaints. Using symbols will cause an error when you try to print encounter forms.

10. From the Location list, select "NVFA."

11. From the *Pos* (Place of Service) list, select "OFFICE."

12. Do not link the appointment to an open recall for the patient.

13. Do not link the patient's appointment to a specific case.

14. Do not select recurring appointment.

15. Click *Save.* The application schedules the appointment (**Figure 4-4**).

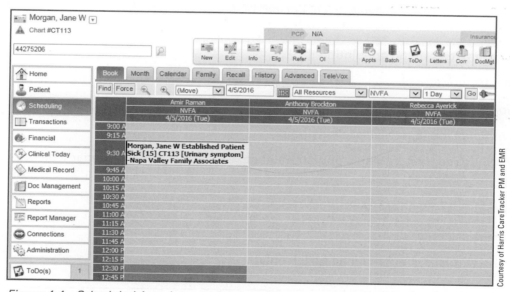

Figure 4-4   Scheduled Appointment for Jane Morgan

 Print the Schedule/Booking screen for each patient scheduled (from Table 4-1), label them "Activity 4-1," and place them in your assignment folder.

Activity 4-2
Book an Appointment Using the Find Button

Building upon your previous scheduling practice (see Activity 4-1), schedule an appointment on the most appropriate date for the following patient using the *Find* button (**Table 4-2**). Record the date and time of the appointment scheduled for future reference.

Table 4-2 Patient Appointment to Be Scheduled Using Find

PATIENT NAME *PROVIDER*	CHIEF COMPLAINT	TYPE OF APPOINTMENT: RECORD DATE/TIME SELECTED
Barbara Watson *Dr. Raman*	Fever—103F	1st available appointment next week/Est. Pt. Sick Date/Time: _____

1. Pull patient Barbara Watson into context.

2. Click the *Scheduling* module. Harris CareTracker PM displays the *Book* application.

3. Click the *Find* button in the top left corner of the *Book* application. Harris CareTracker PM displays the *Appointment Criteria* window (**Figure 4-5**).

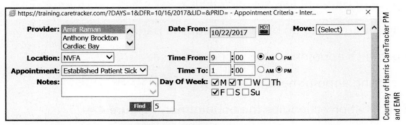

Figure 4-5 *Appointment Criteria Window*

4. Select the parameters of the appointment:

   a. *Provider* (Amir Raman)

   b. *Location* (NVFA)

   c. *Appointment* type (Established Patient Sick)

   d. *Date From* (select first available appointment next week, using the calendar icon or by using *Move*)

   e. *Time From* (select 9:00AM)

   f. *Time To* (select 1:00PM)

   g. *Day of Week* (place check mark by M, T, F only)

 TIP You can select multiple providers by holding down the [Ctrl] key on your keyboard while clicking on each provider name.

5. *Find* will default to display the first 20 appointments that match the search criteria. Change the number to "5" and click *Find* (see **Figure 4-5**).

6. To select an available appointment, click in the *Appointment/Task Class* column or anywhere on the row that corresponds to the desired date and time for that particular appointment. Harris CareTracker PM re-displays the *Book* application for the selected appointment date, highlighting the selected time in red (**Figure 4-6**).

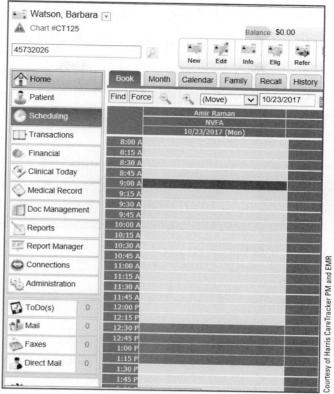

Figure 4-6   Find Appointment—Red Highlight

7. Click the selected time slot. The application displays the *Book Appointment* window.

8. Select the *Appointment Type* (Established Patient Sick). When you select an *Appointment Type*, the application automatically populates the *Resource*, *Task*, and *Duration* fields.

9. Enter the *Complaint* by entering the free text description (Fever 103F).

10. From the *Location* list, select the location "NVFA."

11. From the *Pos* list, select the place of service (OFFICE).

12. Click *Save*. The application schedules the appointment (**Figure 4-7**).

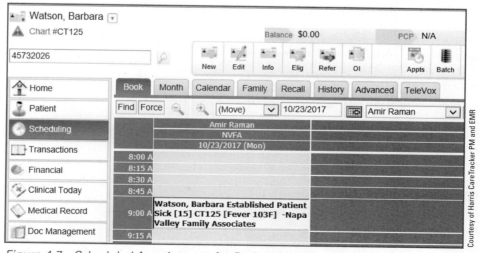

Figure 4-7   Scheduled Appointment for Barbara Watson

🖳 **Print the Booked Appointment screen, label it "Activity 4-2," and place it in your assignment folder.**

Activity 4-3

Book an Appointment Using the Force Button

Using *Force* allows you to double-book appointments and to book an appointment during a different appointment-type time slot. Using the patient in **Table 4-3**, force an appointment at the same time slot as the previous patient in Activity 4-2, Barbara Watson.

Table 4-3 Patient Appointment to Be Scheduled Using Force		
PATIENT NAME / ***PROVIDER***	**CHIEF COMPLAINT**	**TYPE OF APPOINTMENT: RECORD DATE/TIME SELECTED**
Thomas Barret / *Dr. Raman*	Fall—swollen wrist	Same date/time as Barbara Watson's appointment scheduled in Activity 4-2/Est. Pt. Sick Date/Time: _____

1. Before you start, refer back to the appointment you just booked for Barbara Watson in Activity 4-2. You will need the date and time of the appointment to complete this activity. Once you have that information in hand, continue with step 2.

2. Pull patient Thomas Barret into context.

3. Click the *Scheduling* module. Harris CareTracker PM displays the *Book* application.

4. Click the *Force* button in the top left corner of the *Book* application. Harris CareTracker PM displays the *Book Appointment* window.

5. From the *Appointment Type* list, select the appointment type "Established Patient Sick." When you select an appointment type, Harris CareTracker PM automatically populates the *Task* and *Duration* fields (**Figure 4-8**).

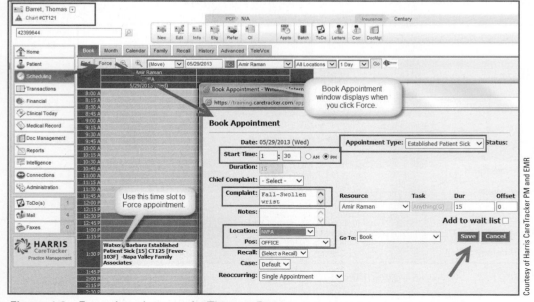

Figure 4-8   Force Appointment for Thomas Barret

6. From the *Resource* list, select the resource needed for the appointment (Dr. Raman).

7. In the *Start Time* field, enter the start time for the appointment. (Use the same date and time as for the patient booked in Activity 4-2, Barbara Watson.)

8. Enter *Complaint* by entering free text (Fall—swollen wrist).

9. From the *Location* list, select "NVFA."

10. From the *Pos* list, select "OFFICE."

11. Click *Save.* The application schedules the appointment (**Figure 4-9**).

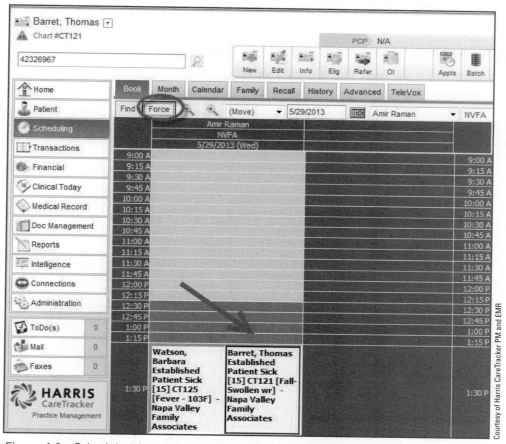

Figure 4-9   Scheduled Appointment Using Force for Thomas Barret

 Print the Booked Appointment using Force screen, label it "Activity 4-3," and place it in your assignment folder.

PROFESSIONALISM CONNECTION

There are times that you may feel compelled to double book appointments. Oftentimes, this occurs during flu season, or when you have a patient that is acutely ill and needs to be seen the day of the appointment request. When this is the case, always check with the provider first. Make certain the provider is on board with being double-booked. If you are unable to accommodate the patient, weigh all other options before discontinuing the call. Check to see if any other providers are available to see the patient, or when possible, refer the patient to an urgent care facility connected with your organization. Always demonstrate a caring attitude toward the patient, and when unable to accommodate the patient's specific preferences, offer an apology while you work to explore additional options for the patient

Activity 4-4

Reschedule Appointments

Reschedule an appointment to the following day:

1. Before you start, begin by booking an appointment for patient Galah Piccerelli approximately two weeks from today using the following information (refer to Activity 4-1 if you need help):

   a. *Appointment Type*: Follow up

   b. *Complaint*: Follow up labs

   c. *Resource*: Amir Raman

2. When finished scheduling the appointment in Step 1, with finished scheduling the appointment in Step 1, with the patient in context, click the *Scheduling* module. The application displays the *Book* application by default.

3. From the date of Galah's current appointment, *Move* to "Next Day," same provider, and same location (**Figure 4-10**).

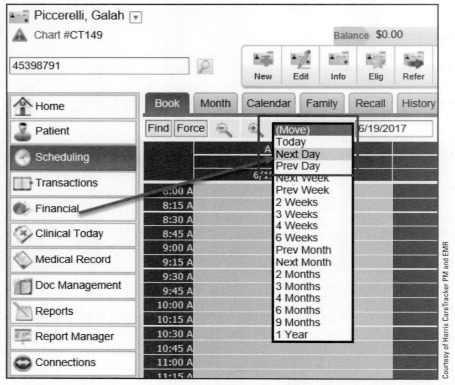

Figure 4-10   Reschedule Appointment for Galah Piccerelli

4. Click on the time slot in which you want to reschedule the appointment (same time slot as previous appointment). The application displays the patient's existing appointment(s) (**Figure 4-11**). (**Note:** You cannot reschedule an appointment that has an encounter created or that has already passed.)

5. From the *Action* list, select "Reschedule" and then click *Go*. The application displays the *Reschedule Appointment* window.

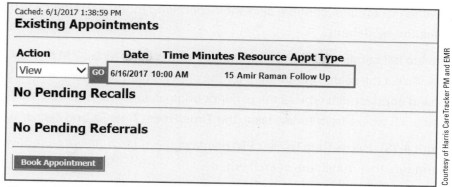

Figure 4-11   Existing Appointments Window

 TIP Do not click the *Book Appointment* button. If you do, you will book an additional appointment instead of rescheduling the existing appointment.

6. From the *Reschedule* list, (*Select a Reason*) for rescheduling the appointment (**Figure 4-12**). (Select "Entry Error.")

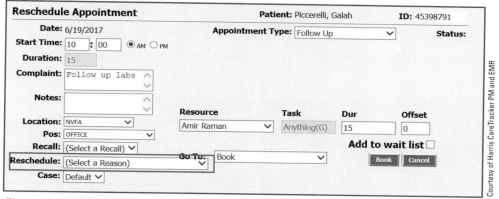

Figure 4-12   Reschedule Reason for Galah Piccerelli

 Print the Rescheduled Appointment screen, label it "Activity 4-4," and place it in your assignment folder.

7. Click *Book.* The application cancels the original appointment and adds the rescheduled appointment to the calendar. Record the date/time of Galah's appointment here: _____.

Activity 4-5
Reschedule Appointments Using the Find Button

Using Galah Piccerelli, reschedule the appointment from Activity 4-4 using the *Find* button.

 ALERT! If Galah's appointment date has already passed, you will need to first enter a new appointment for the patient scheduled out one week from today, as appointment dates that have already passed cannot be rescheduled.

1. With patient Galah Piccerelli in context, click the *Scheduling* module. Harris CareTracker PM displays the *Book* application by default.

2. Click *Find* in the top left corner of the *Book* application. Harris CareTracker PM displays the *Appointment Criteria* window. Select the search parameters for the appointment you want to find. Select the same provider, location, and appointment type as the patient's original appointment (from Activity 4-4). Change the *Date From* to three (3) weeks from today; leave the *Time From*, *Time To*, and *Day of Week* as is.

3. Click *Find* (**Figure 4-13**). Harris CareTracker PM displays the *Search Results* window containing the first 20 appointments that match the search criteria.

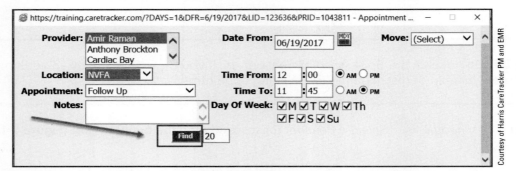

Figure 4-13   Reschedule Appointment for Galah Piccerelli Using Find

4. Click on an appointment in the *Appointment Task Class* column to select it. (Select any time slot for the next available day.) The application then displays the selected appointment in the *Book* application.

5. A red bar on the schedule marks the available appointment time you selected from the *Search Results* list. Click on the red bar in the selected time slot. Harris CareTracker PM displays the patient's existing appointment(s) (**Figure 4-14**).

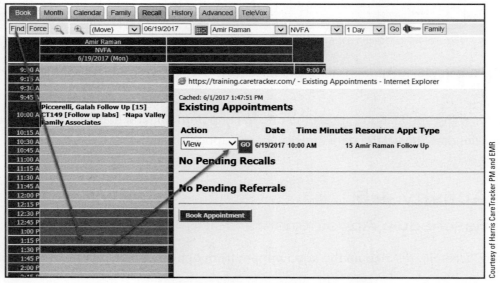

Figure 4-14   Existing Appointments Window for Galah Piccerelli

6. From the *Action list* select "Reschedule" and then click *Go*. The application displays the *Reschedule Appointment* window. Do <u>not</u> click the *Book Appointment* button. If you do, you will book an additional appointment instead of rescheduling the existing appointment.

7. From the *Reschedule* list, select a reason for rescheduling the appointment (**Figure 4-15**). (Select "Entry Error.")

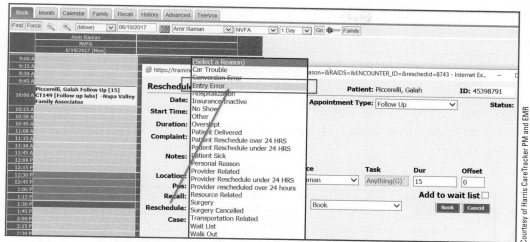

Figure 4-15   *Reschedule Reason for Galah Piccerelli*

 Print the Rescheduled Appointment screen, label it "Activity 4-5," and place it in your assignment folder.

8. Click *Book*. Harris CareTracker PM cancels the original appointment and adds the rescheduled appointment to the calendar (**Figure 4-16**). Record the date/time of Galah's appointment here: _____.

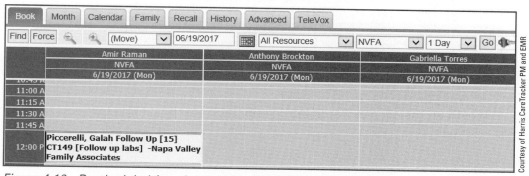

Figure 4-16   *Rescheduled Appointment for Galah Piccerelli Using Find*

Activity 4-6
Cancel Appointments

Using the appointment you scheduled for Thomas Barret in Activity 4-3, cancel the appointment in the *History* application.

1. Pull the patient for whom you are canceling an appointment into context (Thomas Barret).

2. Click the *Scheduling* module and then click the *History* tab (**Figure 4-17**).

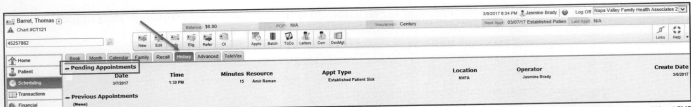

Figure 4-17   *History Tab in Scheduling Module*

Courtesy of Harris CareTracker PM and EMR

3. Under the *Pending Appointments* heading, click on the appointment you want to cancel (the appointment scheduled in Activity 4-3). Harris CareTracker PM displays the *Appointment Detail* window (**Figure 4-18**).

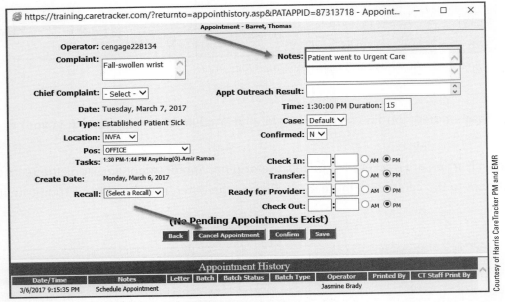

Figure 4-18   *Appointment Detail Window*

Courtesy of Harris CareTracker PM and EMR

4. Enter a note regarding the canceled appointment in the *Notes* box. (Free text note: "Patient went to Urgent Care.")

5. Click the *Cancel Appointment* button.

6. From the *Cancel Reason* list, select the reason for canceling the appointment (**Figure 4-19**). (Select "Hospitalization.")

 TIP A note saved in a canceled appointment will always be linked to that cancellation and appears in the *History* application.

7. The *Go To* field defaults to "(Select)." From the drop-down menu you can select an application so that when the appointment is canceled, Harris CareTracker PM opens that application. (Select "Book.")

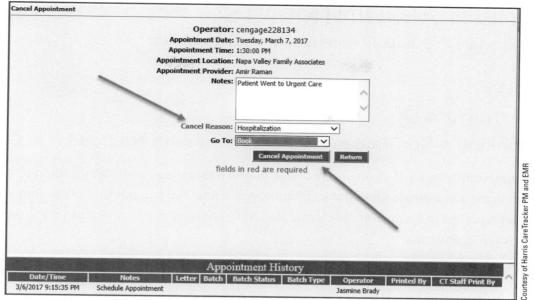

Figure 4-19   Cancel Appointment Window

8. Click *Cancel Appointment*. Harris CareTracker PM cancels the appointment and removes it from the schedule (**Figure 4-20**).

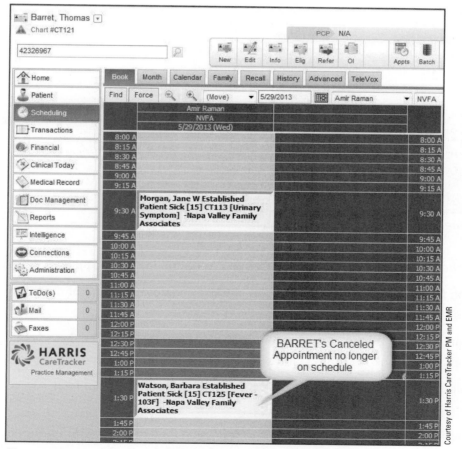

Figure 4-20   Canceled Appointment for Thomas Barret

💾 **Print the Canceled Appointment screen, label it "Activity 4-6," and place it in your assignment folder.**

NON-PATIENT APPOINTMENTS

Learning Objective 2: Schedule non-patient appointments.

Activity 4-7
Booking a Non-Patient Appointment with No Patient in Context

Non-patient appointments, such as meetings or out-of-office times (i.e., provider vacation or training), are scheduled in the *Book* application of the *Scheduling* module. You can book a non-patient appointment with or without a patient in context on the *Name Bar*. A non-patient appointment can be scheduled for multiple providers at one time.

1. Using the drop-down, select "None" from the *Name* list on the *Name Bar* so that there is no patient in context (**Figure 4-21**).

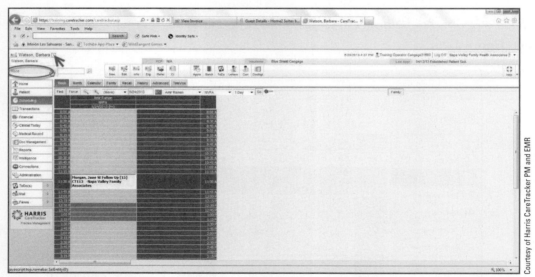

Figure 4-21   No Patient in Context

2. Click the *Scheduling* module. Harris CareTracker PM opens the *Book* application by default.

3. Select "Next Month" (**Figure 4-22**). To display the desired date, use one of the following options:

   a. Select an option from the *Move* list to display the schedule for specific time increments such as Next Day, Next Week, 2 Months, and so on. (Select "Next Month," or do the following.)

   b. Manually enter a date in MM/DD/YYYY format or click the *Calendar* icon ⊞ to display the schedule for a specific date.

4. Select the resources (All Resources), location (All Locations), and the number of days (1 Day) to display and then click *Go* (**Figure 4-23**). If not all providers are showing, move the schedule to the next day until all four provider schedules display.

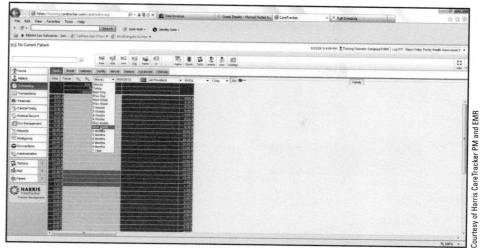

Figure 4-22   Move Schedule to Next Month

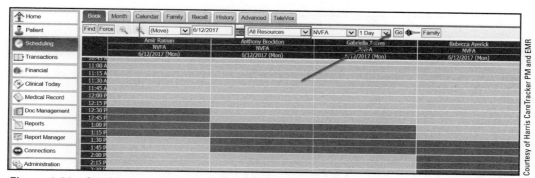

Figure 4-23   Set Schedule for Non-Patient Appointment

5. Click on the time slot in any provider's schedule for which you are booking the appointment (select the 1:00 PM time slot). Harris CareTracker PM displays the *Non-Patient Appointment* window.

6. In the *Description* field, enter a brief description of the appointment. (Enter "Monthly Providers Meeting.")

7. In the *Notes* field, enter any additional information about the appointment. (Enter "Guest Speaker, Cardiology Group.")

8. In the *Resources* field, click on the resource needed for the appointment. You can select multiple resources by holding down the [Ctrl] key on your keyboard and clicking on each resource (select all providers: Amir Raman, Anthony Brockton, Gabriella Torres, and Rebecca Ayerick). If you select *All*, you will include all resources such as lab, cardiac bay, and so on.

9. The *Location*, *Date*, and *Time* fields are automatically populated.

10. The *Duration* defaults to 30 minutes but you can change the duration as needed (change to 60 minutes) (**Figure 4-24**).

11. Click *Save*. The application schedules the appointment for all of the selected resources.

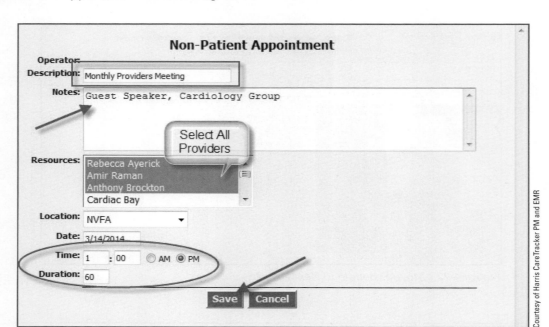

Figure 4-24   Non-Patient Appointment Window

 Print the Book screen with the non-patient appointment scheduled, label it "Activity 4-7," and place it in your assignment folder.

ADD PATIENT TO THE WAIT LIST

Learning Objective 3: Add a patient to the Wait List.

Activity 4-8
Add Patient to the Wait List from the Mini-Menu

Patients who would like an appointment with a provider sooner than their currently scheduled appointment can be added to the *Wait List* in Harris CareTracker PM and EMR. A patient must have a currently scheduled appointment in Harris CareTracker PM and EMR to be added to the *Wait List*.

There are several places you can add a patient to the *Wait List* in Harris CareTracker PM and EMR:
- From the scheduling mini-menu in the *Book* application (see **Figure 4-25** and this activity)
- From the *Book Appointment* window in the *Book* application (**Figure 4-26**)
- From the *Appointments* tab in *Clinical Today, Actions* menu in the *Appointment List* (**Figure 4-27**)

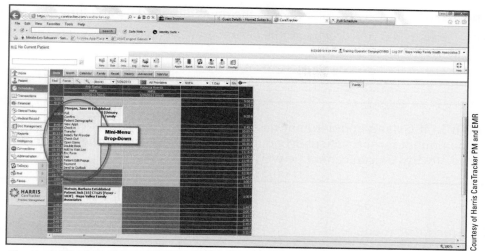

Figure 4-25   Scheduling Mini-Menu

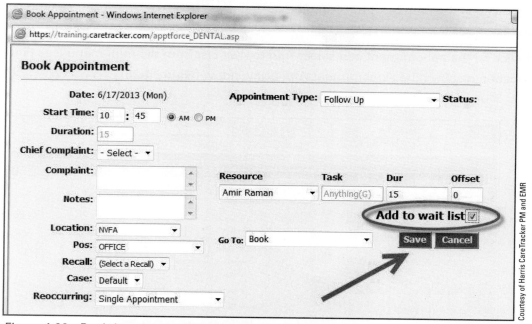

Figure 4-26   Book Appointment Window—Add to Wait List

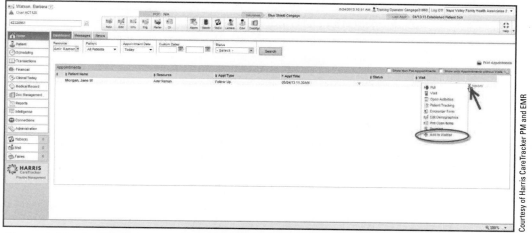

Figure 4-27   Appointments tab in Clinical Today, Appointments Actions Drop-Down

1. Before beginning this activity, refer back to the appointment date and time you scheduled for Galah Piccerelli in Activity 4-5. You will need this information on hand to complete this activity; then proceed to step 2.

 ALERT!   If Galah's appointment date has already passed, you will need to first enter a new appointment for the patient scheduled out one week from today, as appointment dates that have already passed cannot be wait listed.

2. Click the *Scheduling* module. Harris CareTracker PM displays the *Book* application by default.

3. *Move* the schedule to display the appointment for the patient you want to add to the wait list (select the appointment you created for Galah Piccerelli in Activity 4-5). This can be done by manually entering the date in the *Date* box by clicking the *Calendar* icon, or by selecting a time period from the *Move* list.

4. Left-click on the appointment and select *Add to Wait List* from the mini-menu (see **Figure 4-25**). The application displays the *Appointment Wait List* window (**Figure 4-28**).

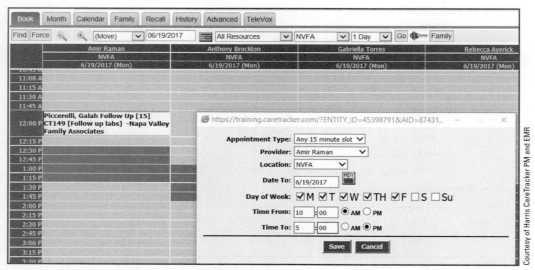

Figure 4-28   Appointment Wait List Window

5. From the *Appointment Type* list, select the type of appointment the patient needs or select "Any 15 minute slot" to book the first available appointment type. (Select "Any 15 minute slot.")

6. From the *Provider* list, select the provider the patient wants to see (select Amir Raman). You would select "Any Provider" to book the first available provider.

7. From the *Location* list, select the location where the patient wants to be seen. (Select "NVFA.")

8. In the *Date To* field, click the *Calendar* ▦ icon and select the last date before which the appointment must fall. Select the day the appointment was scheduled for patient Galah Piccerelli in Activity 4-5.

9. In the *Day of Week* field, select the checkbox next to each day the patient is available for an appointment (select Monday through Friday, unchecking the other days).

10. In the *Time From* and *Time To* fields, select the desired time for the appointment. (Select "10:00 AM" through "5:00 PM.")

11. Click *Save.* The application adds the patient to the *Wait List*. (The *Wait List* is managed from the *Wait List* link in the *Front Office* section of the *Dashboard*, under *Appointments*.)

12. Return to the *Dashboard* (*Home* module) and click on the *Wait List* link (under the *Appointments* header) (**Figure 4-29**).

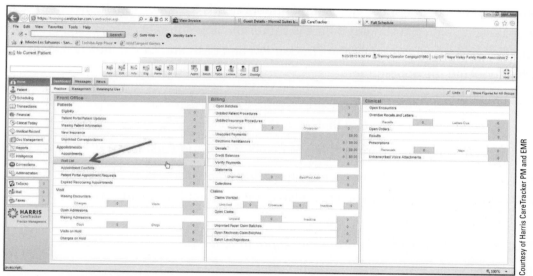

Figure 4-29   *Wait List Link*

13. Select *Resource* (Amir Raman).

14. Review the *Date From* and *Date To* displayed. Enter today's date in the *Date From* field. Enter a date approximately four weeks from today in the *Date To* field.

15. Then click *Go.*

16. The wait-listed appointment will appear with a *Possible Match* (**Figure 4-30**). **Note**: A possible match will not display if there are no dates that meet the specified criteria.

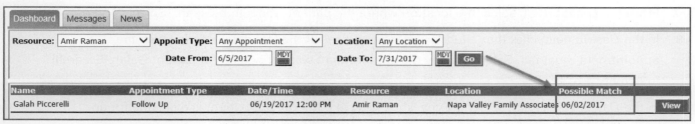

Figure 4-30   *Wait List Dashboard Display*

Courtesy of Harris CareTracker PM and EMR

Print the Patient Wait List screen, label it "Activity 4-8," and place it in your assignment folder.

Activity 4-9
Enter an Appointment Recall

Recalls are reminders to patients that an appointment needs to be booked. Rather than scheduling a future appointment, a recall (reminder) date is set for the appointment. You can generate patient recall letters for any recall tracked in Harris CareTracker PM and EMR and can manually link an appointment to recalls when booking the appointment.

1. Pull patient Edith Robinson into context.

2. Click the *Scheduling* module and then click the *Recall* tab.

3. Click *+ New Recall*. Harris CareTracker PM displays the *Add Patient Recall* box (see **Figure 4-31**).

4. Select the time frame for the recall from the *Time Frame* list (select "1 Year"). When Days, Weeks, Months, or Years is selected, you must also enter a numeric value to correspond to the selected time unit.

5. Select the type of appointment from the *Appointment Type* list. (Select "Lab.")

6. Select the provider from the *Resource* list. (Select "Amir Raman.")

7. Select the location from the *Location* list. (Select "Napa Valley Family Associates.")

8. If the recall appointment needs to be linked to a case, select the appropriate case from the *Case* list (not applicable here).

9. Select an alert type from the *EMR Alert Status* list. (Select "Soft Alert.")

10. Enter a note about the recall in the *Recall Notes* field. (Free text note: "Annual CPE Labs.")

11. Leave the *Active* field "Yes."

12. Leave the *Go To* field as (Select).

13. Click *Save* (**Figure 4-31**).

14. When you receive the "Success" box, click on "X" to close.

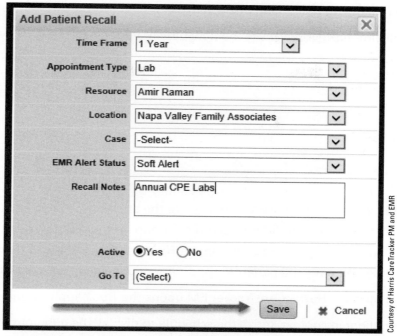

Figure 4-31   Entering an Appointment Recall

 Print the Patient Recalls screen, label it "Activity 4-9," and place it in your assignment folder.

CHECK IN PATIENTS

Learning Objective 4: Check in patients.

Activity 4-10
Check in Patient from the Mini-Menu

For a patient encounter to be generated in the electronic medical record (EMR), the patient must be checked in when he or she arrives for an appointment. Checking in a patient changes his or her Harris CareTracker PM and EMR status to "Checked in," and Harris CareTracker PM and EMR verifies that the patient's billing and demographic information is complete. Harris CareTracker PM and EMR will display the *Patient Alert* dialog box if the patient is missing important billing or demographic data.

> **✓ TIP** *Patient Alerts* will only display if the *Show Alerts* feature is activated in your batch.

You can check in a patient in Harris CareTracker PM and EMR in the following places:

- In the *Book* application of the *Scheduling* module, using the mini-menu drop-down feature (see **Figure 4-32**)
- From the *Appts* button in the *Name Bar*
- From the *Appointments* list on the *Dashboard*
- From the *Appointments* tab in *Clinical Today*

1. You will check in the following patients in this activity:

   a. Francisco Powell Jimenez (**Note:** This is the new patient you registered in Activity 3-4.)

   b. Craig X. Smith

   c. Jane Morgan

   d. Ellen Ristino

   e. Adam Thompson

   f. Edith Robinson

   g. Barbara Watson

   Before you begin this activity, refer back to the dates of the appointments you scheduled for each of them in Activities 4-1 and 4-2. If you did not record their appointment dates, pull the patient into context, click on the *Scheduling* module, and click on the *History* tab. All of the patient's appointments will be displayed. Once you have the patients' appointment dates in hand, continue to step 2.

2. Click the *Scheduling* module. Harris CareTracker PM opens the *Book* application by default.

3. With or without the patient in context, move the schedule to display the appointment for the patient you want to check in. This can be done by manually entering in the date in the *Date* box, by clicking the *Calendar* icon, or by selecting a time period from the *Move* list. Be sure that "All Resources" and "All Locations" display. If not, use the drop-down, change the parameters and click *Go*.

4. Left-click the name of the patient you want to check in and select *Check In* from the mini-menu (see **Figure 4-32**). Harris CareTracker PM and EMR changes the patient's status to "Checked In" and highlights the patient's appointment in green in both the *Book* application and the *Appointments* link in the *Front Office* section of the *Dashboard* (*Home* module). Checking in a patient from the mini-menu will pull the patient into context. **FYI:** Harris CareTracker PM and EMR records the check-in time and displays the patient's wait time in the *Appointments* link (**Figure 4-33**). For all the patients to appear in the *Appointments* link, be sure to change the *Resource* to *All*, enter the date you want to check status for, and select *All* from the *Status* drop-down.

5. Repeat steps 2 through 4 until you have all patients from step 1 checked in.

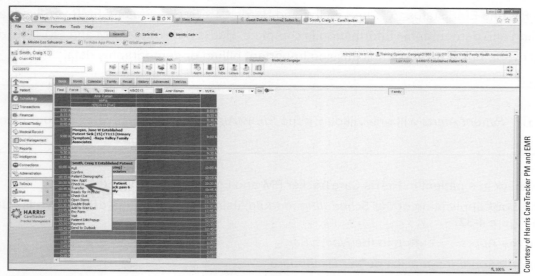

Figure 4-32   Mini-Menu Check-In

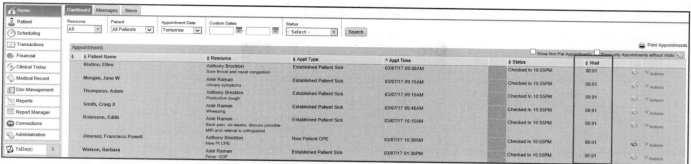

Figure 4-33   Check-in Wait Time Noted in the Dashboard, Appointments link.

Courtesy of Harris CareTracker PM and EMR

🖨 **Print the Schedule screen for each day that patients were checked in, label it/them "Activity 4-10," and place it/them in your assignment folder.**

CREATE A BATCH

Learning Objective 5: Set Operator preferences, create a batch, accept payments, print patient receipts, run a journal, and post the batch.

Activity 4-11

Setting Operator Preferences

The *Batch* application is used for setting defaults for both "Financial" and "Clinical" components. The "Financial" portion of the batch establishes defaults and assigns a name to a batch (group) of financial transactions you will be entering into Harris CareTracker. A new financial batch is created daily to enter financial transactions into Harris CareTracker; for example, charges, payments, and adjustments. This helps identify transactions linked to the batch, the date of each transaction, and the operator who entered it into the system. Setting up the financial batch helps identify a group of charges or payments and helps run reports to balance against the actual charges or payments entered.

The "Clinical" batch settings are typically set up only once and are used to set preferences and pre-populate fields common to your workflow (**Figure 4-34**). The "Clinical" batch settings are in the middle and lower sections of the *Operator Encounter Batch Control* dialog box. Setting the defaults here can speed up scheduling by having default *Resource* and *Location* defined.

The *Batch* application enables you to set up operator preferences based on the workflow for your role. This reduces the number of clicks required to get from one application to the other, making navigation through Harris CareTracker PM and EMR easy.

The first time you log in to Harris CareTracker you will be prompted to create a batch. Activities related to searching for a patient or scheduling a patient do not require that a batch be created and you may simply close out the batch prompt. For the activities related to financial and clinical workflows, you will need to have a batch open. You begin by setting your operator preferences (Activity 4-10).

The available batch redirects are described in **Table 4-4.** These are located in the lower section of *the Operator Encounter Batch Control* dialog box (**Figure 4-35**).

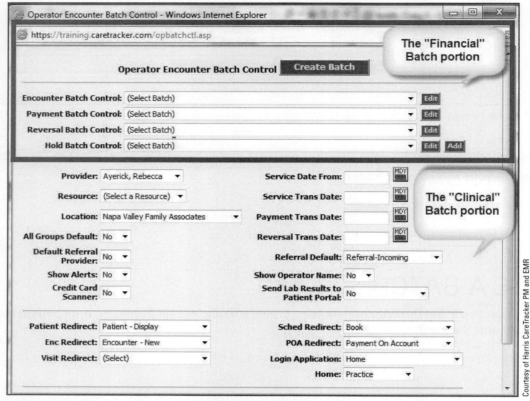

Figure 4-34 *Financial and Clinical Components of a Batch*

Table 4-4 Batch Redirects

REDIRECTS *FIELD*	DESCRIPTION
Patient Redirect	Launches the selected application after editing a *Demographic* record in the *Patient* module. You can also change this setting in the *Demographic* application if necessary.
Enc Redirect	Launches the selected application after saving a *Charge* in the *Transactions* module.
Visit Redirect	Launches the selected application after a visit is saved in the *Visit* application.
Sched Redirect	Launches the selected application after an appointment is booked via the *Book* application of the *Scheduling* module.
POA (Payment on Account) Redirect	Launches the selected application after a payment is entered via the *Payment on Account* application of the *Transaction* module.
Login Application	Launches the selected application when you log in to Harris CareTracker PM and EMR.
Home	If the *Log in Application* is set to "Home," you can select which *Home* module application to display by default. For example, the *Management, Meaningful Use, Messages,* or *News* applications.
When finished with redirects, click *Save*	Your screen will be saved with selections made.

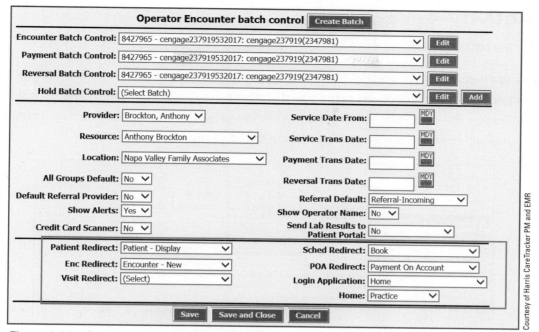

Figure 4-35   Operator Encounter Batch Control

1. With no patient in context, click on the *Batch* icon on the *Name Bar*. Harris CareTracker PM and EMR displays the *Operator Encounter Batch Control* dialog box.

2. If there is an open batch, by default the batch will display. Harris CareTracker PM and EMR assigns redirects, making it easy to navigate from different applications within Harris CareTracker PM and EMR. The default redirects are based on the most commonly used workflow. Redirect means to change the path or direction; for example, changing a redirect allows the operator to select the most efficient workflow.

3. Click *Edit* if the fields are grayed out. Otherwise, enter (or confirm if already populated) the information for each of the fields in the *Operator Encounter Batch Control* dialog box (see **Figure 4-36**) as follows:

   a. Patient Redirect: (Select "Patient – Display")

   b. Enc Redirect: (Select "Encounter – New")

   c. Visit Redirect: (Select "Select")

   d. Sched Redirect: (Select "Book")

   e. POA (Payment on Account) Redirect: (Select "Payment on Account")

   f. Login Application: (Select "Home")

   g. Home: (Select "Practice")

4. Click *Save*. Screen will be saved with selections made.

5. Click *Close* to close out the batch control box.

📭 **Print the Operator Encounter Batch Control screen, label it "Activity 4-11," and place it in your assignment folder.**

Activity 4-12

Create a Batch

A provider's paperless desk is incorporated in the *Clinical Today* module. Therefore, selecting the *Clinical* module from the *Login Application* list takes you directly to the *Clinical Today* module each time you log in to Harris CareTracker PM and EMR, streamlining workflow (**Figure 4-36**). When you begin clinical activities in Chapter 6, you will change your *Login Application* to the *Clinical* setting.

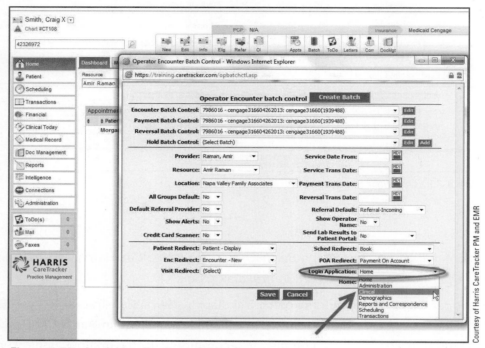

Figure 4-36   Login Application—Clinical

Courtesy of Harris CareTracker PM and EMR

Table 4-5 outlines the fields and related instructions to complete your batch details. You will finish creating a batch in this activity, referencing instructions in **Table 4-5**. After entering the copayments as assigned in Activity 4-13, you will print a receipt (see Activity 4-14), run a journal (see Activity 4-15), and post your batch (see Activity 4-16). Posting a batch permanently stores all financial transactions linked to it in Harris CareTracker PM and EMR. The application is updated in real time.

Having set up your operator preferences in the *Operator Encounter Batch Control* in Activity 4-10, you will now create a batch. Reference the instructions in **Table 4-5** when creating your batch.

1. Before creating a batch, make sure your fiscal period and fiscal year are open for the month(s) in which patient appointments are scheduled (refer to Activities 2-5 and 2-6 if you need to refresh your memory). For example, if Jane Morgan's appointment is in March 2017, make sure the fiscal period March 2017 is open. Once you have confirmed the fiscal period and year are open, proceed to step 2. **Note**: If you are working at the month's end and are booking appointments in the following month, you would need to open the current <u>and</u> next month in fiscal period. This would also apply to the fiscal period selected in your batch.

2. Click on the *Batch* icon on the *Name* Bar. Then click *Edit* and then click *Create Batch*. The *Batch Master* dialog box displays (**Figure 4-37**).

3. By default, the *Batch Name* box displays a batch identification name. The name consists of your user name followed by the current date. (**Note:** You can edit the batch name if necessary and change the

Table 4-5 Batch Details Field and Instructions

BATCH DETAILS FIELD	INSTRUCTIONS
Provider	From the *Provider* list, select the name of the billing provider associated with the batch. **Note:** The *Admissions* application accessed via the *Dashboard* and the *Charges* application in the *Transaction* module display the billing provider set up in the batch.
Resource	From the *Resource* list, select the servicing provider. In most instances, the billing provider and the resource are the same. **Note:** The *Book* application in the *Scheduling* module and the *Appointment* application in the *Clinical Today* module display the resource set up in the batch.
Location	From the *Location* list, select the location associated with the batch. **Note:** The *Admissions* application accessed via the *Dashboard* and the *Book* application in the *Scheduling* module display the location set up in the batch.
All Groups Default	By default, the *All Groups Default* list is set to "No." Change the list to "Yes" if necessary. This displays patient financial information for the current group or all groups in the practice based on the setting selected. If *Yes* is selected, you can only see the financial transactions for the groups that you have access to as an operator. This setting mostly benefits multi-group practices and also determines the default value in the *Open Items* application of the *Financial* module and *Edit* application of the *Transactions* module.
Default Referral Provider	By default, the *Default Referral Provider* list is set to "No." Change the field to "Yes" if there is no referring provider in the patient's demographics or if there is no active referral/authorization for the patient. This sets the billing provider as the referring provider.
Show Alerts	In the *Show Alerts* field, select "Yes" to enable Harris CareTracker PM to display the *Patient Alert* window; otherwise select "No." The *Patient Alerts* window notifies users when key information is missing from a patient's demographics or when there are other issues with a patient's account.
Credit Card Scanner	The *Credit Card Scanner* field is set to "No" by default. Your student version of Harris CareTracker will NOT have this feature. In a real practice setting, select "Yes" if your group uses a credit card scanner to process payments by credit card.
Service Date From	Click the *Calendar* icon ▦ and select the start of the service dates included in the batch.
Service Trans Date	Click the *Calendar* icon ▦ and select the service transaction date included in the batch.
Payment Trans Date	Click the *Calendar* icon ▦ and select the payment transactions date included in the batch.
Reversal Trans Date	Click the *Calendar* icon ▦ and select the reversal transactions date included in the batch.
Referral Default	By default, the *Referral Default* list is set to "Referral-Incoming." Select a referral type based on your practice specialty. The selected option will display as the default option when the *Ref/Auth* application is accessed via the *Name Bar* or *Patient* module.
Show Operator Name	Select "Yes" to display the operator's name on the Harris CareTracker PM and EMR interface. Select "No" if you do not want the operator's name displayed.

Click *Save*. The batch information is saved.

Note: Click *Edit* to make changes if necessary.

Click *X* on the right-hand corner to close the dialog box.

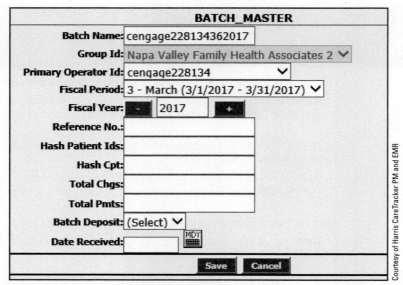

Figure 4-37   Batch Master Dialog Box

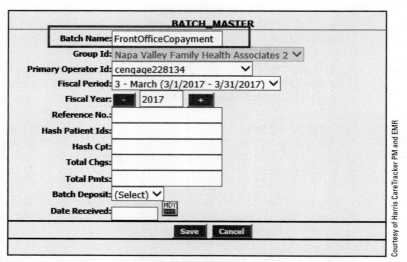

Figure 4-38   Rename Batch "FrontOfficeCopayment Batch"

batch name to identify the types of financial transactions associated with the batch; for example, "copayment5132017.") Do not use symbols when editing the name. Change the Batch Name to "FrontOfficeCopayment" (**Figure 4-38**).

4. By default, the *Group Id* displays the name of your group.

5. By default, the *Primary Operator Id* displays your user name.

6. In the *Fiscal Period* field, click the month in which patients from Activity 4-1 have appointments. The list will only display fiscal periods that are currently open.

7. By default, the *Fiscal Year* displays the current financial year set up for your company in Activity 2-5.

8. *Hash Patient Ids* box—Leave blank for this activity. (**FYI**) The *Hash Patient Ids* box is where the person entering the batch data would enter the sum of all patient Harris CareTracker PM and EMR ID numbers pertaining to the charges associated with the batch. This is to ensure that a charge is entered for all patients associated with the batch.

9. *Hash Cpt* box—Leave blank for this activity. (**FYI**) The *Hash Cpt* box is where you enter the sum of all CPT® codes pertaining to the charges associated with the batch. This is to ensure that a charge is entered for all procedures. Example: If two patients are seen for the day, and the CPT® codes selected on the encounter form for the first patient are 71101 and 99213, and the second patient are 71101 and 99203, calculate the *Hash CPT* by adding 71101+ 99213+ 71101+ 99203 = 340618.

10. *Total Chgs* box—Leave blank for this activity. (**FYI**) The *Total Chgs* box is where you enter the sum of all charges that are associated with the batch.

11. *Total Pmts* box—Leave blank for this activity. (**FYI**) The *Total Pmts* box is where you enter the sum of check(s) that are associated with the batch.

12. *Batch Deposit* list—Leave blank for this activity. (**FYI**) The *Batch Deposit* list is where you would select the *Deposit ID* to link to a deposit number, if using the *Batch Deposit* application. (This feature is not active in your student version.)

13. *Date Received* box—Leave blank for this activity. (**FYI**) You could enter the date the encounter was received in MM/DD/YYYY format or click the *Calendar* icon 📅 and select the date. (**Figure 4-39**).

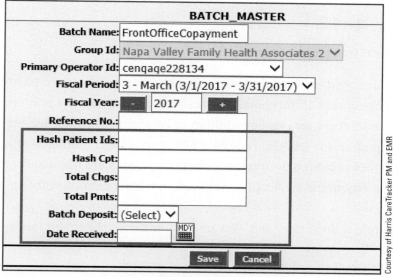

Figure 4-39   *Batch Master Selections for "FrontOfficeCopayment"*

14. Click *Save*. You may receive a message box asking if you are sure you want to select the fiscal period. After confirming the correct fiscal period is displaying, click *OK*. Harris CareTracker PM and EMR displays the *Operator Encounter Batch Control* dialog box with the new batch information (**Figure 4-40**).

15. Now, further edit your batch by updating the provider, resource, location, and so on (the middle section of the *Operator Encounter Batch Control box*). Select the *Provider* (Amir Raman), *Resource* (Amir Raman), and *Location* (Napa Valley Family Associates).

16. Click *Save*.

17. Write down your "Encounter Batch Control No." for future reference. (Should include "FrontOfficeCopayment") _____.

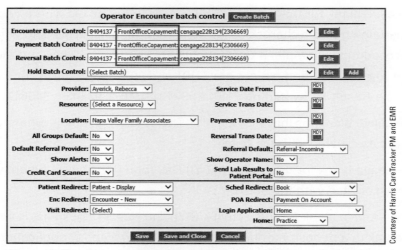

Figure 4-40   Operator Encounter Batch Control Dialog Box

 Print the Batch screen, label it "Activity 4-12," and place it in your assignment folder.

18.   Click "*X*" in the right-hand corner to close the *Batch* dialog box.

Activity 4-13
Accept/Enter a Payment

The *Payments On Account* (*Pmt on Acct*) application is used to record patient payments. Typically, you will accept a patient's copayment at the check-in process. A copayment is a predetermined (flat) fee than an individual pays for health care services in addition to what the insurance covers. For example, some health maintenance organizations (HMOs) require a $25 "copayment" for each office visit, regardless of the type or level of services provided during the visit. Copayments are not usually specified by percentages. You can access the *Payments on Account* application from locations within practice management, as outlined below.

- *Scheduling* module > *Book* tab > left-click on a patient's *appointment* to display the Mini-Menu > Select *Payment* link
- *Name Bar* > *Appts* button > *Actions* menu > *Payment* link
- *Transactions* module > *Pmt on Acct* tab
- *Transactions* module > *Charge* tab

1.   Pull patient Jane Morgan into context.

2.   In the *Transactions* module, click on the *Pmt on Acct* tab.

3.   From the drop-down list at the top of the screen, select whether the payment is being made by the *Patient* or *Responsible Party*. (Select "Patient.")

4.   If a patient is paying a portion of his or her balance (or copayment), enter the dollar amount of the payment in the *Amount* box. (Enter "$20.00.")

    (FYI) If the patient was paying his or her entire balance, you would click *Pay Bal*. Harris CareTracker PM and EMR automatically pulls the patient's balance into the *Amount* box.

5. From the *Payment Type* list, select the payment method. (Select "Payment - Patient Check.") **Note:** If the payment type was a credit card, you would select the *Process Credit Card* checkbox.

6. If the payment method is a check, enter the check number in the *Reference #* box. (Enter "5013" as the check number.) The reference number will print on the patient's receipt.

7. From the *Method* list, select how to apply the payment to the patient's account:

   a. If you are collecting a copayment for a patient who does *not* have an outstanding balance, select <u>only</u> "Force Unapplied." Harris CareTracker PM and EMR creates an unapplied balance for the patient that is applied to the patient's private pay balance when their charges are saved.

   b. Because Ms. Morgan has a scheduled appointment, select "Force Unapplied" and check the *Copay?* Box.

   (FYI) If the patient has an outstanding balance you would:

   • Select *Today's First* in the *Method* field to apply the money starting with the most current balance and then back toward the oldest date of service for which the patient has an outstanding balance.

   • Select *Oldest to Newest* in the *Method* field to apply the money to the oldest date of service for which the patient has an outstanding balance and then forward toward the most current date of service.

8. In the *Trans. Date* box, enter the transaction date to which you want to link the payment. Because you are entering a copayment for a patient visit, select the date of the patient's appointment. (You scheduled Jane Morgan's appointment in Activity 4-1.) **Note:** If you had selected dates in your batch defaults when you set up your batch, they would prepopulate. **Hint:** If you are working at the month's end and are booking appointments in the following month, you would need to open both the current and next month in fiscal period. This would also apply to the fiscal period you selected in your batch.

   (FYI) The following are the various Transaction Date Defaults:

   • If a transaction date was selected when you created your batch, Harris CareTracker PM and EMR pulls that date into the *Trans. Date* box.

   • If a transaction date was not selected, the transaction date defaults to the date in your batch name.

   • If there is no date in your batch name, the transaction date defaults to the date the payment is entered in Harris CareTracker PM and EMR.

9. Because this is a copay:

   a. Select the *Copay?* checkbox.

   b. In the *Appt* field, select the appointment date to which the copay applies (the appointment scheduled in Activity 4-1), if possible. (**Note:** You cannot link a copay to a future appointment date. If your appointment is in the future, you won't be able to select it, and you can skip this step.)

   c. **FYI:** The *Plan Name* and *Copay Amt* fields display the insurance plan and copay amount saved in the patient's demographics, if applicable. These fields are read-only.

10. The *Go To* field defaults to the redirect option selected in the operator's batch. You can select a different option if needed (**Figure 4-41**). (Select "Payment on Account.")

11. To view a summary of the transaction prior to saving, click *View Trans* (**Figure 4-42**).

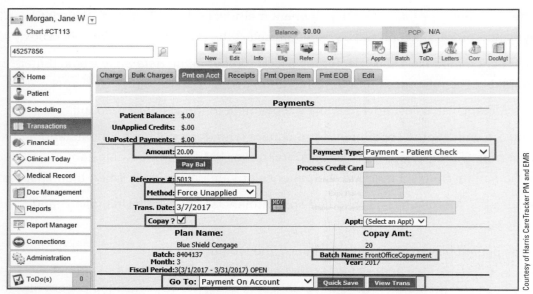

Figure 4-41   Enter Payment on Account

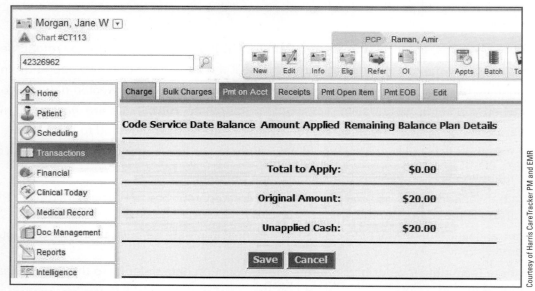

Figure 4-42   View Transaction

Note: If you do not need to view the transaction, you can click directly on *Quick Save* to save the transaction.

12. After clicking *View Trans*, then click *Save*. Harris CareTracker PM and EMR saves the payment information and launches the application selected in the *Go To* field. (You selected the *Go To* of *Payment on Account*, which brings you back to the original *Pmt on Acct* tab.)

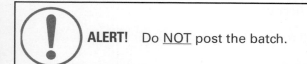

ALERT!   Do <u>NOT</u> post the batch.

13. Click on the *Home* module and the *Open Batches* link under the *Billing* header on the *Dashboard* (**Figure 4-43**) to view your batch with the payment recorded. **Note:** Only view the batch, do not post it.

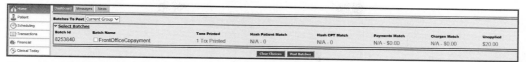

Figure 4-43   Open Batches

Courtesy of Harris CareTracker PM and EMR

14. You will later print a receipt from the *Receipts* tab in the *Transactions* module (Activity 4-13).

💾 **Print the Open Batch screen, label it "Activity 4-13," and place it in your assignment folder.**

PROFESSIONALISM CONNECTION

Some patients feel that medicine and money should never mix; however, a medical office is a business and must conduct itself as such. This means that collecting the copayment prior to the visit makes the most business sense. Once the appointment is completed, the services have been rendered and the patient may not be as willing to meet his or her financial obligations. When possible, the collection of payments should be performed outside of the reception area; however, when this is not possible, the collection of payments should be handled in a discreet manner. You may use a phrase such as the following: "Mrs. Barrett, what method of payment will you be using today to meet your co-payment requirement?" This sentence illustrates that payment is expected, but you are willing to work with the patient by accepting a mode of payment that works best for her.

Activity 4-14
Print Patient Receipts

After entering the payment information in Activity 4-13, print a receipt from the *Receipts* tab in the *Transaction* module. Receipts in Harris CareTracker PM and EMR identify a patient's previous balance, the activity of charges and payments for that date of service, and the new patient balance.

1. With the patient in context (Jane Morgan), click the *Transactions* module. **Note:** You will still be working in the *Batch* you created in Activity 4-12. **Hint:** If you are working at the month's end and are booking appointments in the following month, you would need to open the current <u>and</u> next month in fiscal period. This would also apply to the fiscal period selected in your batch.

2. When the *Transactions* module opens, click on the *Receipts* tab.

3. From the drop-down list at the top of the screen, select who you would like to view the receipt from, *Patient* or *Responsible Party*. (Select "Patient.")

4. Select the date of service for which you need to print a receipt from the *Receipts* list. (Select the date of the payment received, which should also be the same date as your batch and the date that matches the patient's appointment.) When a date of service is selected, the receipt displays on the screen.

5. Click on the *Print* button (**Figure 4-44**), or right-click on the receipt.
   - When you right-click, a gray pop-up menu appears; select *Print*, and the receipt will print.

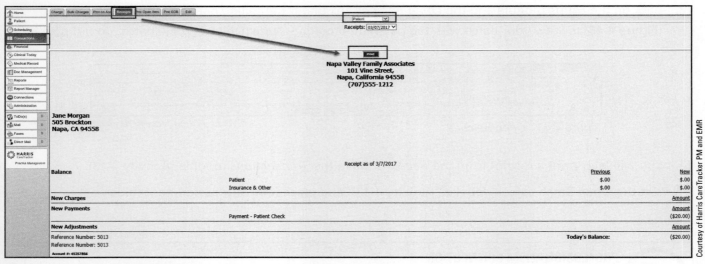

Figure 4-44   Print Patient Receipt

 Print the Patient Receipt, label it "Activity 4-14," and place it in your assignment folder.

 # Activity 4-15

Accept/Enter a Payment and Print Receipt

1. Using the information below and steps 2 through 17, accept/enter a payment and print a receipt for each of the following patients:

   a. Ellen Ristino; $20.00 copay paid by CHECK # 4452.

   b. Barbara Watson; $20.00 copay paid by CHECK # 11247.

2. Pull patient into context.

3. In the *Transactions* module, click on the *Pmt on Acct* tab.

4. From the drop-down list at the top of the screen, select whether the payment is being made by the *Patient* or *Responsible Party*. (Select *Patient*.)

5. Enter the amount of copay for each patient listed in steps 1a and 1b.

6. From the *Payment Type* list, select the payment method listed in steps 1a and 1b.

7. If the payment method is a check, enter the check number in the *Reference #* box.

8. From the *Method* list, select how to apply the payment to the patient's account. For this activity, select "Force Unapplied" and check the *Copay?* box for each of the patient's noted in steps 1a and 1b.

9. In the *Trans. Date* box, enter the transaction date to which you want to link the payment. Select the date of the appointment you scheduled previously in the chapter for each patient. (**Note:** This date must be a date within the fiscal period of the batch you created in Activity 4-14.)

10. In order to record or override the copayment amount noted in the patient's demographic record for a specific appointment:

    a. Select the *Copay?* checkbox.

b. In the *Appt* box, select the appointment date to which the copay applies. If possible, select the appointment date for the patient(s) you created previously in the chapter. **Note:** This is not an option for an appointment date that is after the date you are completing this activity.

11. In the *Go To* field, select "Payment on Account" (see **Figure 4-41**).

12. Click *Quick Save*. Harris CareTracker PM and EMR saves the payment information and launches the application selected in the *Go To* field of the batch.

13. With the patient in context, click the *Transactions* module.

14. When the *Transactions* module opens, click on the *Receipts* tab.

15. From the drop-down list at the top of the screen, select "Patient" or "Responsible Party" as noted in step 4.

16. Select the date of service for which you need to print a receipt from the *Receipts* list. (Select the date of the payment received, which should be the same as the date of the patients' appointments scheduled previously in the chapter.)

17. Click on the *Print* button (see **Figure 4-44**), or right-click on the receipt. When you right-click, a gray pop-up menu appears; select *Print*, and the receipt will print.

🖳 **Print the Patient Receipt for each of the patients, label them "Activity 4-15," and place them in your assignment folder.**

Activity 4-16
Run a Journal

Now that you have entered copayments, you will complete the process by running a journal and posting your batch as part of your "end-of-day" workflow. You must run a journal prior to posting your batch to verify that you have entered all the financial transactions correctly in Harris CareTracker PM and EMR. Journals provide a summary of financial transactions, for example, charges, payments, and adjustments.

It is important to identify any errors before a batch is posted. Once a batch has been posted, the transactions linked to it are locked in the system and cannot be changed. To be corrected, the charges must be reversed. Posted errors can only be corrected by reversing the transaction on the patient's account, which occurs in the *Edit* application of the *Transaction* module. It is highly recommended as a best practice, that you run a journal before posting your batch to make sure that your transactions for the day are correct and balance.

Posted batches are accessible at any time so you can always access an old journal from the *Historical Journals* link (**Figure 4-45**) under the *Financial Reports* section of the *Reports* application, which alleviates the need to save paper copies of journals.

1. Click the *Reports* module.

2. Click the *Todays Journals* link under the *Financial Reports* section (**Figure 4-46**). Harris CareTracker PM displays the *Todays Journal Options* screen (**Figure 4-47**). All of your group's open batches are listed in the *Todays Batches* box.

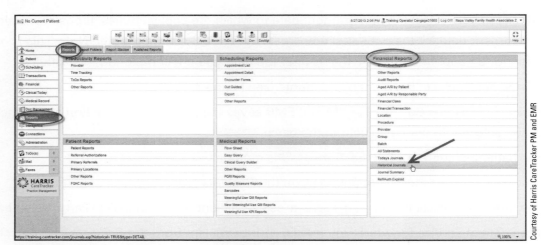

Figure 4-45   Historical Journals Link

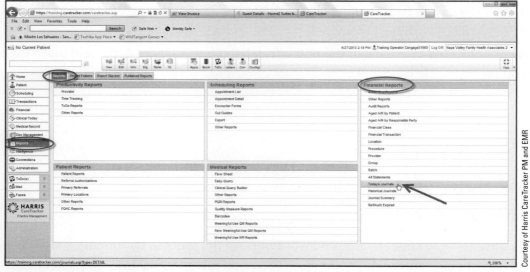

Figure 4-46   Todays Journals Link

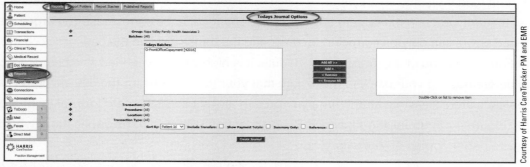

Figure 4-47   Todays Journal Options

3.   Select a batch to include in the journal either by double-clicking on the batch name or by clicking on the batch and then clicking *Add* (**Figure 4-48**). Harris CareTracker PM and EMR adds the selected batches to the box on the right. (Add batch "FrontOfficeCopayment.")

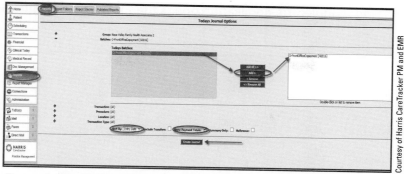

Figure 4-48 Select a Batch for the Journal

4. From the *Sort By* list drop-down, select "Entry Date."

5. Select the *Show Payment Totals* checkbox (see **Figure 4-48**).

6. Click *Create Journal*. Harris CareTracker PM generates the journal (**Figure 4-49**).

7. To print, right-click on the journal and select *Print* from the shortcut menu.

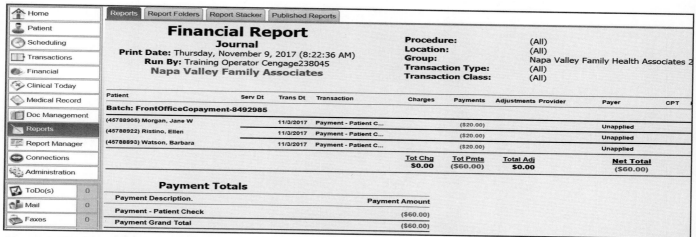

Figure 4-49 Create Journal

Courtesy of Harris CareTracker PM and EMR

🖫 **Print the Journal screen, label it "Activity 4-16," and place it in your assignment folder.**

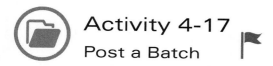

Activity 4-17
Post a Batch

After reviewing the transactions in your journal for accuracy, you will post your open batch. Batches should only be posted after a journal has been generated and you have verified your journal balances. Posting batches locks the transactions permanently in Harris CareTracker. All transactions will show on reports generated in Harris CareTracker, and any corrections to posted transactions must be made via the *Edit* application in the *Transactions* module. *Open Batches* can also be viewed and posted by clicking on the *Open Batches* link under the *Billing* section of the *Dashboard* on the *Home* page.

After generating a journal for the batch(es), you would like to post, review, identify, and correct transactions errors, if any, prior to posting the batch.

1. Click the *Administration* module. The application opens the *Practice* tab (**Figure 4-50**).

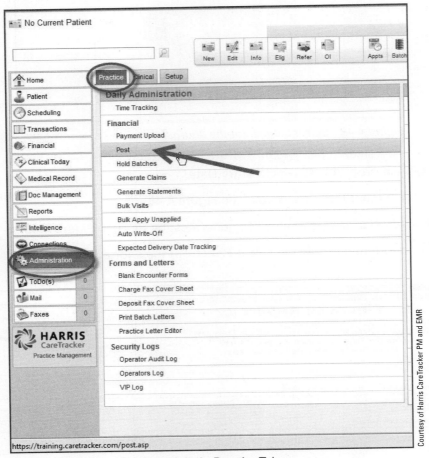

Figure 4-50   Post Link from Admin Practice Tab

2. Click the *Post* link under the *Daily Administration > Financial* header (see **Figure 4-50**). Harris CareTracker PM displays a list of all open batches for the group.

3. Select the checkbox next to the batch you want to post. (Select batch "FrontOfficeCopayment.")

🖫 **Print the Post Batch screen, label it "Activity 4-16," and place it in your assignment folder.**

4. Click *Post Batches* (**Figure 4-51**).

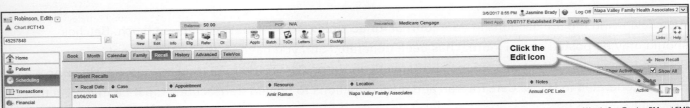

Figure 4-51   Post Batches

CRITICAL THINKING   Now that you have completed this chapter's activities, how do you feel about the scheduling and financial responsibilities of a medical assistant? Were you able to follow instructions and accurately schedule patients, receive and post copayments, and create and post a batch? Were there any activities or steps that seemed to be difficult and challenging? If so, which ones? What measures did you take to accurately complete the activities and move forward? What are your impressions of the front office administrative staff that must balance their responsibilities? If you become a front office medical assistant, what skills and key attributes can you comfortably say you can offer to your employer?

An alternative way of posting batches is via the *Open Batches* link on the Home>*Dashboard*, under the *Billing* header. Although not required, it is recommended to only post a batch after a journal has been generated and balances verified. The total number of open batches for your group displays next to the *Open Batches* link.

CASE STUDIES

To complete Case Study 4-1, you must have completed Case Study 3-1 in Chapter 3. If you have not completed Case Study 3-1, you may use Case Study 4-2 instead. For Case Studies 4-1 and 4-2, you will not be able to link the copay to a visit if the appointment you booked is on a future date. For example, if you are entering data on the weekend and the first available appointment was scheduled on Monday, you will not be able to link the copay to a "future visit date" but you will be able to complete the rest of the steps as instructed.

Case Study 4-1

1. Book the following appointment for James M. Smith. Refer to Activity 4-1 for help).

   • Provider: Dr. Ayerick

   • Time: Book today or first available (Record date/time here: _____)

   • Appointment Type: Follow Up

   • Complaint: Follow-up exam/consultation; review lab and EKG

2. Check in patient James Smith from the mini-menu. Refer to Activity 4-10 for help.

3. Create a batch. Name the batch "CaseStudyCopayment4-1." Refer to Activity 4-12 for help.

4. Accept/Enter a cash payment for James Smith. Refer to Activity 4-13 for help. (**Hint:** Look in his patient demographics to confirm the amount of his copay.)

5. Print the patient receipt for James Smith. Refer to Activity 4-14 for help.

6. Run a journal for the "CaseStudyCopayment4-1" batch created in this case study. Refer to Activity 4-16 for help.

7. Post the batch "CaseStudyCopayment4-1" created in this case study. Refer to Activity 4-17 for help.

   📧 **Print the Post Batch Screen, label it "Case Study 4-1," and place it in your assignment folder.**

(continues)

CASE STUDIES *(continued)*

Case Study 4-2

1. Book an Appointment for Kimberly Johnson using the following criteria. Refer to Activity 4-1 for help.

    *   Provider: Dr. Ayerick
    *   Time: Book today or first available (Record date/time here: _____)
    *   Appointment Type: Follow Up
    *   Complaint: Follow-up exam/consultation; review lab and EKG

2. Check in Patient Kimberly Johnson from the mini-menu. Refer to Activity 4-10 for help.

3. Create a batch. Name the batch "CaseStudyCopayment4-2." Refer to Activity 4-12 for help.

4. Accept/Enter a payment by check# 4478 for Kimberly Johnson. (**Hint:** look in her patient demographics to confirm the amount of her copay.) Refer to Activity 4-13 for help.

5. Print a patient receipt for Kimberly Johnson. Refer to Activity 4-14 for help.

6. Run a journal for the "CaseStudyCopayment4-2" batch created in this case study. Refer to Activity 4-16 for help.

7. Post the batch "CaseStudyCopayment4-2" created in this case study. Refer to Activity 4-17 for help.

💾 **Print the Post Batch Screen, label it "Case Study 4-2," and place it in your assignment folder.**

MODULE 3
Clinical Skills

This module includes:

- Chapter 5: Preliminary Duties in the EMR
- Chapter 6: Patient Work-Up
- Chapter 7: Completing the Visit
- Chapter 8: Other Clinical Documentation

As a health care professional you may use Harris CareTracker PM and EMR to perform clinical duties. Once a patient is registered in the database and has an appointment scheduled, you will perform the steps to activate care management registries, check in and track patients throughout their visits, record vital signs, update the patient's medical record, create progress notes, and capture the visit to create a billable encounter. All the activities you will complete in this module mimic a real-world setting using the clinical features of electronic health records.

QUICK START

Because Harris CareTracker is a live EMR, you will need to complete several tasks to simulate a live clinic where patient accounts are ready for a clinical work-up. The following activities are required in order to complete the activities in this module. **If you have been following along in this book from the beginning and have completed all the Required** 🚩 **activities as you've moved sequentially through the text, then you have already completed the activities below and can move forward. If you are beginning with this module, then you will need to complete the activities given below *before* you can complete any other activities in this module.**

Be sure you are working in a supported browser (Internet Explorer 11 or Safari for iPad) before you begin. Other browsers (such as Chrome and Firefox) are not supported. Review Best Practices, included on page xiv of this text.

- ❏ Activity 1-1: Disable Toolbars
- ❏ Activity 1-2: Set Up Tabbed Browsing
- ❏ Activity 1-3: Turn Off Pop-Up Blocker
- ❏ Activity 1-4: Change Page Setup
- ❏ Activity 1-5: Add Harris CareTracker to Trusted Sites
- ❏ Activity 1-6: Clear Your Cache
  - *Note: Remember that you should clear your cache each time before you being working in CareTracker.*
- ❏ Activity 1-8: Disable Download Blocking
  - *Note: Once you have completed the system set-up requirements (Activities 1-1, 1-2, 1-3, 1-4, 1-5, and 1-8), you will not need to repeat these activities unless you change the device you are using or the settings automatically default back to prior settings.*

❑ Activity 1-9: Register Your Credentials and Create Your Harris CareTracker PM and EMR Training Company
 • *Note: It will take up to 24 hours for your CareTracker "Student Company" to be created. Plan accordingly.*

❑ Activity 2-1: Log in to Harris CareTracker PM and EMR
 • *Note: Be sure to write down your new password inside the front cover of your workbook for easy reference.*

❑ Activity 2-5: Open a New Fiscal Year
 • *Note: Every January 1, you will need to open a new fiscal year.*

❑ Activity 2-6: Open a Fiscal Period
 • *Note: Every first of the month, you will need to open a new fiscal period.*

❑ Activity 3-1: Searching for a Patient by Name
 • *Complete steps 1 and 2 only.*
 • *Note: You will search for patients throughout the text using the steps in Activity 3-1.*

❑ Activity 3-4: Register a New Pediatric Patient and Print Demographics
 • *You can complete only steps 1 through 6, 31, and 33. However, if you complete Chapter 3 later in your studies, you should complete the rest of the steps in Activity 3-4 by editing the patient's demographics.*

❑ Activity 4-1: Book an Appointment
 • *The directions for this activity state to book the appointment for one week from today. Instead, book the appointment for today (the day you are working). If no appointments are available today, then book the appointment for a day within the past week.*
 • *Also book an "Established Patient Sick" appointment for today for Barbara Watson with Amir Raman. Her chief complaint is "Fever—103F."*

❑ Activity 4-10: Check in Patient from the Mini-Menu
❑ Activity 4-12: Create a Batch
 • *Note: At various times throughout the activities, you will be directed to create batches.*

❑ Activity 4-13: Accept/Enter a Payment
❑ Activity 4-15: Accept/Enter a Payment
 • *Complete steps 1 through 12 only. You do not need to print receipts for this activity at this time.*

❑ Activity 4-17: Post a Batch
 • *Note: At various times throughout the activities, you will be directed to post batches.*

Once you have completed these activities as part of this Quick Start, you will not need to complete them again if you come across the activities while working in Chapters 1–4.

PREREQUISITES FOR CASE STUDIES

In addition to the activities listed in the Quick Start, you will need to complete these case studies if you plan to complete case studies in the Clinical Module:

❑ Case Study 3-1
 • *You can complete an abbreviated registration by only entering the patient's name, address, phone number, date of birth, social security number, sex, and insurance information.*

❑ Case Study 4-1
 • *You may complete steps 1 and 2 only.*

Preliminary Duties in the EMR

Learning Objectives

1. Describe tools within Harris CareTracker PM and EMR that assist with meaningful use.
2. View the meaningful use dashboard in Harris CareTracker PM and EMR.
3. Activate the care management registries in Harris CareTracker PM and EMR.
4. Navigate throughout the Medical Record module.
5. View the patient's encounter information, medications, allergy information, and problem list.
6. State the three types of alerts in Harris CareTracker PM and EMR.
7. View, change, and print a chart summary in Harris CareTracker EMR.
8. Perform routine maintenance functions in Harris CareTracker PM and EMR such as adding a room, editing a room, adding a custom resource, and managing immunizations.

Real-World Connection

In the first four chapters, you learned a great deal about the practice management side of the Harris CareTracker software. This chapter introduces you to the EMR component. This chapter focuses on the utilization of EMRs in ambulatory care settings. For providers to obtain full reimbursement from governmental agencies such as Medicare and Medicaid, they must be in full compliance with specific guidelines set forth by those agencies.

EMRs have been in use for the past couple of decades, but their widespread adoption skyrocketed largely due to Medicare and Medicaid financial incentives offered by the federal government for practices that meet meaningful use as well as the penalties that come about for not instituting and meaningfully using the EMR. As you work in this chapter, keep in mind how your position as a medical assistant may be impacted by meaningful use, and how you will be able to assist both providers and patients in meeting these goals.

Before you begin the activities in this chapter, refresh your memory on working with Harris CareTracker by referring back to the Best Practices list on page xiv of this workbook. Following best practices will help you complete work quickly and accurately.

TOOLS WITHIN HARRIS CARETRACKER TO ASSIST PROVIDERS WITH MEANINGFUL USE

Learning Objective 1: Describe tools within Harris CareTracker PM and EMR that assist with meaningful use.

Learning Objective 2: View the meaningful use dashboard in Harris CareTracker PM and EMR.

Activity 5-1

Viewing the *Meaningful Use Dashboard*

The *Meaningful Use Dashboard* within Harris CareTracker PM tracks a provider's progress toward meeting the Medicare and Medicaid EHR Incentive Program reporting requirements for the core and menu set items. The dashboard displays a progress bar next to each of the measures that has a reporting requirement. **Figure 5-1A** illustrates a graphing screen of the core requirements for Dr. Olivia Sherman and **Figure 5-1B** illustrates the graphing features of the menu set requirements for Dr. Olivia Sherman. (Dr. Sherman is not a provider in our NVFHA environment.)

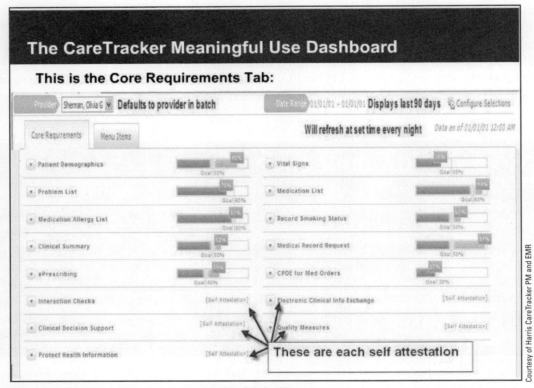

Figure 5-1A Core Requirements for Dr. Olivia Sherman

The dashboard's default date range is determined by when the provider begins the attestation period, or the date that begins the 90-day reporting period of meeting the core and menu measures listed previously. The dashboard calculates these measures over the previous 90 days.

From the dashboard, you can

- customize the requirements displayed on the dashboard for each participating provider,
- view a status of a provider's progress for the last 90 days (percentages updated nightly),
- hover over the percentage bar to review the data used to calculate the provider's percentage,
- click the *Menu Items* tab and then the drop-down arrow to download reference documents or run Key Performance Indicator (KPI) reports

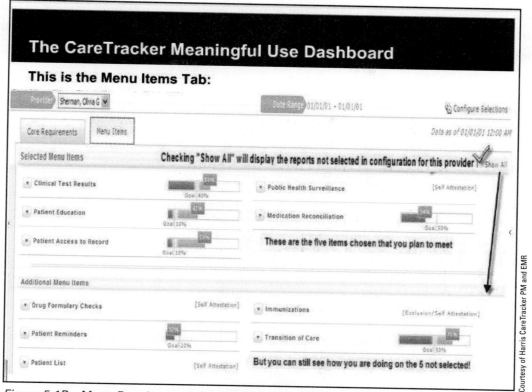

Figure 5-1B   Menu Requirements for Dr. Olivia Sherman

Note: Any time you are working in the EMR side of Harris CareTracker, you need to make sure that "Compatibility View" is turned off in your Internet Explorer browser. If you experience any functionality issues, please check your settings. (Refer to Best Practices for help.)

1. Click the *Home* module.

2. Click the *Meaningful Use* tab under the *Dashboard* tab (**Figure 5-2**). Harris CareTracker PM displays the *Meaningful Use Dashboard*.

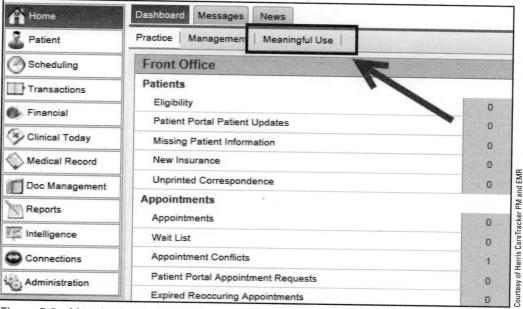

Figure 5-2   Meaningful Use Tab

3. From the *Provider* list, select the name of the provider whose data you want to view. In this case, click on "Brockton, Anthony." Harris CareTracker PM displays the provider's percentages on the *Core Requirements* tab (**Figure 5-3**).

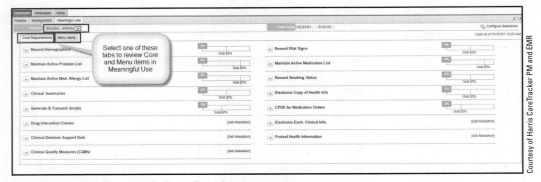

Figure 5-3   Dr. Brockton's Core Requirements

 Print the Core Requirements screen, label it "Activity 5-1A," and place it in your assignment folder.

4. Click the *Menu Items* tab to view the *Menu Items* requirements. On the *Menu Items* tab, select the *Show All* checkbox on the right-hand side of the screen to view any excluded requirements.

Print the Menu Items screen, label it "Activity 5-1B," and place it in your assignment folder.

FYI   Because this is a training environment, you are only able to see the shell; no meaningful use statistics are available. **Figure 5-4** illustrates what a *Core Requirements* tab looks like in a fully functional environment.

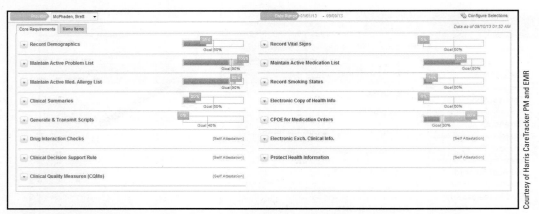

Figure 5-4   *Core Requirements in a Fully Functional Environment*

ACTIVATING CARE MANAGEMENT

Learning Objective 3: Activate the care management registries in Harris CareTracker PM and EMR.

Activity 5-2

Activating Care Management Items

The *Care Management* feature in Harris CareTracker PM and EMR allows practices to set clinical measures for health maintenance and disease management registries. The registries will assist with early identification of disease and early treatment. Keeping up-to-date with immunizations will help to prevent future disease and control costs associated with those diseases. This feature also assists in meeting some of the standards of meaningful use.

By default, clinical measures are turned off in Harris CareTracker PM and EMR. You need to activate the registries and measures you want to make available to the providers in your group. As you will observe, these registries will check to determine if the patient is up-to-date with preventive testing and immunizations. After activation, the registries and measures selected are included in the *Pt Care Management* application of the *Medical Record* module and the *Care Management* application of the *Clinical Today* module. Registries are repopulated with the *Clinical Today/Population Management* tab. Once activation occurs, anytime you open the patient's chart, you can see where he or she falls within the registries and help the patient to come into compliance with testing or procedures.

1. Click on the *Administration* module and then click the *Clinical* tab.

2. Click the *Care Management Activation* link under the *Maintenances* heading (**Figure 5-5A**). Harris CareTracker PM and EMR launches the *Care Management Activation* application.

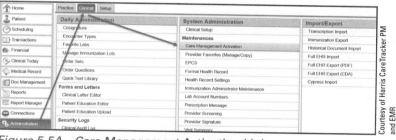

Figure 5-5A   *Care Management Activation Link*

3. Select all of the measures and registries listed by selecting/clicking on all of the boxes. The check-boxes are dynamic and will auto-save on a single click. (A green "Saved" message appears briefly when each box is clicked to indicate the settings are saved [**Figure 5-5B**].)

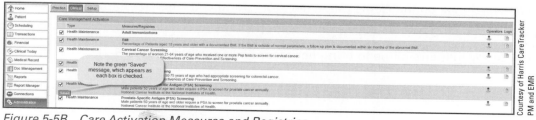

Figure 5-5B   *Care Activation Measures and Registries*

📇 **Print the Care Management Activation screen, label it "Activity 5-2," and place it in your assignment folder.**

PROFESSIONALISM CONNECTION

In case you did not make the connection, many of the disease prevention goals that you set for the patient are directly connected to meaningful use and the provider's core requirement percentages. When you are unable to get the patient to agree to these goals, it not only impacts the patient's health but also the provider's meaningful use statistics. Because we are a "Pay for Performance" facility, it impacts the practice's bottom line as well.

NAVIGATING THE MEDICAL RECORD MODULE

Learning Objective 4: Navigate throughout the Medical Record module.

Activity 5-3
Viewing a Summary of Patient Information

The *Medical Record* module is designed to mimic a paper chart and to follow the provider's normal work-flow, facilitating effective EHR documentation for a patient. The module is accessed by pulling the patient into context on the *Name Bar* and then clicking the *Medical Record* module. If a patient has an appointment scheduled, you can click the patient name in the *Appointments* application (tab) of the *Clinical Today* module to launch the *Medical Record* module.

The *Medical Record* module consists of four main components: *Patient Detail Bar, Patient Health History* pane, *Clinical Toolbar*, and *Chart Summary*.

Patient Detail Bar

The *Patient Detail Bar* (**Figure 5-6**) can be found at the top of the window once you open the patient's medical record.

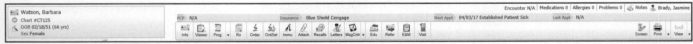

Figure 5-6   Patient Detail Bar

Courtesy of Harris CareTracker PM and EMR

1. In the *ID* search box on the *Name Bar*, enter "tol" (for the last name "Tolman" and hit [Enter]. The *Patient Search* dialog box displays with a list of patients matching the search criteria you entered.

2. Click on Gabby Tolman's name to bring her record into context (**Figure 5-7**).

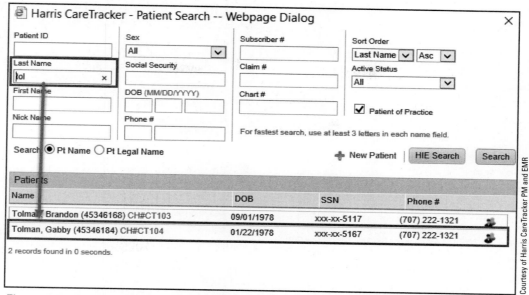

Figure 5-7   Click on Gabby Tolman's Name to Bring Up Her Medical Record

3. Click on the *Patient* module, which will open the *Demographics* tab.

4. You will notice that in Gabby's demographics window, no primary care provider (PCP) has been selected. Click on *Edit*, then scroll down to *PCP*, click on the drop-down list, and select "Anthony Brockton" as her PCP.

5. Scroll down and click *Save*. The *Patient Alerts* dialog box will display after saving. Close out of the *Patient Alerts* dialog box. You will see the update you made to the patient's PCP in her *Patient Details* screen.

6. Click on the *Medical Record* module.

7. A clinical alert comes up alerting you that the patient is allergic to codeine. Click on *Close* to exit the box.

8. To view Gabby's summary information, click the *Patient Information* icon ![icon] to the left of the patient's name. **Figure 5-8** illustrates what the summary looks like once you click on the *Patient Information* icon.

9. To view additional patient information details, click the *View complete Patient Information* link on the lower right of the window. **Figure 5-9** illustrates what the window should like once you click on the *View complete Patient Information* link.

🖻 **Print the View complete Patient Information screen by right-clicking on the screen and selecting the Print function. Label it "Activity 5-3" and place it in your assignment folder.**

10. Close out of the *Complete Patient Information* screen by clicking "X" on the browser window.

11. Close out of Gabby Tolman's *Chart Summary* by clicking "X" on the browser window.

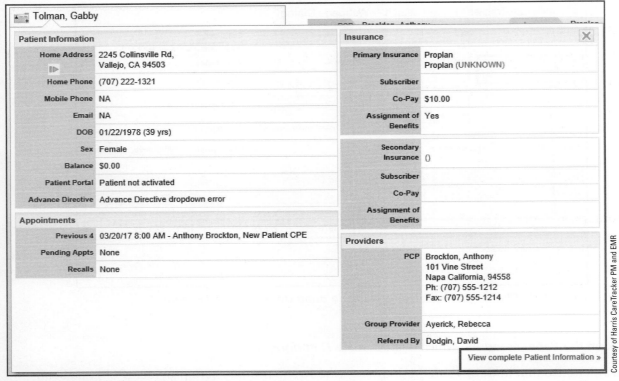

Figure 5-8   Patient Information Screen

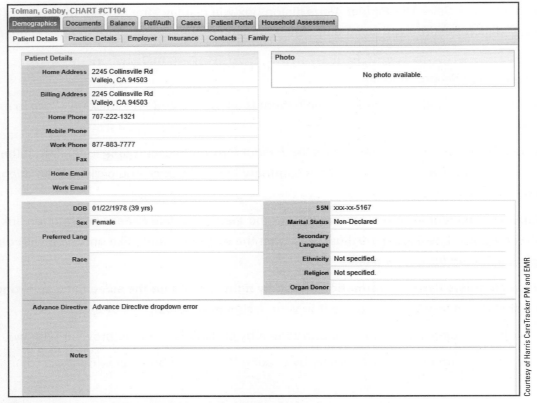

Figure 5-9   View Complete Patient Information Link

Viewing Encounter Information

Learning Objective 5: View the patient's encounter information, medications, allergy information, and problem list.

Learning Objective 6: State the three types of alerts in Harris CareTracker PM and EMR.

Activity 5-4

Viewing the Encounters Application, Active Medications, Allergies, and Problems

An encounter is an interaction with a patient on a specific date at a specific time and includes visits, phone calls, renewal requests, results, and more. Each patient can have many encounters, each encounter can have many services, and each service can have many CPT® codes associated with it.

1. Pull patient Gabby Tolman into context.

2. Click on the *Medical Record* module. The *Clinical Alerts* dialog box will display. Close out of the *Clinical Alerts* dialog box and proceed with the activity.

3. To view Gabby Tolman's encounter information, click on the word *Encounter* (which appears blue) in the detail bar (at the top right of the screen). A box with a listing of the patient's previous encounters will pop up as well as an option to create a new encounter (**Figure 5-10**). Make a note of the date of the patient's only encounter that displays in your screen: _____.

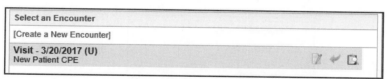

Figure 5-10   Creating a New Encounter   Courtesy of Harris CareTracker PM and EMR

4. Close the encounter window by clicking on the "X" in thetop right corner of the window.

5. View clinical information for the patient, such as the active medications, allergies, and problems, by clicking the corresponding links in the *Patient Detail* bar (located in the upper-right portion of your screen on the same line following *Encounter*) and record this information.

📠 **On a blank sheet of paper write down the date of the patient's only encounter, a listing of the patient's active medications, and any problems listed for the patient. Label the page "Activity 5-4" and place it in your assignment folder.**

6. Close out Gabby Tolman's chart summary by clicking "X" on the *Medical Record* browser window.

Activity 5-5

Viewing Patient Alerts in the Patient's Medical Record

You can view clinical alert information for a patient by clicking on the *Alert* ⚠ icon next to the chart number in the *Medical Record* module. Harris CareTracker PM and EMR displays the *Clinical Alerts* dialog box with three patient alert types; *Clinical Alerts*, *Patient Care Management Alerts*, and *Clinical Notes*.

1. Pull patient Gabby Tolman into context.

2. Click on *Medical Record.*

3. When you open the *Medical Record*, the alert box automatically pops up. Review the information in the box before closing it out. Close out of the box by clicking on *Close.*

4. Click on the *Alert* ⚠ icon to the left of the chart number. Notice that the information that pops up here is the same clinical alert information that popped up when you opened the medical record.

💾 **Write down any alerts listed for Gabby on a piece of paper. Label the page "Activity 5-5" and place it in your assignment folder.**

5. Click *Close* on the *Clinical Alerts* box.

6. Close Gabby Tolman's *Chart Summary* screen by clicking "X" on the *Medical Record* browser window.

Patient Health History Pane

The *Patient Health History* pane (**Figure 5-11**) is a series of panes located to the left of the *Chart Summary* content in the *Medical Record* module that you can use to access different applications for reviewing, entering, and editing patient information such as diagnoses, medications, and more. The function of each pane is described in **Table 5-1**.

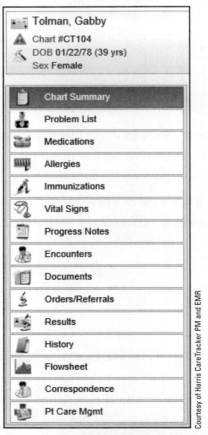

Figure 5-11   Patient Medical History Pane

Table 5-1   Patient Health History Panes

PATIENT HEALTH HISTORY PANE	FUNCTION
Chart Summary	A view-only window displaying a summary of patient medical information.
Problem List	A list of chronic and ongoing patient problems.
Medications	Displays all prescribed medications for the patient.
Allergies	A list of patient allergies.
Immunizations	A list of immunizations given to the patient.
Vital Signs	Displays patient statistics such as height, weight, and blood pressure taken during each office visit or at home.
Progress Notes	Displays information about patient visits documented via quick text, point and click, dictation, or a combination of methods.
Encounters	Displays all patient encounters.
Documents	Displays all scanned or uploaded documents and voice recordings for the patient; for example, clinical documents, insurance cards, or identification cards.
Orders/Referrals	Displays test orders and referrals for the patient.
Results	Displays patient test results. Abnormal results display in red to help identify issues needing immediate attention.
History	Displays patient information such as the family, past medical, and social history.
Flowsheet	Most commonly used for tracking vital statistics, diabetic insulin dosages, pain assessment, lab results, blood pressure, medication start and stop dates, physical assessment, and drug frequency.
Correspondence	Displays all *To Do*(s) for the patient and other communications such as patient education, recall, or collection letters provided or mailed to the patient.
Pt Care Mgmt	Displays a list of overdue preventive or maintenance items such as screening plans that need to be completed for the patient.

Courtesy of Harris CareTracker PM and EMR

To familiarize yourself with these panes, go into Gabby Tolman's medical record, click out of the alert box, and click on each of the panes in the *Patient Health History Pane* (e.g., click on *Chart Summary, Problem List, Medications*, etc.). You will learn the specifics of each pane in future activities.

Clinical Toolbar

The *Clinical Toolbar* (**Figure 5-12**) is a convenient workflow tool that you can use to record information during a patient appointment. The toolbar can be found in *Medical Record* module and contains a series of tool buttons. The function of each button is described in **Table 5-2**.

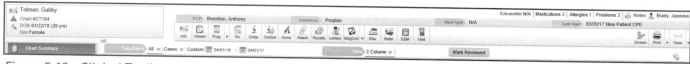

Figure 5-12   Clinical Toolbar

Courtesy of Harris CareTracker PM and EMR

Table 5-2 The Clinical Toolbar

CLINICAL TOOL BUTTON	FUNCTION
Patient Information (Info)	The *Patient Information* window provides access to a patient's demographic, appointment, and other information.
Chart Viewer (Viewer)	The *Chart Viewer* provides a quick and easy way to access other applications when documenting a clinical encounter at the point of care.
Progress Note (Prog)	The *Progress Notes* application helps you document the patient visit in various methods that include diagnosis-specific guidelines, provider-specific templates, quick-pick templates, dictation, or a combination of all.
Prescriptions (Rx)	The *Rx Writer* application (Surescripts® certified for prescription routing), uses the Surescripts® network to transmit electronic prescriptions directly to a selected pharmacy.
Order	The *Orders* application enables you to enter new orders and process orders by printing and sending to a clinical lab or by sending electronically via the Health Level 7 (HL7) interface.
Order Set (OrdSet)	The *Order Set* application enables you to group patient orders for a specific diagnosis or condition.
Immunizations (Immu)	The *Immunization* application facilitates documenting immunizations administered during a patient visit. Additionally, the application helps administer vaccinations from a "lot" and helps you manage information on immunization lots that pertain to the group.
Attachments (Attach)	The *Document Management Upload* application helps upload or scan documents that include anything from a letter to a medical report for the patient.
Recalls	The *Recall* application helps create patient reminders and letters for events such as annual physical exams, follow-up consultations, and lab tests.
Letters	The *Letters* application helps generate and print anything from a letter to a label for a patient by extracting information from the patient medical record.
Message Center (MsgCntr)	The *Messages* application facilitates patient-related communications with patients (if the patient is registered in Harris CareTracker's Patient Portal), office staff, and Harris CareTracker PM and EMR Support Department staff without having to pull or file a chart. There are three components in the Message Center: (1) New ToDo, (2) New Fax, and (3) New Mail.
Patient Education (Edu)	The *Patient Education* application gives you access to a comprehensive library of education material provided by Krames StayWell.
Referral (Refer)	The *Referral* application helps manage inbound and outbound referrals and authorizations.
E&M Evaluator (E&M)	The *E&M Evaluator* application helps identify the most appropriate E&M procedure (CPT®) code to use when charging for office visits and consultations.
Visits (Visit)	The *Visits* application helps capture information such as CPT® and ICD codes for the patient encounter.
Screen	The *Screen* feature enables you to check for drug interactions in real time for the patient in context.
Print	The *Print* feature export patients data into a PDF format in one- or two-column layout.
View	The *View* feature enables you to view the Clinical Log and the Continuity of Care Document (CCD) of the patient.

Courtesy of Harris CareTracker PM and EMR

You will be using these tools throughout your training activities.

Chart Summary

Learning Objective 7: View, change, and print a Chart Summary in Harris CareTracker EMR.

Activity 5-6
Accessing a Patient Chart Summary Using the Name Bar

The *Chart Summary* is a paperless format of a patient's medical record. It is a proprietary display that serves as a medical and legal record of a patient's clinical status, care history, and caregiver involvement.

The information on the *Chart Summary* is taken from various applications within Harris CareTracker PM and EMR. Information available in the *Chart Summary* includes contact and personal information, problem and medication lists, lab results, patient history, and other information. You can access the *Chart Summary* by clicking on the *Medical Record* module.

1. Pull patient Gabby Tolman into context.

2. Click the *Medical Record* module.

3. Review the *Clinical Alerts* dialog box and then close.

4. By default, the *Chart Summary* tab displays from the *Patient Health History* pane. (Your screen should look like **Figure 5-13**.) Review all of the categories in the *Chart Summary* by scrolling up and down using the scroll bar.

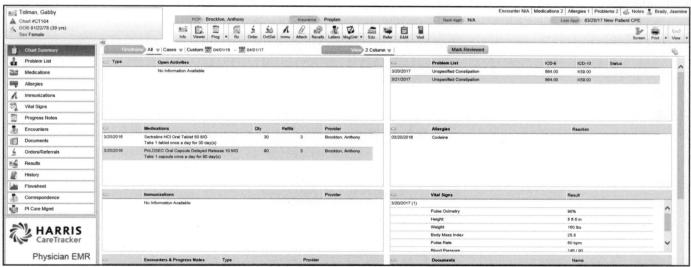

Figure 5-13   Chart Summary   Courtesy of Harris CareTracker PM and EMR

5. To change the look of the *Chart Summary*, find the gray *View* tab in the middle of the page, just below the *Clinical Toolbar* (**Figure 5-14**). Click on the drop-down arrow next to the *View* tab and change the view to "3 Column."

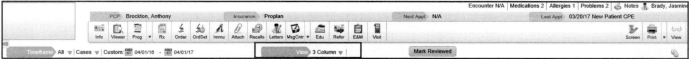

Figure 5-14   View Column Drop-Down Menu   Courtesy of Harris CareTracker PM and EMR

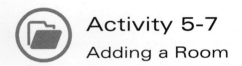 Click on the drop-down arrow next to the Print 🖶 icon and select "Print Chart Summary." Label the printed chart summary "Activity 5-6" and place it in your assignment folder.

6. Now change the *View* using the drop-down arrow and change the view to "1 Column."

7. Change the *View* again using the drop-down arrow and selecting "Chronological."

8. Change the *View* back to the original "2 Column" view as originally set.

9. Close Gabby Tolman's *Chart Summary* screen by clicking "X" on the *Medical Record* browser window.

MAINTENANCE FUNCTIONS THAT AFFECT HARRIS CARETRACKER EMR

Learning Objective 8: Perform routine maintenance functions in Harris CareTracker PM and EMR such as adding a room, editing a room, adding a custom resource, and managing immunizations.

Activity 5-7
Adding a Room

It is important to have an efficient appointment workflow to better serve the patient during an appointment. The *Room Maintenance* feature helps you set up rooms to keep track of a patient appointment by updating a patient's location during his or her stay at your office. Building upon room maintenance activities completed in Chapter 2, continue with Activity 5-7, which illustrates how to add and name rooms within the system.

1. Click the *Administration* module and then click the *Setup* tab.

2. Click the *Room Maintenance* link at the bottom of the *Scheduling* section (**Figure 5-15**).

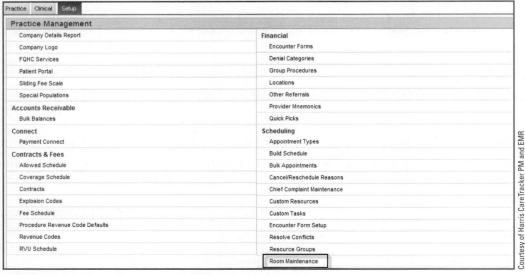

Figure 5-15   Room Maintenance Link

3. Click the drop-down menu beside (*Select*) to see what rooms are already in the system. (You will notice that there are two rooms listed for our environment: "Exam Room # 1" and "Exam Room # 2." You added "Exam Room # 2" in Activity 2-13. Note: If you began your work with the Clinical Module Quick Start, you will not have added Exam Room # 2, and it will not display.)

4. Click *Add* beside the (*Select*) drop-down menu.

5. Enter "Exam Room # 3" in the *Room Name* box (**Figure 5-16**).

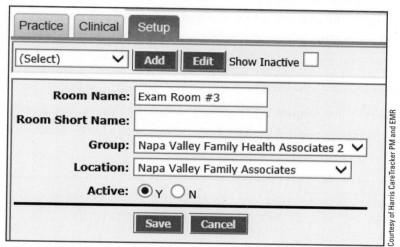

Figure 5-16   Add Exam Room #3

6. A "Room Short Name" field is available, which is not necessary to complete unless a short version or acronym of the room name is often used (leave blank).

7. Select "Napa Valley Family Health Associates 2" from the *Group* list.

8. Select "Napa Valley Family Associates" from the *Location* list. (These lists are useful for multi-location practices.)

9. By default, the *Active* field is set to "Y." This means the room is active.

10. Click *Save*. The application adds the room.

11. Click on the drop-down menu. "Exam Room #1," "Exam Room 2," and "Exam Room #3" should appear in the drop-down list.

12. Now repeat the same procedure, adding the following rooms: "Triage Room" and "Cardiac Bay" with the same *Group* and *Location* as in Steps 7–8.

13. Click on the (*Select*) drop-down menu. All the rooms you added should appear in the drop-down list.

14. Click on the "Cardiac Bay" room listing.

📧 **If you have a screenshot application with a "10-second delay" feature, you will be able to capture the drop-down list. If not, print the information from the Cardiac Bay field to illustrate that it was added to the list. Label it "Activity 5-7" and place it in your assignment folder.**

Activity 5-8
Adding Custom Resources

There may be times where you will need to add *Resources* to the system. Resources can be people, places, or things. Providers are always considered a resource, but an exam room or a piece of equipment can also be considered a resource. Something that requires a schedule is considered a resource because it has specific availability with days and times it can provide certain services. If the resource does not need a set schedule then it is not considered a "resource" in Harris CareTracker PM and EMR.

After a resource is entered in the system, you can customize the resource, assign it to resource classes, and assign it to a resource group for scheduling purposes. Building upon the activities you completed in Chapter 2, add a custom resource (Activity 5-8).

1. Click the *Administration* module and then click the *Setup* tab.

2. Click the *Custom Resources* link (**Figure 5-17**) under the *Scheduling* section. Harris CareTracker PM displays the *Schedule Resource* page. All providers and resources in the practice are listed as *Available Resources*.

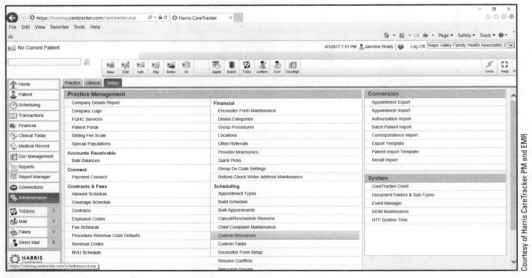

Figure 5-17   Custom Resources Link

3. Click *New* to the right of the *Available Resources* list. Harris CareTracker PM displays a dialog box, prompting you to enter a name for the resource.

4. In the dialog box, enter "Accent Laser Machine" (**Figure 5-18**).

5. Click *OK.* The application adds the resource to the *Available Resources* list (**Figure 5-19**).

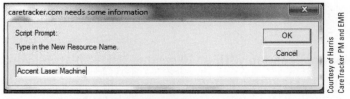

Figure 5-18   Add an Available Resource

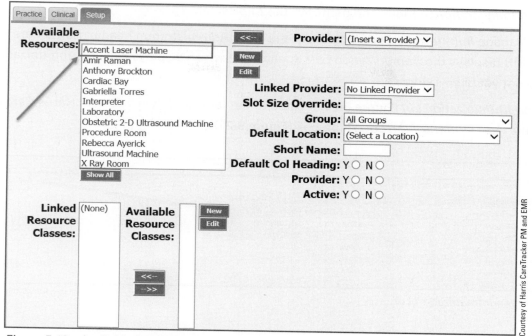

Figure 5-19   Available Resources List

 Print a copy of the Available Resources screen, indicating that the Accent Laser Machine is now in the Available Resources box. Label it "Activity 5-8" and place it in your assignment folder.

Activity 5-9

Adding an Immunization Lot

The *Manage Immunization Lots* application enables you to manage immunization lots that pertain to groups. When immunizations are received, you can add the lot information for the immunizations to the system. After an immunization lot is added, the system keeps track of the inventory and deducts administered immunization from the quantity in the lot. Tracking inventory ensures that required immunizations can be reordered in a timely manner.

The *Manage Immunization Lots* application also enables you to modify lots, make lots inactive, and delete lots as necessary. You can also add and manage immunization lots via the *Add Immunization Lot* and *Edit Immunization Lot* dialog boxes accessed via the *Immunization* application in the *Clinical Toolbar*. Immunization lots are practice-specific and not determined by the provider selected in the *Admin Provider* list. Therefore, lot details recorded display in the *Lots* list for all providers.

PROFESSIONALISM CONNECTION

Whenever possible, lot numbers from immunization shipments should be entered into the EMR as you are checking in the shipment. Because many of these immunizations need to be refrigerated, you often have to stop what you are doing and check in the shipment. You may be tempted to enter vaccination lot numbers at a later time, but failing to enter the information during the check-in process may hamper your ability to remember it later. This will create extra work for the individual that uses the first vial from that particular lot number. If this happens repeatedly, staff members may lose faith in your ability to follow through with assignments.

1. Click the *Administration* module, and then click the *Clinical* tab.
2. Click the *Manage Immunization Lots* link under the *Daily Administration* header. Harris CareTracker PM and EMR displays the *Immunization Lots* application, which displays existing immunization lots that have not yet been exhausted.
3. Click *+ Add Immunization Lot* (**Figure 5-20**) located to the far right of your screen. Harris CareTracker displays the *Add Immunization Lot* dialog box (**Figure 5-21**).

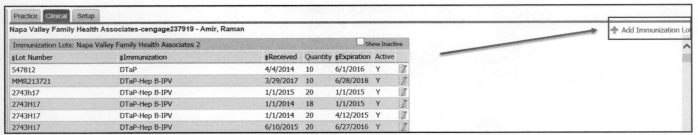

Figure 5-20 Adding an Immunization Lot

Courtesy of Harris CareTracker PM and EMR

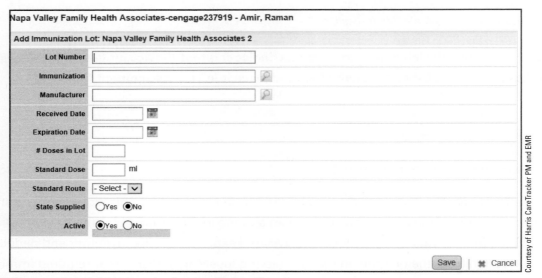

Figure 5-21 Add Immunization Lot Dialog Box

Courtesy of Harris CareTracker PM and EMR

4. In the *Lot Number* box, enter "MMR" followed by your operator number. (For example, if your login username (operator number) is "cengage59290," you would enter the lot number "MMR59290.")
5. In the *Immunization* box, type "MMR" and then click the *Search* icon.
6. Click on the word "MMR" under *Search Results* (**Figure 5-22**).

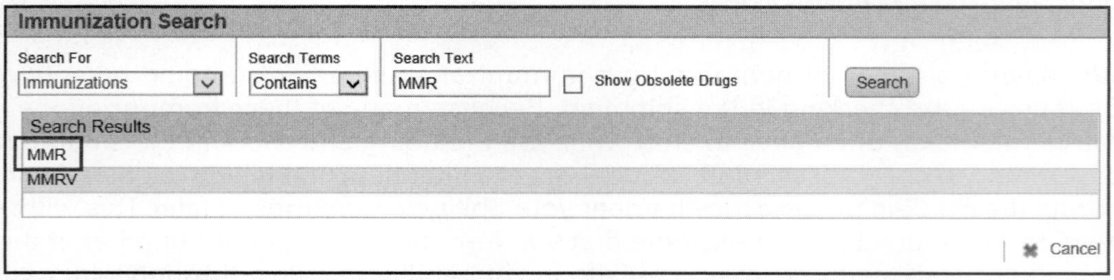

Figure 5-22 Select MMR in the Immunization Search Box

Courtesy of Harris CareTracker PM and EMR

7. In the *Manufacturer* box, type the word "MedImmune" and then click the *Search* 🔍 icon. Select the radio dial (**Figure 5-23**) next to "MedImmune" under *Search Results*.

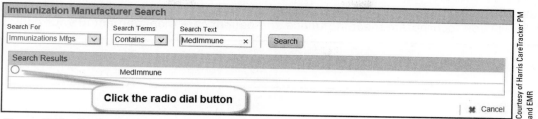

Figure 5-23   Radio Button

8. In the *Received Date* box, click on the calendar and select today's date.

9. In the *Expiration Date* box, type in a date that is 15 months from today's date.

10. In the *# Doses in Lot* box, type "10".

11. In the *Standard Dose* box, type "0.5".

12. In the *Standard Route* box, click the drop-down menu and select "SC" for "subcutaneous."

13. In the *State Supplied* category, click "No."

14. In the *Active* category, select "Yes."

15. Your dialog box should look like **Figure 5-24**. Click on *Save*.

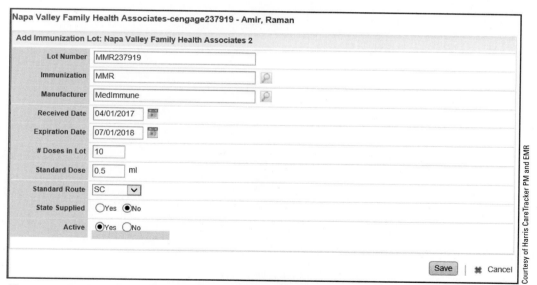

Figure 5-24   Completed Add Immunization Lot Box

💾 **Print the screen listing the Immunization Lots for NVFA to illustrate that the vaccine has been added to the list. Label it "Activity 5-9" and place in your assignment folder. (Hint: In order to find the lot you entered, you may need to scroll down the list in the "Lot Number" column, or it may help to sort the list by "Received" date.)**

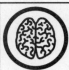

CRITICAL THINKING At the beginning of this chapter, you were asked to keep in mind how your position as a medical assistant may be impacted by meaningful use, and how you will be able to assist both providers and patients in meeting these goals. Having completed your studies and activities, describe how you see your role in the practice as an advocate for both the provider and patients. How will you incorporate meaningful use and patient care management in your daily activities?

CASE STUDIES

CASE STUDY 5-1

Access Donald Schwartz's chart using the *Name Bar*. Change the view of the chart summary it to *Chronological* view. For help completing this activity, refer to Activity 5-6.

📧 **Print the screen with Donald Schwartz's chronological chart view, label it "Case Study 5-1," and place it in your assignment folder.**

CASE STUDY 5-2

Add two new rooms to Harris CareTracker: *X-Ray* and *Laboratory*. For help completing this activity, refer to Activity 5-7.

📧 **Print a copy of the screens that illustrate you added the rooms. Label the *X-Ray* screenshot "Case Study 5-2A" and the *Laboratory* screenshot "Case Study 5-2B." Place each one in your assignment folder.**

Patient Work-Up

6

Learning Objectives

1. Set operator preferences in your Batch applications.
2. List major applications of the Clinical Today module.
3. View daily appointments in Clinical Today.
4. Perform check-in duties and track patients throughout their visits.
5. View prescription renewals and new prescriptions within Clinical Today.
6. Retrieve the patient's EMR and update sections within the patient health history panes.
7. Record vital signs and document the patient's chief complaint.
8. View and create Flowsheets within Harris CareTracker EMR.
9. Create and print a growth chart.
10. Update the Patient Care Management application.
11. Create and print a Progress Note.

Real-World Connection

In this chapter, you are going to learn a great deal about working in the patient's electronic medical record (EMR). You are very fortunate to enter the medical field at a time when technology is flourishing. Electronic medical records organize the patient's information so that you know exactly where each item is stored within the patient's chart. EMRs also help medical assistants stay on task and keep up with lab reports and prescription renewals. Your challenge is to embrace the training in this chapter so that you are able to fully navigate the patient's medical record in Harris CareTracker EMR.

Before you begin the activities in this chapter, refresh your memory on working with Harris CareTracker by referring back to the Best Practices list on page xiv of this workbook. This list is also posted to the student companion website. Following best practices will help you complete work quickly and accurately.

SETTING OPERATOR PREFERENCES IN THE BATCH APPLICATION

Learning Objective 1: Set operator preferences in your Batch applications.

Activity 6-1
Setting Operator Preferences in Your Batch Application

As discussed in previous chapters, the *Batch* application in Harris CareTracker PM and EMR enables you to set up your operator preferences based on the workflow for your role. This reduces the number of clicks required to get from one application to the other, making navigation through Harris CareTracker easy.

As a medical assistant working in a clinical capacity, you will want your screen to open in the *Clinical Today* module each time you log in to Harris CareTracker. Selecting the appropriate setting from the *Login Application* in your *Batch* preferences will take you directly to the *Clinical Today* module after logging in. This activity will assist you in making the appropriate changes to your preferences. Changing your batch settings now is highly recommended to improve workflow.

1. To set up operator preferences, click *Batch* on the *Name Bar*. Harris CareTracker PM and EMR displays the *Operator Encounter Batch Control* dialog box.

2. Click on the *Edit* button.

3. Click on the drop-down arrow beside *Provider* and select "Dr. Raman," if he has not already been selected.

4. Click on the drop-down arrow beside *Resource* and select "Dr. Raman," if he has not already been selected.

5. Click on the drop-down arrow beside *Show Alerts* and select "Yes."

6. In the *Login Application* box, click on the drop-down arrow and select "Clinical."

7. Click on *Save*. Now every time you log in to Harris CareTracker, you will be taken directly to the *Clinical Today* module.

8. Click "X" in the right-hand corner to close the dialog box.

OVERVIEW OF THE CLINICAL TODAY MODULE

Learning Objective 2: List major applications of the Clinical Today module.

Within Harris CareTracker EMR, the *Clinical Today* module is the area where most medical assistants working in a clinical capacity spend their time. The *Clinical Today* module consists of three main applications: *Appointments*, *Tasks*, and *Population Management*. This chapter focuses on the *Appointments* and *Tasks* applications.

Appointments

Learning Objective 3: View daily appointments in Clinical Today.

Learning Objective 4: Perform check-in duties and track patients throughout their visits.

The *Appointments* application (**Figure 6-1**) consists of patient and nonpatient appointments scheduled via the *Book* application in the *Scheduling* module.

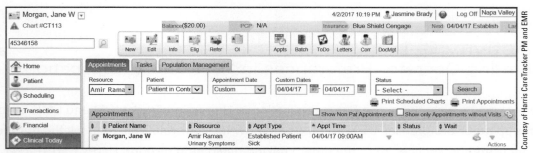

Figure 6-1   Appointment Screen in Clinical Today

Activity 6-2
Viewing Appointments

At the start of each day, you will review the patient appointment list for the current workday. Some workers like to make copies of the schedule and have it close by for easy referencing; however, with Harris CareTracker PM and EMR, this information is just a screen away.

In Chapter 4, you scheduled nine patients for future appointments and cancelled one, leaving eight patients with appointments. Now you will pull up some of these patients in *Clinical Today* and start working in the EMR portion of their records.

> **(!) ALERT!**   When you click on *Clinical Today*, the screen automatically defaults to the patients scheduled for the current date. For Activity 6-2, you will need the dates of the appointments you scheduled for patients in Chapter 4.

1. Click on *Clinical Today*.

2. Click on the drop-down arrow under *Resource* and select "All."

3. Click on the drop-down arrow under *Patient* and select "All Patients."

4. Click on the drop-down arrow under *Appointment Date* and select "Custom."

5. Click on the calendar beside the first box under *Custom Dates* and select the date you scheduled Jane Morgan's appointment in Chapter 4.

6. Click in the second box to the right of the calendar under *Custom Dates*. The date that you inserted in the first box should automatically populate in this box.

7. In the status box, click on the drop-down arrow and select "All" (**Figure 6-2**). **Note:** You may have to click back on the body of the *Status* box field for the drop-down to disappear.

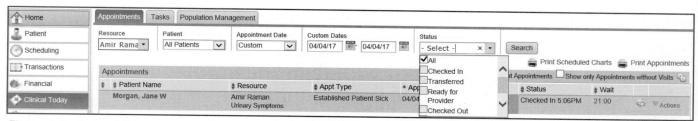

Figure 6-2   Select All   Courtesy of Harris CareTracker PM and EMR

8. Click on *Search*. (The appointment screen with Ms. Morgan's appointment should now appear along with any other appointments scheduled on this day.)

📇 **Print a screenshot of your Appointment screen from Clinical Today. Label it "Activity 6-2" and place it in your assignment folder.**

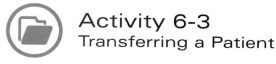

Activity 6-3
Transferring a Patient

In Chapter 4 (Activity 4-10a–g), you practiced checking in patients. Patients are typically checked in upon arrival. This cues the clinical staff that the patient is ready to be taken back to the exam room. Once the patient has been transferred to the exam room, this will alert the staff of the patient's current status. This activity describes how to change a patient's status from "Checked In" to "Transferred." Transfer refers to the status of a patient when he or she has been taken to an exam room.

1. Click on *Clinical Today*.

2. Match the search parameters to those set in Activity 6-2. Click *Search*.

3. Jane Morgan's appointment should be listed in the *Appointments* window. Her current status is green, which means that she has already been checked in. (**Note:** A row highlighted in red means the patient has been checked out. If you completed billing activities prior to this activity, the status would be red.)

4. Change her status by clicking on the drop-down arrow in her *Status* column and selecting "Transfer."

5. The *Patient Location* box will pop up. Select the radio button next to "Exam Room #1."

6. Click *Select* (**Figure 6-3**). (**Note:** If the there is nothing listed in the *Patient Location* box, review your Compatibility View setting (refer to Best Practices), and try again.)

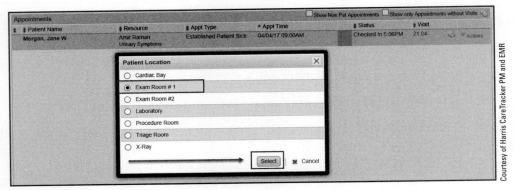

Figure 6-3   Patient Location Box

7. Ms. Morgan's entry line should now be blue, indicating that she has been transferred to the exam room. The appropriate exam room number will now appear in the *Status* column (**Figure 6-4**).

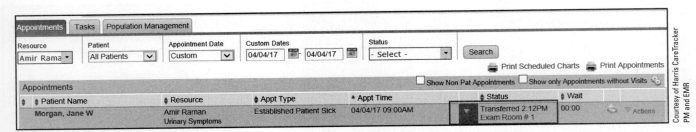

Figure 6-4   Exam Room Status Column

🖫 **Print a screenshot of the Exam Room Status Column. Label it "Activity 6-3" and place it in your assignment folder.**

Viewing Prescription Renewals

Learning Objective 5: View prescription renewals and new prescriptions within Clinical Today.

The *Rx Renewals* application displays a list of renewal requests sent electronically by the pharmacy and patient to the provider set up in your batch. The *Rx Renewal* application can be accessed via the *Tasks* tab in the *Clinical Today* module.

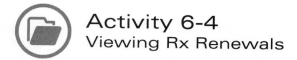

Activity 6-4
Viewing Rx Renewals

1. Click on the *Clinical Today* module.

2. Select the *Tasks* tab.

3. View the *Tasks* panes on the right side of the window.

4. Click on the *Rx Renewals* link (**Figure 6-5**) in the *Tasks* pane.

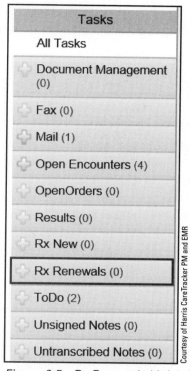

Figure 6-5   Rx Renewals Link in Tasks Pane

5. To set your parameters, click on the word "All" beside *Provider.*

6. Click on the word "All" for *Request Type.*

7. For *Status,* click on "Active."

8. Click on "All" beside the *Dates* tab (**Figure 6-6**). Setting the parameters to "All" in the *Rx Renewals* application allows you to review all active prescription renewals for all providers in the practice.

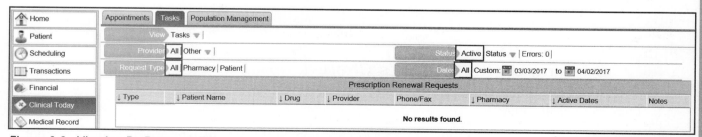

Figure 6-6   Viewing Rx Renewals Tab

Courtesy of Harris CareTracker PM and EMR

📇 **Print this screen, even though it does not show any prescription renewals. Label it "Activity 6-4" and place it in your assignment folder.**

Viewing New Prescriptions

The *Rx New* application displays a list of prescriptions that are not transmitted electronically, printed, or failed transmission that you must review and resolve on a daily basis. Additionally, you can view details for each prescription listed and reorder a prescription, eliminating the need to reenter redundant information, view interactions, and more. Along with prescription renewals, new prescriptions can be viewed from the *Tasks* tab in *Clinical Today*. Instead of clicking on the *Rx Renewal* link, click on *Rx New* on the right-hand side of the screen and follow the prompts.

This chapter has just briefly touched on a few of the available functions in the *Clinical Today* module. Harris CareTracker PM and EMR provides users with an assortment of tools to streamline and organize information so that important tasks are never overlooked. When working in the medical field, you should review electronic tasks throughout the workday and resolve unsettled items in a timely manner.

RETRIEVING AND UPDATING THE PATIENT'S ELECTRONIC MEDICAL RECORD

Learning Objective 6: Retrieve the patient's EMR and update sections within the patient health history panes.

Once the patient has been checked in and transferred to an exam room, you are ready to bring up his or her electronic medical record (EMR). In the case of Jane Morgan, she is an established patient. Napa Valley Family Health Associates has transitioned from paper records to Harris CareTracker PM and Physician EMR. Because Ms. Morgan's has not been seen since the practice converted to electronic health records, her chart has not yet been converted. You will need to build her electronic chart from scratch in this chapter's activities.

PROFESSIONALISM CONNECTION

The status tab in the *Appointment* module within *Clinical Today* allows you to determine exactly where the patient is throughout the visit. It also tracks the length of time the patient spends in each area of the visit. If you happen to notice that the patient has been waiting particularly long in any area, even if it is not your assigned area, do a little investigating to establish the reason for the wait. Someone may have forgotten about the patient or may be tending to an emergency. Once you determine the reason for the wait, alert the patient and apologize for the delay. If the circumstances causing the delay cannot be resolved within a reasonable period of time, offer the patient an opportunity to reschedule the appointment. The entire Napa Valley Family Health Associates staff is on the same team and need to support each other as well as the patient.

Activity 6-5
Bringing Up the Patient's Chart

1. Click on *Clinical Today*.

2. In the *Appointments* screen within *Clinical Today*, bring up the date of Jane Morgan's appointment. Be sure that *Resources* reflect "All." **Hint:** If you don't recall the date of the appointment, click on the *History* tab in the *Scheduling* module to locate the patient's appointment. Do not create a new encounter for this visit, only use the appointment/encounter previously scheduled.

3. Click on Ms. Morgan's name. The patient's *Chart Summary* will open in a new window (**Figure 6-7**).

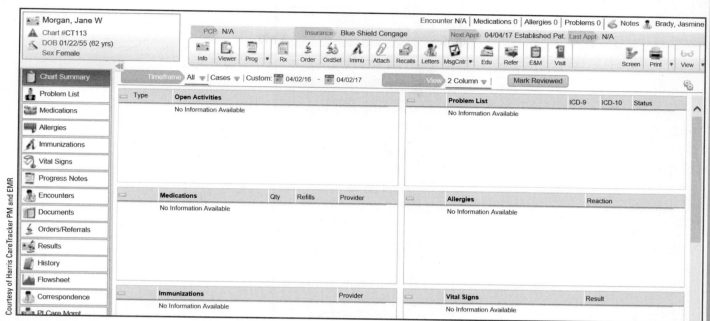

Figure 6-7   *Chart Summary in New Window*

 Print a screenshot of the Chart Summary in new window. Label it "Activity 6-5" and place it in your assignment folder.

The order in which you complete activities in the patient's chart is purely subjective. Some medical assistants start by entering the vital signs and chief complaint, and then adding new medications, allergies, and history information. The order really does not matter as long as you complete the process. We are going to start the process by creating the patient's current medication list.

Activity 6-6
Adding a Medication to a Patient's Chart

1. In the patient's *Chart Summary*, the *Medications* application allows you to manually update the patient's medication list. New prescriptions can also be added here; however, you will only enter the patient's current medications at this time.

    Following the steps used in Activity 6-5, bring up Jane Morgan's patient chart using the *Clinical Today* module:

    - Click on *Clinical Today*.

    - In the *Appointments* screen within *Clinical Today*, bring up the date of Jane Morgan's appointment. Be sure that *Resource* reflect "All." **Hint:** If you don't recall the date of the appointment, with the patient in context, click on the *History* tab in the *Scheduling* module to locate the patient's appointment. Do not create a new encounter for this activity; use only the appointment/encounter previously scheduled.

    - Click on Ms. Morgan's name. The patient's *Chart Summary* will open in a new window (refer to Figure 6-7).

2. In the *Patient Health History* pane, click on the *Medications* link (**Figure 6-8**). The *Medications* window displays.

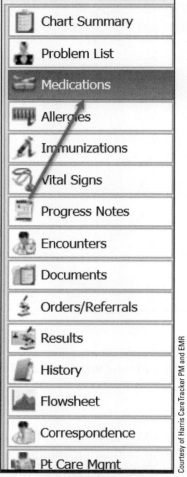

Figure 6-8   Medications Link

3. Click *+ Patient Med*, which is located at the top right side of the screen (**Figure 6-9**). The *Medication* dialog box will display (**Figure 6-10**).

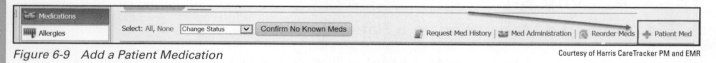

Figure 6-9   Add a Patient Medication

Courtesy of Harris CareTracker PM and EMR

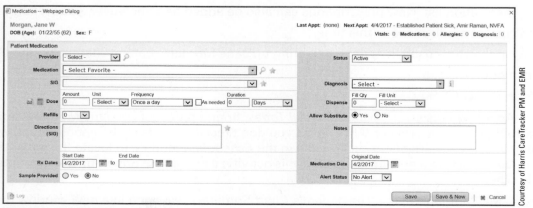

Figure 6-10   Medication Dialog Box

4. In the *Provider* drop-down list, select the patient's provider "Amir Raman." The *Provider* list displays the group providers first, followed by the referring providers.

5. By default, the *Status* list is set to "Active" (**Figure 6-11**), but you can change to another applicable status if necessary. (Leave the *Status* as "Active.")

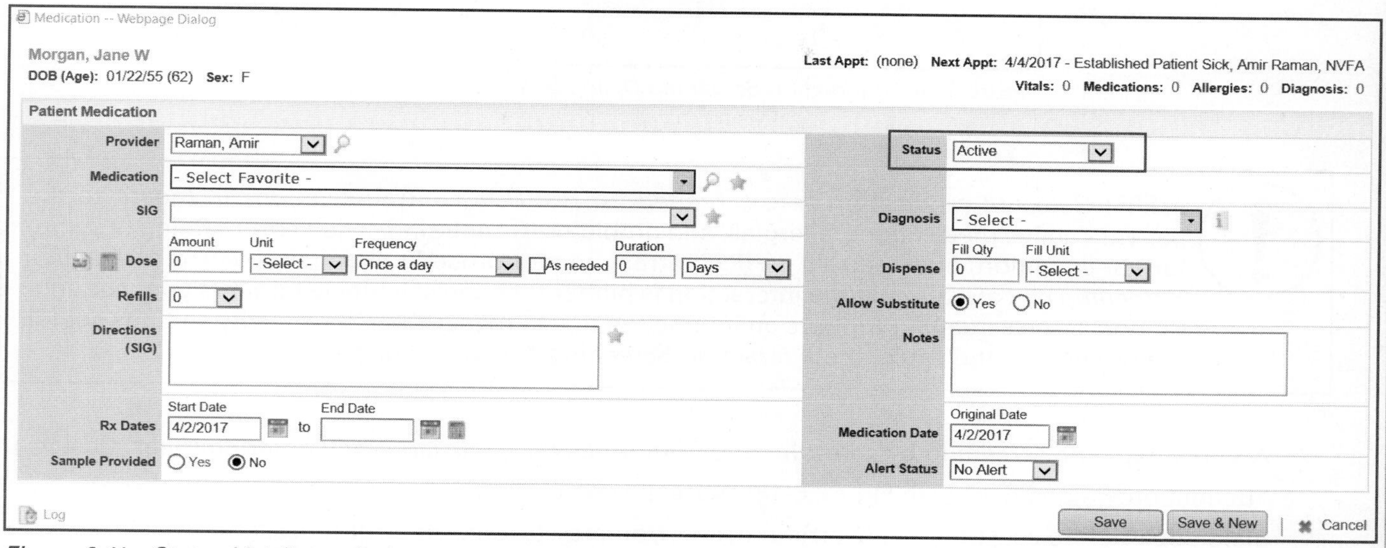

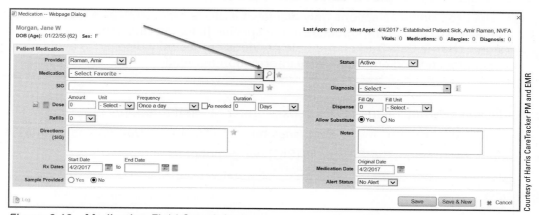

Figure 6-11   *Status List Set to Active*

6. In the *Medication* field, click on the search icon (**Figure 6-12**). The *Medication Search* dialog box opens. In the *Search Text* box, type in "Boniva" and click on *Search* (**Figure 6-13**). The various options display. Click on "Boniva Oral Tablet 150 MG." (Ms. Morgan is currently taking Boniva to help slow down her osteoporosis.) An *Interaction Screening* box will pop up (**Figure 6-14**).

Figure 6-12   *Medication Field Search Icon*

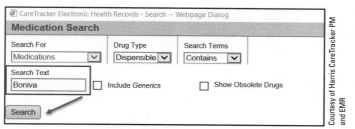

Figure 6-13   *Medication Search Text*

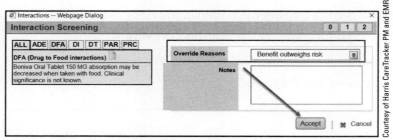

Figure 6-14   *Interaction Screening Dialog Box*

> ⓘ **ALERT!** Selected medications are screened for possible contraindications in regard to the patient's active medications, allergies, and problems. A contraindication is something (a symptom or condition) that makes a particular treatment or procedure inadvisable. The *Interaction Screening* box alerts you if the interaction is higher than the severity level set in your configurations. If the screening triggers an interaction that is higher than the severity settings set for the provider in the batch, the *Interaction Screening* dialog box displays.

7. Acknowledge the screening by selecting one or more *Override Reasons* and entering notes. Select "Benefit outweighs risk" (see Figure 6-14). **Note:** If you click *Cancel* in the *Interaction Screening* dialog box before accepting an override reason, you may receive an error message.

8. Click *Accept* (see Figure 6-14).

9. You will skip over the SIG box for now. Refer to the FYI box below. Once a SIG is saved as a favorite, you will be able to select it from the manage favorites icon. SIG is an abbreviation for *signa* in Latin (meaning "label" or "sign"). SIG refers to specific dosage instructions that are given when prescribing medications.

> 💡 **FYI** The drop-down selections only display if a SIG is associated as a favorite to the medication selected and auto-populates in the specific fields. Because this is a live (educational) version of Harris CareTracker, multiple previous entries may display. To avoid duplication, you will proceed and enter the *Dose* information manually.

10. Enter the dosage information in the *Dose* boxes. Enter "1" in the *Amount* box, "Tablet" in the *Unit* box, and "Once every month" in the *Frequency* box, and "6" in the *Duration* box (**Figure 6-15**). As you enter the *Dose* information, the *Directions* (SIG) will populate.

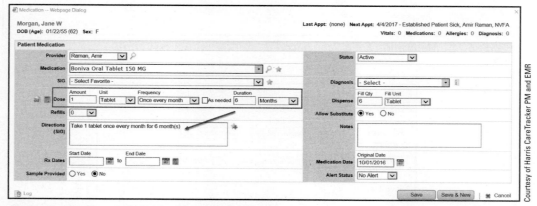

Figure 6-15   *Dose—Amount, Unit, Frequency*

11. Tab down to the *Rx Dates* field. Because the medication is not being renewed, remove any dates that appear in the *Start Date* box. Leave the *End Date* box blank as well.

12. The patient states that she started taking the medication on October 1 of last year. Insert this information in the box titled *Medication Date/Original Date* on the right side of the screen (**Figure 6-16**).

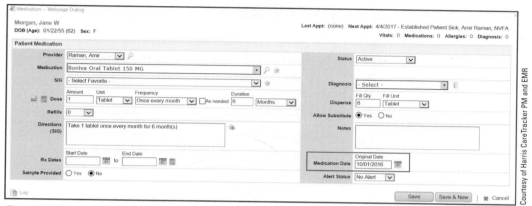

Figure 6-16   *Original Date*

13. Because you are not creating a new prescription, no other information needs to be entered. Click *Save*.

14. "Boniva Oral Tablet 150 MG" should now appear in the *Medications* box of the *Patient Health History* pane (**Figure 6-17**).

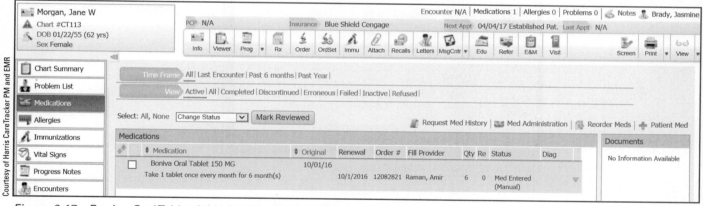

Figure 6-17   *Boniva Oral Tablet Added to Medications Window*

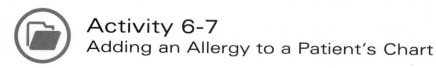

Activity 6-7
Adding an Allergy to a Patient's Chart

The *Allergies* application is where you add new and existing allergies to a patient's medical record. It is important to ensure that all active allergies are recorded for accurate drug–allergy contraindication checks when prescribing medications and ordering immunizations.

1. If you are not in Jane Morgan's medical record, access it using the following steps:
   - Click on *Clinical Today*.

- In the *Appointments* screen within *Clinical Today*, bring up the date of Jane Morgan's appointment. Be sure that *Resource* reflects "All." **Hint:** If you don't recall the date of the appointment, with the patient in context, click on the *History* tab in the *Scheduling* module to locate the patient's appointment. Do not create a new encounter for this activity; use only the appointment/encounter previously scheduled.

- Click directly on the patient's name under *Appointments*, and the *Patient Health History* pane will appear. (**Note:** Close out of the *Clinical Alerts* dialog box if displaying.)

2. In the *Patient Health History* pane, click on *Allergies*. Harris CareTracker EMR displays the *Allergies* window.

3. Click + *Add Allergy* (**Figure 6-18**). Harris CareTracker EMR displays the *Patient Allergy* dialog box (**Figure 6-19**).

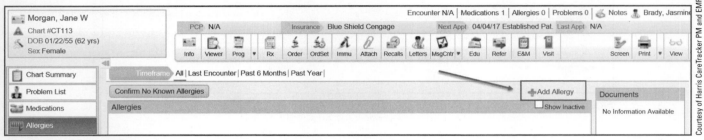

Figure 6-18   Add Allergy

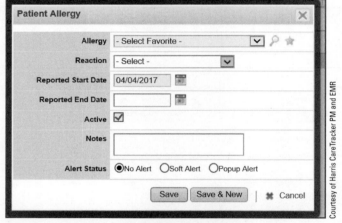

Figure 6-19   Patient Allergy Dialog Box

4. Ms. Morgan is allergic to codeine, so this information will need to be entered in her electronic chart. Search for codeine by clicking on the *Search* 🔍 icon next to the *Allergy* field. (**Note:** If codeine has been previously entered as a favorite in the system, it will appear in the drop-down *Allergy* list. We will mimic searching for it as though it were not saved as a favorite.)

5. In the *Search Text* box, type "Codeine." Click the *Search* button.

6. A list of several medications will pop up that include the word "codeine." If "Codeine" is already on the favorites list, it will be indicated by the *On Favorites* 🔲 icon.

7. Click on the search result "Codeine Phosphate." The *Patient Allergy* window will reappear with "Codeine Phosphate" listed beside *Allergy*.

8. In the *Reaction* box, click on the drop-down arrow and select "Anaphylaxis." (**Note:** Click on the drop-down arrow again to minimize the drop-down list. "Anaphylaxis" is now selected.)

9. In the *Reported Start Date* box, enter the date of onset for the allergy in MM/DD/YYYY format or click the *Calendar* 🗓 icon to select the date. Enter a start date of April 1 of last year.

10. Leave the *Reported End Date* blank.

11. By default, the *Status* is set to *Active* to indicate that the allergy is an active allergy. (**Note:** The active checkbox is read only and is updated based on *Reported End Date* status.)

12. In the *Notes* box, enter additional comments, if necessary. (Leave this section blank.)

13. By default, the *Alert Status* is set to "No Alert." Due to the seriousness of this patient's allergy, click on "Popup Alert" (**Figure 6-20**). The pop-up alert will now pop up whenever Ms. Morgan's medical record is launched and will stop displaying when the alert is closed. You can also click the Alert ⚠ icon next to the patient's chart number on the *Patient Detail* bar to view both soft alerts and pop-up alerts.

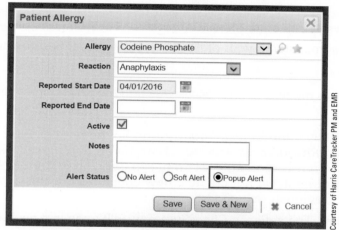

Figure 6-20   *Patient Allergy Popup Alert*

14. Click *Save & New* to save and add another allergy without exiting the *Patient Allergy* dialog box.

15. Add "Peanuts [NS]" as a new allergy for Ms. Morgan.

    a. In the *Reaction* box, scroll down the list and select both "Diarrhea" and "Vomiting."

    b. Click back on the *Reaction* field drop-down arrow to close the list of options.

    c. In the *Reported Start Date* box, enter a date that is 10 years prior to the date of the appointment.

    d. Leave the *Reported End Date* box blank.

    e. In the *Notes* section, type the following: "The reported start date is just an estimate. Patient doesn't know the actual day or year she had the reaction."

    f. Select "Soft Alert" in the *Alert Status* category.

16. Click *Save.* "Peanuts" and "Codeine" will now be listed in the *Allergies* pane (**Figure 6-21**).

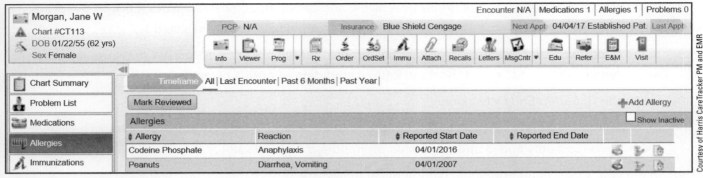

Figure 6-21   Allergies Pane

Activity 6-8
Entering Past Immunizations in a Patient's Chart

The *Immunizations* module allows you to enter history information regarding the patient. It also allows you to enter immunizations you administer in your office. This activity describes how to enter a patient's past immunizations.

1. If you are not in Jane Morgan's medical record, access it using the following steps:

   - Click on *Clinical Today*.

   - In the *Appointments* screen within *Clinical Today*, bring up the date of Jane Morgan's appointment. Be sure that *Resource* reflects "All." **Hint:** If you don't recall the date of the appointment, with the patient in context, click on the *History* tab in the *Scheduling* module to locate the patient's appointment. Do not create a new encounter for this activity; use only the appointment/encounter previously scheduled.

   - Click on Ms. Morgan's name. The patient's *Chart Summary* will open in a new window (refer to Figure 6-7).

2. In the *Patient Health History* pane, click on *Immunizations*. Harris CareTracker EMR displays the *Immunizations* window.

3. Click on the + *Add Past/Refused Immunization* link (**Figure 6-22**).

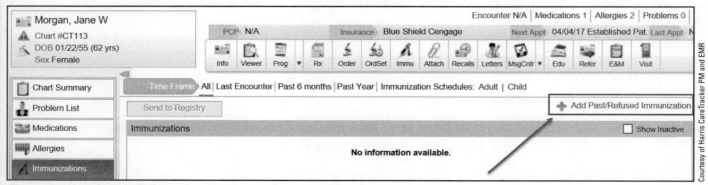

Figure 6-22   Add Past/Refused Immunization Link

4. Type in the word "Tetanus" in the *Immunization* field and then click on the *Search* ◯ icon.

5. An *Immunization Search* dialog box will pop up. Click on "tetanus toxoid, adsorbed" under *Search Results.* The selected immunization will now appear in the *Immunization* field.

6. Because Ms. Morgan's tetanus immunization was not administered at Napa Valley Family Health Associates, the only other information that can be entered is when she received the immunization and where she received it. Ms. Morgan stated that she received the shot on March 3 of last year. Type this information in the *Admin Date* box.

7. Enter a description in the *Administration Notes* field. Ms. Morgan stated that she received the tetanus shot at America's Urgent Care. Enter the following description: "Pt. received Tetanus shot at America's Urgent Care after stepping on a nail."

8. Click *Save.* Your *Immunizations* pane should match **Figure 6-23**.

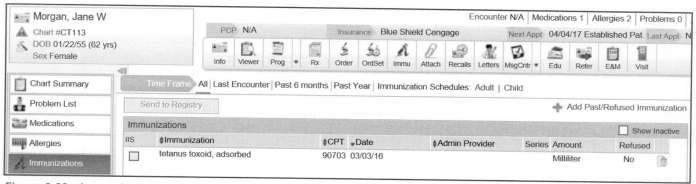

Figure 6-23   *Immunizations Pane*   Courtesy of Harris CareTracker PM and EMR

Print your chart summary using the following instructions, which will illustrate the work you did in the last three activities.

*   Click on *Chart Summary* in the *Patient Health History* pane.
*   Click on the drop-down arrow beside the printer 🖨 icon in the upper-right corner of the screen.
*   Click on *Print Chart Summary.* A new window will pop up.
*   Click the *Print* button. Label this "Activities 6-6, 6-7, and 6-8" and place it in your assignment folder.
*   After printing, close out of the *Formal Health Record* screen.

Activity 6-9
Entering a Patient's Medical History

The *History* application helps capture and review a patient's past medical, family, and social history information from one central location using different data entry methods. It is important to record and review history data because they enable the provider to form a diagnosis and treatment plan together with the clinical examination. The *History* application provides quick and easy data entry methods, such as checkboxes, drop-down lists, text boxes, and more, to record information. In addition, you can also click *Mark Reviewed* for each category to ensure that historical information presented is reviewed to provide better analysis in diagnoses. This information is automatically made available in the *History* section of each progress note, improving documentation quality and patient care.

An alternative method to document history information is directly via the patient *Progress Note.* History information recorded here is also recorded in the *History* application, including addition of family members to the *Family History* section.

1. If you are not in Jane Morgan's medical record, access it using the following steps:

   • Click on *Clinical Today*.

   • In the *Appointments* screen within *Clinical Today*, bring up the date of Jane Morgan's appointment. Be sure that *Resource* reflects "All." **Hint:** If you don't recall the date of the appointment, with the patient in context, click on the *History* tab in the *Scheduling* module to locate the patient's appointment. Do not create a new encounter for this activity; use only the appointment/encounter previously scheduled.

   • Click on Ms. Morgan's name. The patient's Chart Summary will open in a new window (refer to Figure 6-7).

2. Click on the *History* tab in the *Patient Health History* pane. Harris CareTracker EMR displays the *History* window (**Figure 6-24**).

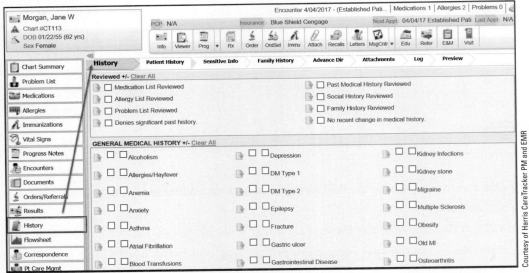

Figure 6-24   *History Window*

3. In the *General Medical History* section of the *Patient History* screen, click on "Y" (for "Yes") on the conditions listed in **Table 6-1**. Click on the *Findings Details* icon to the left of the "Y" boxes and follow the instructions in Table 6-1 regarding information to insert in the *Comments* box (**Figure 6-25**). Click the "X" on the top right of the *Comments* box to close and save each comment. (**Note:** It may take a few moments for the dialog box to activate to be able to enter text.)

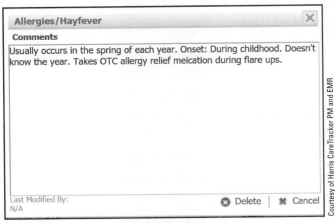

Figure 6-25   *Allergies/Hayfever Comments Box*

Table 6-1   General Medical History Information for Jane Morgan

CONDITION	DETAILS
Allergies/Hay Fever	*Comment:* Usually occurs in the spring of each year. Onset: During childhood. Doesn't know the year. Takes OTC allergy relief medication during flare-ups. (Refer to Figure 6-25.)
Asthma	Under *Severity*, click the box beside "mild." *Comment:* Diagnosed 10 years ago. Has had 2–3 attacks in the past 10 years. Last attack approximately five years ago. Not taking any meds for this condition.
Depression	*Comment:* Has not been formally diagnosed. Has periods of sadness and crying. Doesn't want to do anything during these bouts. Onset: About one year. Occurs a couple of times a month and lasts for a few days.
Joint Pain	*Comment:* Intermittent pain (flare-ups approx. 2–3 times per year). Never been formally diagnosed. Mainly in fingers and toes. Onset date approx. three years ago.

4. Enter the following information in the *Hospitalizations* box:

   a. Tonsillectomy at age 3. Doesn't know which hospital.

   b. Hospitalized for the birth of her three children at County General. No complications.

   c. Left breast lumpectomy in May 2010. Negative for cancer cells.

   d. No other hospitalizations.

5. Enter the following information in the *Other Medical History* box: "Five-year history of UTIs. Approximately 1–2 episodes/year. Treatment: Antibiotics."

6. In the *Tobacco Assessment* section, click on the drop-down menu next to the blank box/field to the right of *Smoking Status* and select "Never Smoker." Beside *Tobacco User* click on the "N" for No. Leave everything else in this section blank. (Note that the *Tobacco Assessment* section supports Stage 1 Meaningful Use.)

7. Enter the following information in the *Social History* section:

   a. Click on the drop-down menu next to the blank box/field to the right of *Alcohol Use* and select "Non-Drinker."

   b. Click on the drop-down menu next to the blank box/field to the right of *Caffeine Use* and select "2 servings per Day." Click on the *Finding Details* icon next to *Caffeine Use* and put a check mark beside "coffee" and "tea" in the "Type" column. In the *Comments* box state the following: "Drinks 1 cup of coffee and 1 glass of iced tea daily." Click the "X" to close out of the box.

   c. *Drug Use*: Click on the "N" for No.

   d. *Sun Protection*: Click on the "Y" for Yes. Click on the *Findings Details* icon. Place a check mark in the "sunglasses" and "sunscreen" boxes. Click on *SPF* and select the "30" box. Click on the "X" to close out of the *Sun Protection* box.

   e. *Tattoos*: Click on the "N" for No.

   f. *Sexually Active*: Click on the "Y" for Yes.

   g. Click on the drop-down menu next to the blank box/field to the right of *Race* and select "Caucasian."

h. Click on the drop-down menu next to the blank box/field to the right of *Native language* and select "English."

i. *Physical Abuse*: Click on the "N" for No.

j. *Domestic Violence*: Click on the "N" for No.

k. Click on the drop-down menu next to the blank box/field to the right of *Education Level* and select "Bachelor's Degree."

l. Click on the drop-down menu next to the blank box/field to the right of *Marital Status* and select "Married."

m. Click on the drop-down menu next to the blank box/field to the right of *Exercise Habits* and select "moderate >3 x/wk."

n. *Seatbelts*: Click on the "Y" for Yes.

o. *Body Piercings*: Click on the "N" for No.

p. *Birth Control Method*: Leave all boxes blank in this section.

q. Click on the drop-down menu next to the blank box/field to the right of *Religion* and select "Christian."

r. *Occupation*: Enter "Nurse."

s. *Other Social History* box: Leave blank.

8. In the *Depression Screening* section, click on the drop-down box next to the blank box/field beside the *Little interest or pleasure in doing things* line and select "Occasionally." Click on the drop-down box next to the blank box/field beside *Feeling down, depressed, or hopeless* and select "Occasionally." Leave the *Date of Last Depression Screening* field blank.

9. Enter the following information in the *OB/GYN History* section:

    a. *LMP*: Leave blank.

    b. *Menopause has occurred*: Click on the "Y" for Yes.

    c. *History of abnormal pap smears*: Click on the "N" for No.

    d. *Sexually Active*: Click on the "Y" for Yes.

    e. *Ectopic Pregnancy*: Click on the "N" for No.

    f. *Menarche Age*: Enter "13."

    g. *Birth Control*: Leave these boxes blank.

10. Enter the following information in the *Pregnancy Summary* section:

    a. *Gravida*: Select "4" from the drop-down menu next to the blank box/field.

    b. *Term*: Select "2" from the drop-down menu next to the blank box/field.

    c. *Preterm*: Select "1" from the drop-down menu next to the blank box/field.

    d. *AB*: Skip over this category.

    e. *Live Children*: Select "3" from the drop-down menu next to the blank box/field.

    f. *Miscarriage*: Select "1" from the drop-down menu next to the blank box/field.

11. Leave the *Other OB-GYN History* box blank.

12. In the *Surgical/Procedural* section, select the box for *Breast Lumpectomy* and click on the associated *Finding Details* icon. In the *Breast Lumpectomy* box, select "left" for the *Location.* In the *Comments* section, enter: "Had lumpectomy in May of 2010. Biopsy negative for cancer cells." Click the "X" to close out of the box. Leave all other boxes in this section blank.

13. Leave the *Other Surgical History* box blank.

14. Enter the following information in the *Preventive Care* section (for all dates, use the previous year unless otherwise indicated):

    a. *Colonoscopy*: Enter 03/12/20XX

    b. *Dilated Eye Exam*: Enter 01/04/20XX

    c. *Flu Vaccine*: Enter 10/12/20XX

    d. *Mammography*: 05/12/20XX

    e. *Pap Smear*: 05/15/20XX (three years ago)

15. In the *Self-Management Goal* box, enter: "Lose 10 pounds this year and start exercising 3x/week."

16. Click *Save*.

🖫 **Go to the top right of the History pane. Click on the drop-down arrow beside the Print icon. Click on Print Patient History. When the box opens, you should see the patient's history form. Print this form, label it "Activity 6-9A," and place it in your assignment folder.**

> **SPOTLIGHT**   There are times a patient will refuse to answer questions outlined on the template. If so, leave the field blank. Do not check "Y" or "N." There is no option of "patient refused," but you could free text a comment in the notes box by clicking the *Finding Details* icon.

17. Click on the *Sensitive Info* tab. Your screen should match **Figure 6-26** (though no selections will have been made yet).

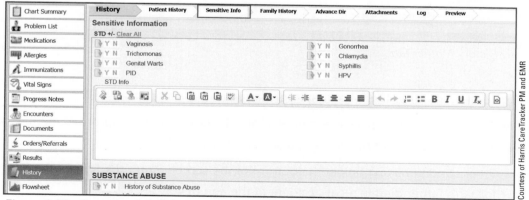

Figure 6-26   *Sensitive Info Tab*

18. In the *STD* section, click "N" for each disease listed. (**Note:** An easy way to mark all categories with the same response is to click on the [+/−] sign between *STD* and *Clear All*. For this scenario, click on the [−] sign. All diseases should now have a red "X" [indicating "No"] beside their names.)

19. Ms. Morgan has no history of substance abuse, so click on the "N" beside *History of Substance Abuse*.

20. Ms. Morgan is not seeing any mental health providers, so click on the "N" beside *Seeing mental health provider*.

21. Ms. Morgan has never had an HIV test. Enter the following comment in the text box below *HIV Status*: "Patient has never had an HIV test but states that she has been in a monogamous relationship with her husband over the past 30 years."

22. Leave the *Medicare High Risk Criteria* section blank because Ms. Morgan is not enrolled in Medicare.

23. Click *Save*.

🖫 **Click on the drop-down arrow beside the Print icon. Select Print Sensitive Information. When the box opens, you should see the Sensitive Information Form. Print this form and label it "Activity 6-9B." Place it in your assignment folder.**

24. Click on the *Family History* tab.

25. Select the *Mother* tab (**Figure 6-27**). Enter the following information in this section:

    a. Ms. Morgan's mother is still alive. Click on the drop-down menu next to the blank box/field to the right of *Status* and select "Alive."

    b. In the *Age* box, enter "85."

    c. Select the checkbox next to *In good health* to indicate the general health status of Ms. Morgan's mother.

    d. Ms. Morgan's mother suffers from GERD and hypertension. Click on the "Y" for Yes next to these two diseases.

    e. Click *Save*.

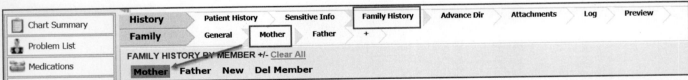

Figure 6-27   Family History/Mother Tab

Courtesy of Harris CareTracker PM and EMR

26. Select the *Father* tab. Enter the following information in this section:

    a. Ms. Morgan's father died in a car accident at age 40. Click on the drop-down menu next to the blank box/field to the right of *Status* and select "Deceased."

    b. In the *Other conditions* text box at the bottom of the screen, enter the following comment: "Ms. Morgan's father died in a car accident at the age of 40."

    c. Click *Save*.

🖫 **Click on the drop-down arrow beside the Print icon. Select Print Family History. When the box opens, you should see the Family History By Family Member form. Print this form, label it "Activity 6-9C," and place it in your assignment folder.**

Recording a Patient's Vital Signs and Chief Complaint

Learning Objective 7: Record vital signs and document the patient's chief complaint.

Activity 6-10

Recording a Patient's Vital Signs

The *Vital Signs* application allows you to record the patient's vital data at every encounter in the office and includes the patient's blood pressure, temperature, pulse respiration, height, weight, oxygen saturation reading, and pain level. This helps to guide clinical decisions about treatment and to identify the need for additional diagnostic measures. This activity describes how to record a patient's vital signs.

1. If you are not in Jane Morgan's medical record, access it using the following steps:
   - Click on *Clinical Today*.
   - In the *Appointments* screen within *Clinical Today*, bring up the date of Jane Morgan's appointment. Be sure that *Resource* reflects "All." **Hint:** If you don't recall the date of the appointment, with the patient in context, click on the *History* tab in the *Scheduling* module to locate the patient's appointment. Do not create a new encounter for this activity; use only the appointment/encounter previously scheduled.
   - Click on Ms. Morgan's name. The patient's Chart Summary will open in a new window (refer to Figure 6-7).

2. In the *Patient Health History* pane, click on *Vital Signs*. Harris CareTracker EMR displays the *Vital Signs* window with vital data taken during the current and past encounters at the office or at home. Because this is Ms. Morgan's first visit since the EMR was instituted, no vital signs have been entered yet.

3. Click on *Record Vital Signs* in the lower-left pane of the screen (**Figure 6-28**). If an encounter is in context, the *Record Vital Signs* dialog box will display.

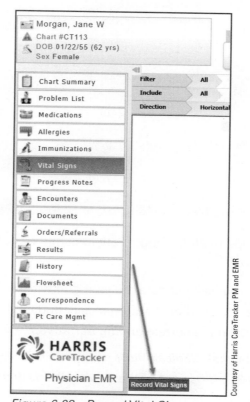

Figure 6-28   Record Vital Signs

TIP If an encounter is not in context, the *Select Encounter* dialog box displays (**Figure 6-29**), and you must create an encounter. Use only the encounter that already exists for this patient because you previously scheduled an appointment and went in through the *Appointment* application in *Clinical Today*; however, if the patient was not coming in for an appointment, but rather just stopping by to have his or her vital signs monitored, you would need to create an encounter to record your measurements. Proceed with step 4 if you do not see the *Select Encounter* dialog box.

Courtesy of Harris CareTracker PM and EMR

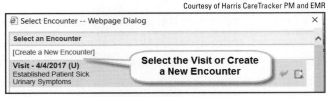

Figure 6-29   Select Encounter Dialog Box

4. Using the information in **Table 6-2**, enter the appropriate values in the *Record Vital Signs* dialog box (**Figure 6-30**).

Table 6-2   Vital Signs for Jane Morgan

MEASUREMENT CATEGORY	READING
Height	5 ft 6 in
Weight	160 lb
Body Mass Index	This will automatically populate.
Blood Pressure	146/90
Pulse Rate	84 bpm
Temperature	98.4°F
Respiratory Rate	16
Pulse Oximetry	97%
Pain Level	7/10

5. In the *Chief Complaint* box, type the following: "Patient complains of urinary symptoms over the last three days."

6. Click *Save*. The vital data automatically update the vital grid with the measurements and the date the vitals are recorded. (**Note:** The vital data automatically update the progress note for the same encounter and display the data in the corresponding narrative.)

7. If previously checked to display, the *Clinical Alerts* dialog box will display, including the *Health Maintenance* items (**Figure 6-31**). Close out of the *Clinical Alerts* dialog box by clicking on the "X" in the upper-right-hand corner.

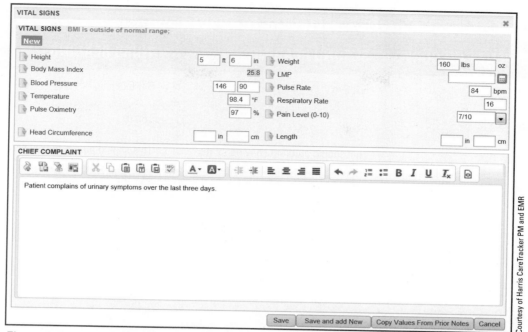

Figure 6-30   Record Vital Signs Dialog Box

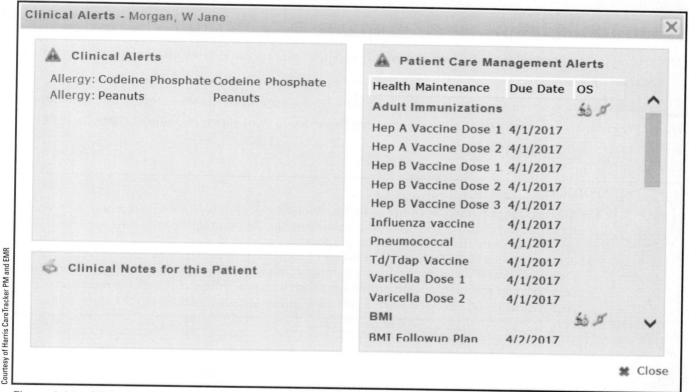

Figure 6-31   Clinical Alerts

8. In Activity 6-12, you are going to be working with flowsheets, which graph a variety of different measurements. Because we can add multiple iterations in one visit for vital signs, click back on *Record Vital Signs* at the bottom left corner of the window pane.

9. Click on *New*. Using the information in **Table 6-3**, record two more sets of readings so that you can graph your results in the flowsheet activity (Activity 6-12).

Table 6-3   Additional Vital Sign Readings for Jane Morgan

MEASUREMENT CATEGORY	SECOND READING	THIRD READING
Height	5 ft 6 in	5 ft 6 in
Weight	160 lb	160 lb
Body Mass Index	This should automatically populate.	This should automatically populate.
Blood Pressure	148/92	144/90
Pulse Rate	84 bpm	80 bpm
Temperature	98.8°F	97.8°F
Respiratory Rate	16	16
Pulse Oximetry	99%	98%
Pain Level	6/10	5/10

10. Click *Save and add New* to add the additional reading.

11. Once you are finished with the two additional readings, click on *Save*. Now all three measurements should appear.

 Click on the drop-down arrow beside the Print icon. Of the options available, select "Print Vital Signs Form." When the box opens, you should see the Vital Signs form. Print this form, label it "Activity 6-10," and place it in your assignment folder.

SPOTLIGHT
- You can record vital data such as height, weight, temperature, head circumference, and length using metric and standard measurements. By default, the vital data are converted from one unit of measure to another.
- You can record multiple iterations (the act of repeating) of vital data by clicking *Save and Add New.* When you record multiple iterations, the *Chart Summary* and *Progress Note* display the date and the iteration number for each instance. When vital data are recorded via the progress note, the *Vital Signs* application automatically updates with the same data.

Activity 6-11
Recording a Pediatric Patient's Vital Signs

Note: You must have completed Activity 3-4 (steps 1-6 and 33) and booked an appointment for Francisco Powell Jimenez in Activity 4-1 prior to completing this activity. If you have not already completed those activities, complete them now, before beginning this activity.

1. If you are not in Francisco Powell Jimenez's medical record, access it using the following steps:
    - Click on *Clinical Today*.

- In the *Appointments* screen within *Clinical Today*, bring up the date of Francisco's appointment. Be sure that *Resource* reflects "All." **Hint:** If you don't recall the date of the appointment, with the patient in context, click on the *History* tab in the *Scheduling* module to locate the patient's appointment. Do not create a new encounter for this activity; use only the appointment/encounter previously scheduled.

- Click on Francisco's name. The patient's *Chart Summary* will open in a new window (refer to Figure 6-7).

2. In the *Patient Health History* pane, click on *Vital Signs*. Because this is Francisco's first visit at NVFHA, no vital signs have been entered yet.

3. Click on *Record Vital Signs* in the lower-left pane of the screen (see Figure 6-28).

4. Using the information in **Table 6-4**, enter the values in the *Record Vital Signs* dialog box (see Figure 6-30).

Table 6-4   Vital Signs for Francisco Powell Jimenez

MEASUREMENT CATEGORY	READING
Height	2 ft 0 in
Weight	18 lb 3 oz
Body Mass Index	This will automatically populate.
Blood Pressure	(leave blank)
Pulse Rate	112 bpm
Temperature	98.3°F
Respiratory Rate	34
Pulse Oximetry	(leave blank)
Pain Level	(leave blank)

5. In the *Chief Complaint* box, type the following: "Well-Baby checkup."

6. Click *Save*.

📠 **Click on the drop-down arrow beside the Print icon. From the options, select "Print Vital Signs Form." When the box opens, you should see the Vital Signs form. Print this form, label it "Activity 6-11," and place it in your assignment folder.**

Filtering Vital Data

The *Vital Signs* application enables you to filter vital data based on the location the vitals are monitored and the date the vitals are recorded. Additionally, you can filter to view vitals pertaining to a specific case.

To filter vital data:

- Access the *Medical Record* module using one of the following methods:
  - Pull the patient into context, and click the *Medical Record* module.
  - If the patient has an appointment, click the patient's name in the *Appointments* tab of the *Clinical Today* module.

- In the *Patient Health History* pane, click *Vital Signs*. Harris CareTracker EMR displays the *Vital Signs* window with vital data taken during the current and past encounters at the office or at home.

- Do one of the following:
  - To filter vitals based on the location recorded, click either the *Recorded at Home* or the *Recorded in the Office* tabs.
  - To filter vitals based on the date the vitals are recorded, click on the *Last Encounter*, *Past 6 months*, or *Past Year* tabs (**Figure 6-32**).

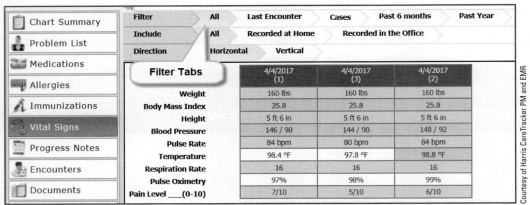

Figure 6-32   Filtering Vital Data-Horizontal View

- To filter vitals pertaining to a specific case, click the *Cases* tab. In the *Select Cases* dialog box, select the checkbox for the case you want and click *Select*.

Viewing Flowsheets

Learning Objective 8: View and create Flowsheets within Harris CareTracker EMR.

Activity 6-12
Viewing a Flowsheet

The *Flowsheet* application provides electronic management of clinical data entry and review of patient progress over time using different flowsheet templates. A flowsheet template is a profile with selected items. Data in a patient medical record can be pulled into a flowsheet, eliminating the need for double entry. It accommodates multidisciplinary documentation requirements and is linked to *Progress Notes*, *Vital Signs*, and *Results* applications. The application displays patient information that includes lab results, medications, vitals, and other medical data in a table or graph view.

The table view includes two formats: vertical grid (**Figure 6-33**) and horizontal grid. In a vertical grid, the columns represent vitals taken, and rows represent an interval of time. The horizontal grid represents the data in the reverse layout. The different formats enable you to analyze data over time from a variety of viewpoints on a single display screen.

1. If you are not in Jane Morgan's medical record, access it using the following steps:
   - Click on *Clinical Today*.

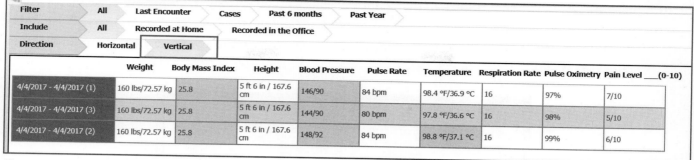

	Weight	Body Mass Index	Height	Blood Pressure	Pulse Rate	Temperature	Respiration Rate	Pulse Oximetry	Pain Level ___(0-10)
4/4/2017 - 4/4/2017 (1)	160 lbs/72.57 kg	25.8	5 ft 6 in / 167.6 cm	146/90	84 bpm	98.4 °F/36.9 °C	16	97%	7/10
4/4/2017 - 4/4/2017 (3)	160 lbs/72.57 kg	25.8	5 ft 6 in / 167.6 cm	144/90	80 bpm	97.8 °F/36.6 °C	16	98%	5/10
4/4/2017 - 4/4/2017 (2)	160 lbs/72.57 kg	25.8	5 ft 6 in / 167.6 cm	148/92	84 bpm	98.8 °F/37.1 °C	16	99%	6/10

Figure 6-33   Vital Signs Vertical Grid

Courtesy of Harris CareTracker PM and EMR

- In the *Appointments* screen within *Clinical Today*, bring up the date of Jane Morgan's appointment. Be sure that *Resource* reflects "All." **Hint:** If you don't recall the date of the appointment, with the patient in context, click on the *History* tab in the *Scheduling* module to locate the patient's appointment. Do not create a new encounter for this activity; use only the appointment/encounter previously scheduled.

- Click on Ms. Morgan's name. The patient's *Chart Summary* will open in a new window (refer to Figure 6-7).

2. In the *Patient Health History* pane, click on *Flowsheet*. Harris CareTracker EMR displays the *Flowsheet* window.

3. Generally, you can select a template from the *Saved Views* drop-down list, but the template you will need for this activity has not been saved yet. Click the *Search* 🔍 icon to the right of *Saved Views* (**Figure 6-34**). Harris CareTracker EMR displays the *Manage Flowsheet Templates* dialog box.

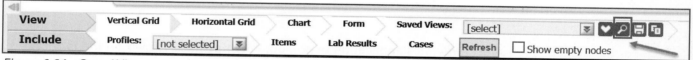

Figure 6-34   Saved Views

Courtesy of Harris CareTracker PM and EMR

4. Enter "Vital Signs" in the *Template* box, and then click on the plus sign (**Figure 6-35**).

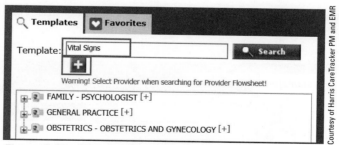

Figure 6-35   Enter Vital Signs in Template Box

5. The *Flowsheet Template* dialog box will appear. In the *Name* box, type "Vital Signs."

6. In the *Specialty* box, click on the drop-down arrow and select "FAMILY MEDICINE."

7. In the *View* box, click on the drop-down arrow and select "Chart."

8. Next to the *Scope* box, click on the drop-down arrow and select "COMPANY."

9. Click on the checkbox next to *In Favorites* to make this a favorite you can select for further activities.

10. Click on the drop-down arrow in the *Flowsheet Profile* box, scroll down, and select "Vital Signs."

11. A list of flowsheet items comes up that you can select for your profile (**Figure 6-36**). Click on the checkboxes next to *Blood Pressure, Body Mass Index, Height, Pain Level, Pulse Oximetry, Pulse Rate, Respiration Rate,* and *Weight.* **Note:** You will need to scroll down the screen to view all options of the *Flowsheet Profile.*

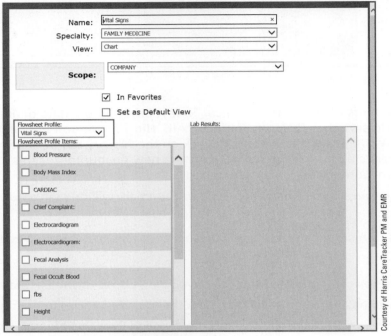

Figure 6-36   Flowsheet Profiles

12. Click *OK.*

13. For the *Manage Flowsheet Templates* application to pop up, you may need to click on the *Favorites* tab and then back on the *Templates* tab and then the new specialty heading *Family Medicine.* (**Note:** Alternatively, you may need to click the *Search* button for your screen to refresh with the new template.)

14. Click on the [+] sign beside *Family Medicine.* You should now see the *Vital Signs* heading (**Figure 6-37**).

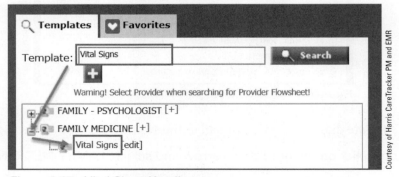

Figure 6-37   Vital Signs Heading

15. Click on the *Vital Signs* heading, which will take you back to the original *Flowsheet* application box (**Figure 6-38**).

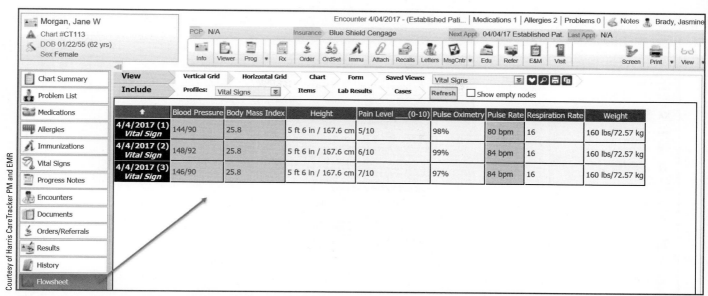

Figure 6-38   *Flowsheet Application Showing Vital Signs*

16.   Change the view by clicking on the *Horizontal Grid* tab.

🖫 **Click on the Print icon in the top right corner of the screen. Select Flowsheet. The vital signs flowsheet should open. Print this flowsheet, label it "Activity 6-12," and place it in your assignment folder.**

17.   Click "X" to close out of the *Vital Signs Flowsheet*.

Pediatric Growth Chart

Learning Objective 9: Create and print a growth chart.

Activity 6-13
Creating a Growth Chart

Harris CareTracker EMR allows users to create, view, and print pediatric growth charts from the *Flowsheet* application in the patient's EMR. Harris CareTracker PM and EMR houses the standard growth charts available from the Centers for Disease Control and Prevention (CDC) and World Health Organization (WHO).

1.   Pull patient Alex Brady into context.

2.   Click on the *Medical Record* module.

3.   Click on the *Flowsheet* tab in the *Patient Health History* pane.

4.   Click on the drop-down arrow beside *Profiles* and select "Boys Length/Weight for Age 0–36 months" (**Figure 6-39**).

5.   Click on the *Items* tab (**Figure 6-40**).

6.   The *Select Flowsheet Items* box displays. Check the boxes for "Weight" and "Length" and then click on *Select*.

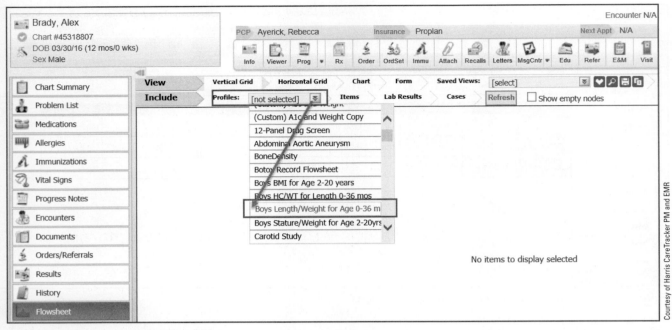

Figure 6-39   Flowsheet Profiles—Boys

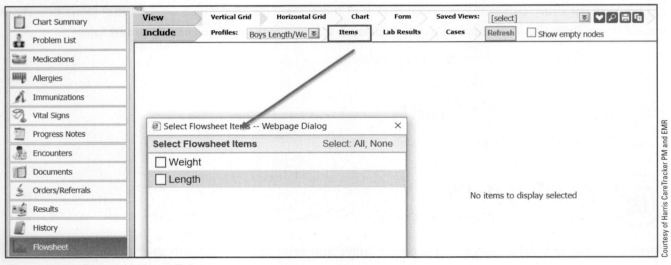

Figure 6-40   Flowsheet Items Tab

7. Notice that three different weights and lengths are already entered for Alex at different age intervals. The current view is set on *Vertical Grid*. Click on *Horizontal Grid* (**Figure 6-41**).

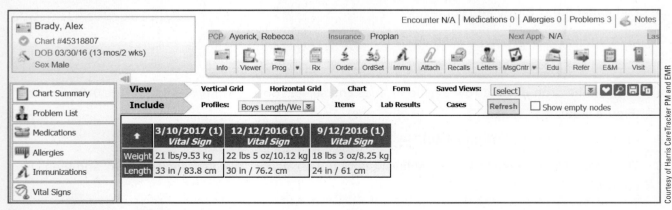

Figure 6-41   Horizontal Grid

8. To bring up Alex Brady's growth chart, click on the *Chart* tab in the *View* row. **Note:** If you receive an error when you click on the *Chart* tab, then print a *Horizontal Grid* view of the flowsheet instead and see Figure 6-50 for an example of what the chart would look like.

💾 **Click on Print in the View row. Label the growth chart "Activity 6-13" and place it in your assignment folder.**

Accessing the Patient Care Management Application

Learning Objective 10: Update the Patient Care Management application.

Activity 6-14
Accessing and Updating Patient Care Management Items

The *Patient Care Management* application is used as a proactive reminder tool to improve the care management process. The patient is evaluated and moved to specific health maintenance and disease management registries based on measures that are activated within your group. The application helps manage the recurring preventive care items pertinent to a patient, flags overdue items, enables you to manually move the patient to a high-risk registry, and more. Additionally, you can view a list of care management items that are complete and pending for the patient by clicking the *Pt Care Mgt* link on the *Patient Health History* pane of the *Medical Record* module.

The care recommendations in the *Health Maintenance* and *Disease Management* registries are based on CDC and National Committee for Quality Assurance/Healthcare Effectiveness Data and Information Set (NCQA/HEDIS) guidelines.

Table 6-5 provides a description of each section within the *Patient Care Management* application.

Table 6-5   Sections within the Patient Care Management Application

SECTION	DESCRIPTION
Health Maintenance	This section displays all tests/exams that a patient is due for that are part of *Health Maintenance* registries.
Disease Management	This section displays all tests/exams that a patient is due for OR is required to have according to disease management measures. Click the *Expand* icon in the *Disease Management* section to view all items that are part of the disease management measure.

Courtesy of Harris CareTracker PM and EMR

1. If you are not in Jane Morgan's medical record, access it using the following steps:

    • Click on *Clinical Today*.

    • In the *Appointments* screen within *Clinical Today*, bring up the date of Jane Morgan's appointment. Be sure that *Resource* reflects "All." **Hint:** If you don't recall the date of the appointment, with the patient in context, click on the *History* tab in the *Scheduling* module to locate the patient's appointment. Do not create a new encounter for this activity; use only the appointment/encounter previously scheduled.

    • Click on Ms. Morgan's name. The patient's *Chart Summary* will open in a new window (refer to Figure 6-7).

2. In the *Patient Health History* pane, click on the *Pt Care Mgmt* tab. Harris CareTracker EMR displays the *Patient Care Management* window with all health maintenance and disease management items for the patient (**Figure 6-42**). The list includes both pending and completed items. **Hint**: You must have completed Activity 5-2 for this feature to display.

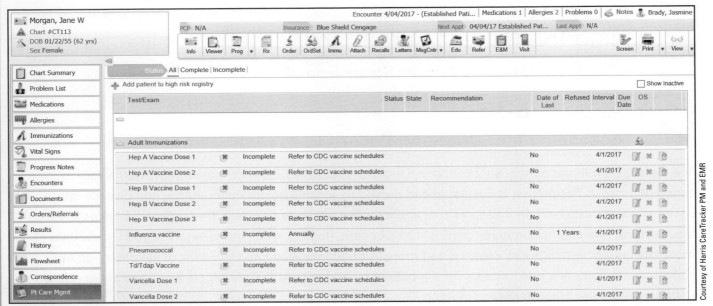

Figure 6-42   Patient Care Management Window

3. As you are reviewing the registry, note that the information collected during the history phase automatically populated in this section, such as the dates of the patient's last colonoscopy and Pap test. While reviewing the registry information with Ms. Morgan, she states that she just remembered that she received an influenza vaccine on October 12 of last year. The patient received the immunization at America's Urgent Care. Click the *Edit* icon in the row in which Influenza appears. Harris Care-Tracker EMR displays the *Edit Test/Exam* dialog box (**Figure 6-43**).

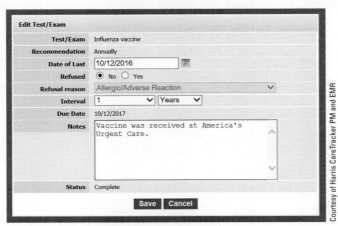

Figure 6-43   Edit Test/Exam Dialog Box

4. In the *Edit Test/Exam* box, enter October 12 of last year in the *Date of Last* field.

5. Leave the other fields blank because the vaccine was not administered at the Napa Valley Family Health Associates facility. Type the following in the *Notes* box: "Vaccine was received at America's Urgent Care."

6. Click *Save.* (**Note:** You may have to close out of the *Patient Care Management* window and re-open it before the influenza entry is updated on the screen. Click on *Status*, which will update as "Complete.")

 Print the updated Patient Care Management list, label it "Activity 6-14," and place it in your assignment folder.

CREATING PROGRESS NOTES

Learning Objective 11: Create and print a Progress Note.

 ## Activity 6-15
Accessing and Updating the Progress Notes Application

Progress notes are the heart of the patient record. They serve as a chronological listing of the patient's overall health status. Data pertaining to the findings from the visit are entered into the progress note. Most EMR software programs, including Harris CareTracker EMR, have progress note templates, copy and paste features, and automatic population tools, which make creating progress notes simplistic and efficient. The software also assists in promoting consistency from one provider to the next.

The *Progress Notes* application displays a list of notes recorded during each patient appointment and is required for medical, legal, and billing purposes. The note includes information such as the patient's history, medications, and allergies as well as a complete record of all that occurred during the visit. The application provides a quick and easy way to review and sign notes and helps identify notes that must be signed by a cosigner.

Note: Updating the *Progress Note* is typically a provider's responsibility and function; however, it is in the medical assistant's best interest to have knowledge and understanding of the *Progress Note*. Some practices use scribes. It is entirely possible that the medical assistant will then be responsible for recording the provider's findings. Although the entire activity is not required, the creation of the *Progress Note* (steps 1–6) is required and must be completed in order to complete later activities.

1. If you are not in Jane Morgan's medical record, access it using the following steps:
   - Click on *Clinical Today*.
   - In the *Appointments* screen within *Clinical Today*, bring up the date of Jane Morgan's appointment. Be sure that *Resource* reflects "All." **Hint:** If you don't recall the date of the appointment, with the patient in context, click on the *History* tab in the *Scheduling* module to locate the patient's appointment. Do not create a new encounter for this activity; use only the appointment/encounter previously scheduled.
   - Click on Ms. Morgan's name. The patient's *Chart Summary* will open in a new window (refer to Figure 6-7).

2. In the *Clinical Toolbar*, click the drop-down in the *Progress Notes* 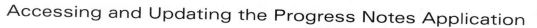 tab and select the encounter in context. If an encounter is in context, which in this case it is, Harris CareTracker EMR displays the *Progress Notes* template window (**Figure 6-44**). (**Note:** If documenting a progress note that is not based on an appointment, the *Encounter* dialog box displays, enabling you to create a new encounter. If you are getting an *Encounter* dialog box, it means that you did not have an encounter in context. Repeat step 1 if necessary.)

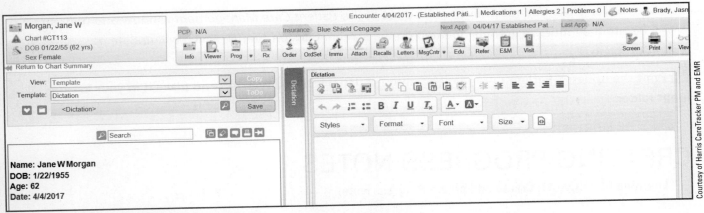

Figure 6-44   Progress Notes Template Window

3. Alternatively, if the *Progress Notes* template window does not display, click on the date of the *Encounter* you want to make a progress note for. Then, beneath the *Progress Note* window, click *Edit.*

4. By default, the *View* field displays "Template." (Skip this box at this time.)

5. In the *Template* field, click on the drop-down arrow and select "IM OV Option 4 (v4) w/A&P" (**Figure 6-45**). Complete the note by navigating through each tab. (The provider would ordinarily work in the progress note, but because the provider is not available or you are the designated scribe, you will be entering the information for the provider.)

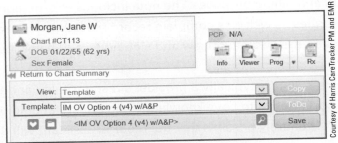

Figure 6-45   IM OV Option 4 (v4) w/A&P Template

6. All the information you entered regarding Ms. Morgan's medical history, allergy information, medication list, vital signs, and preventive care are now populated within the progress note. The *CC/HPI* tab will be showing on the right side of the screen (Figure 6-45). Review the note you wrote regarding the patient's chief complaint. The provider will expand a bit on the complaint by developing the History of Present Illness (HPI). Scroll down to the *History of Present Illness* box and type the following:

   "Patient has a five-year history of UTIs (1-2 infections/year). Current episode includes frequency, urgency, and pain upon urination (7/10). Pt. denies fever, blood, or pus in urine, or the presence of vaginal symptoms. No back or abdominal pain. Patient drinks very little water and has at least two beverages per day which include caffeine. Last UTI was approximately three months ago. Treatment included a 10-day treatment of Bactrim DS. Patient states she completed the treatment and was free of urinary symptoms. Patient did not follow up for a post check." Your documentation should match **Figure 6-46**.

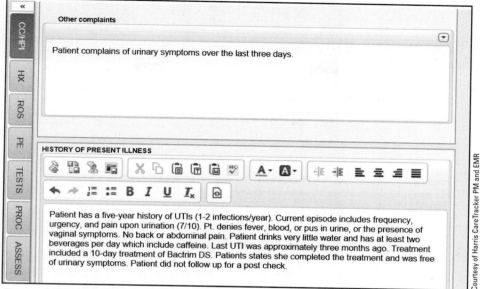

Figure 6-46   Jane Morgan HPI

7. Click on *Save*, located in the template box in the middle of the screen (**Figure 6-47**).

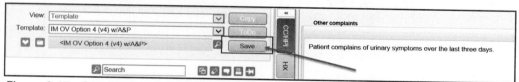

Figure 6-47   Save Button for Template Screen

Courtesy of Harris CareTracker PM and EMR

8. Click on the *HX* tab on the right side of the progress note (center of screen). Review the information that you entered while collecting the patient history. Because you are acting as the provider or the scribe in this section, indicate that you reviewed each section of the history by clicking on the plus sign [+] next to *Reviewed* at the top of the screen. Check marks will now appear next to each box in the *Reviewed* section (**Figure 6-48**).

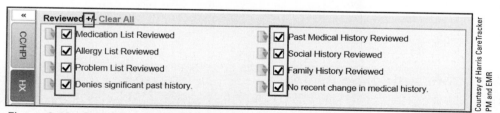

Figure 6-48   Reviewed Check Marks

9. Click on *Save* to update the note.

10. Click on the *ROS* tab. Refer to **Table 6-6** to complete this section of the progress note.

11. Click *Save* to update the progress note with the ROS findings.

12. Click on the *PE* tab. Use **Table 6-7** to complete this portion of the note.

13. Click *Save* to update the progress note with the PE findings.

14. Skip the *TESTS* and *PROC* tabs.

Table 6-6   Completing the ROS Tab

SECTION	ENTRY
Constitutional	Check the box beside *No constitutional symptoms*.
Eyes	Check the box beside *No eye symptoms*.
ENMT	No entry.
Neck	Check the box beside *No neck symptoms*.
Breasts	No entry.
Respiratory	Check the box beside *No respiratory symptoms*.
Cardiovascular	Click on the minus symbol so that *N* for No is selected for each box. Now click on the *Y* beside "cold hands or feet."
Gastrointestinal	Check the box beside *No GI symptoms*.
Genitourinary	Select *Y* for Yes for the following categories: "dysuria," "burning on urination," "urgency," and "frequency." Select *N* for No for all other genitourinary (GU) symptoms.
Skin	No entry.
Musculoskeletal	No entry.
Neurological	No entry.
Psychiatric	Select *Y* for Yes for depression and *N* for No for all other symptoms.
Hematologic	No entry.
Endocrine	No entry.

Table 6-7   Completing the PE Tab

SECTION	ENTRY
General	Click the plus sign beside *General* so that a check mark is placed beside each box in the section.
HEENT	*Head*: Check the box beside *Negative head exam*. *Eyes*: Click on the *Y* for Yes next to "PERRL." Click on the *N* for No next to "EOMI" and "scleral icterus." *ENT*: No entry.
Neck	Check the box beside *Negative neck exam*.
Lymphatics	No entry.

Chest	Chest: Check the box beside *Negative chest exam.*
	Breasts: No entry.
	Lungs: Check the box beside *Negative lung exam.*
Heart	Check the box beside *Negative heart exam.*
Abdomen	Click on the minus sign beside *Abdomen* so that a red "X" is placed beside each box in the section. Click the *Y* for Yes beside "soft" and "tenderness."
	In the *Other abdomen findings* section, enter: "The abdomen was soft with minimal tenderness to palpation in the left periumbilical and left lower quadrant. There was no guarding or rebound."
Genitourinary	Check the box beside *Negative genitourinary exam.*
Musculoskeletal	No entry.
Neurologic	No entry.
Mental Status Exam	No entry.
Skin	No entry.

15. Click on the *ASSESS* tab. By default, the *ASSESS* tab defaults to "Template." The other quick view tabs are the "Problem List" tab and the "Visit" tab (**Figure 6-49**).

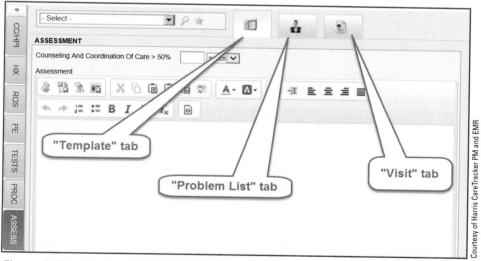

Figure 6-49   *Progress Note ASSESS Tab Icons*

16. It was discovered during the exam that the patient has hypertension. The provider also diagnosed the patient with a urinary tract infection (UTI) and dysuria. You will be selecting only ICD-10 codes associated with the provider's diagnoses, as directed in steps 17 through 19.

17. Click on the *Search* icon to the right of the *-Select-* drop-down menu at the top of the screen. In the *Diagnosis Search* window that pops up, enter "urinary tract infection" in the *Search Text* field and click the *Search* button. Click on "urinary tract infection" (ICD-10 code N39.0) in the results section of the *Diagnosis Search* window (note that it may have already been marked as a favorite diagnosis).

18. Search for and select "essential hypertension" (ICD-10 code I10).

19. Search for and select "recurrent and persistent hematuria" (ICD-10 code N02.9) and "dysuria" (ICD-10 code R30.0) as well. After selecting each diagnosis, scroll down to the bottom of the *ASSESS* tab, and see all selected codes listed under *Today's Selected Diagnosis*. Both the ICD-9 and ICD-10 versions of the code are listed (**Figure 6-50**).

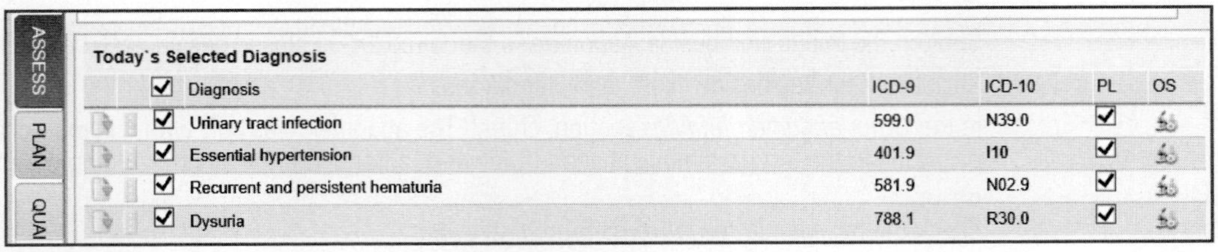

	Today's Selected Diagnosis	ICD-9	ICD-10	PL	OS
☑	Diagnosis				
☑	Urinary tract infection	599.0	N39.0	☑	
☑	Essential hypertension	401.9	I10	☑	
☑	Recurrent and persistent hematuria	581.9	N02.9	☑	
☑	Dysuria	788.1	R30.0	☑	

Courtesy of Harris CareTracker PM and EMR

Figure 6-50   Today's Selected Diagnosis

20. Click *Save* to update the progress note with the *Assessment* information.

21. Click on the *PLAN* tab to record the provider's plans. Document the following in the *Additional Plan Details* box (**Figure 6-51**):

   a. Stat lab test—"Urinalysis dipstick panel by Automated test strip"

   b. Send urine out for lab test "Urinalysis microscopic panel [#volume] in urine by automated count"

   c. Give patient educational handouts (1) Urinary Tract Infections in Women, and (2) What is Hematuria? (**Note:** You will search for and select Patient Educational handouts in Chapter 7, Activity 7-10.)

   d. Bactrim DS Oral Tabs (80–160 mg), Sig 1 tab bid for 5 days, No refills

   e. Enter Order for 3-phase CT cystourethrogram

   f. Patient to return in 10 days for a Follow-Up UA

   g. Set patient up for a referral with a urologist

   PREVENTION GOALS

   a. Patient to have her first Hepatitis B shot today

   b. Set patient up for a mammogram

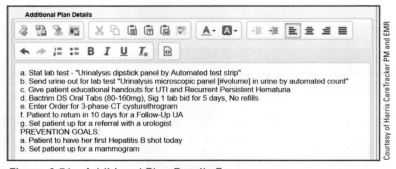

Figure 6-51   Additional Plan Details Box

22. Click *Save*.

💾 **Click the orange Print 💾 icon in the middle of the screen. The Clinical Note dialog box will open. Click the Print button and select your printer to print a copy of the progress note. Label it "Activity 6-15" and place it in your assignment folder.**

23. Close out of the Printed Progress Note by clicking on the "X" in the upper-right-hand corner.

24. Click on the *Return to Chart Summary* link (in blue) at the top left of the screen just under the patient's name and chart number to return to the patient's medical record.

Activity 6-16

Creating a Progress Note with Pediatric Template (abbreviated version only)

1. If you are not in Francisco Powell Jimenez's medical record, access it using the following steps:

   - Click on *Clinical Today*.

   - In the *Appointments* screen within *Clinical Today*, bring up the date of Francisco's appointment. Be sure that Resource reflects "All." **Hint:** If you don't recall the date of the appointment, with the patient in context, click on the *History* tab in the *Scheduling* module to locate the patient's appointment. Do not create a new encounter for this activity; use only the appointment/encounter previously scheduled.

   - Click on Francisco's name. The patient's *Chart Summary* will open in a new window (refer to Figure 6-7).

2. In the *Clinical Toolbar*, click the drop-down in the *Progress Notes* tab and select the encounter in context. If an encounter is in context, Harris CareTracker EMR displays the *Progress Notes* template window (**Figure 6-52**). (**Hint:** Be sure the encounter is displaying above the name bar for the appointment you booked in Chapter 4.) (**Note:** If documenting a progress note that is not based on an appointment, the *Encounter* dialog box displays, enabling you to create a new encounter. If you are getting an *Encounter* dialog box, it means that you did not have an encounter in context. Repeat step 1 if necessary.)

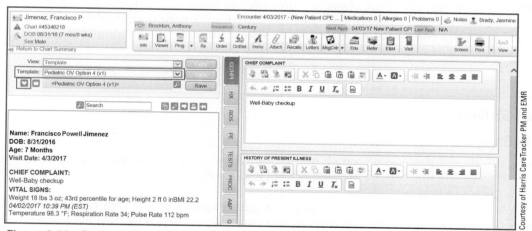

Figure 6-52   Pediatric Progress Note Template

3. Alternatively, if the *Progress Notes* template window does not display, click on the date of the *Encounter* you want to make a progress note for. Then, beneath the *Progress Note* window, click *Edit*.

4. By default, the *View* field displays "Template." (Skip this box at this time.)

5. Below the *Template* field, click on the *Search* icon. The *Search Template* dialog box will display.

6. Scroll down and click on the + sign next to PEDIATRICS.

7. Scroll down and select "Pediatric OV Option 4 (v1)" by clicking on the template.

8. Click on the *Favorite* icon (the heart) to save this template as a favorite.

9. Complete the note by navigating through each tab. **Note**: Because you are only creating an "abbreviated" progress note, you will not be entering additional information at this time.

10. Any information you would have entered regarding Francisco's medical history, allergy information, medication list, vital signs, and preventive care would now be populated within the progress note.

11. The *CC/HPI* tab will be showing on the right side of the screen. Review the note you wrote regarding the patient's chief complaint. The provider will expand a bit on the complaint by developing the History of Present Illness (HPI).

12. Scroll down to the *History of Present Illness* box and type the following:

    "Patient here for Well-Baby Check."

13. Click on *Save*, which is located in the template box in the middle of the screen.

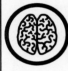 **Click the orange Print icon in the middle of the screen. The Clinical Note dialog box will open. Click the Print button and select your printer to print a copy of the progress note. Label it "Activity 6-16" and place it in your assignment folder.**

14. Close out of the printed progress note.

15. Click on the *Return to Chart Summary* link (in blue) at the top left of the screen to return to the patient's medical record.

CRITICAL THINKING At the beginning of this chapter, you were challenged to embrace the EMR training in this chapter so that you are able to fully navigate the patient's medical record in Harris CareTracker EMR. Now that you have completed many detailed clinical tasks, did you find the transition from administrative to clinical duties seamless? Were there any particular activities that were challenging? What steps did you take to work through the tasks? Does the amount of information needed to accurately record patient information and patient care help with your understanding of the roles of health care providers and the health care system overall? Explain your thoughts and conclusions.

CASE STUDIES

Case Study 6-1

(**Note**: You must have completed all of the prior chapter Case Studies for patient James Smith in order to complete this activity. If you have not previously completed the James Smith case studies, skip to Case Study 6-2.)

Using the steps you learned throughout this chapter and the information packet for James Smith, update Mr. Smith's medical record and create a progress note. See the steps below for more information.

1. Click on *Clinical Today*.

2. In the *Appointments* screen within *Clinical Today*, bring up the date of James Smith's appointment scheduled in Chapter 4. Be sure that *Resource* reflects "All." **Hint**: If you don't recall the date of the appointment, with the patient in context, click on the *History* tab in the *Scheduling* module to locate the patient's appointment. Do not create a new encounter for this activity; use only the appointment/encounter previously scheduled.

3. Click on Mr. Smith's name. The patient's *Chart Summary* will open in a new window (refer to Figure 6-7).

4. Complete the following activities/entries using information from **Table 6-8**:

   - Add medications (refer to Activity 6-6 for help). **Note:** Select "Benefit outweighs risk" in the *Interaction Screening* dialog box when entering medication(s).

   - Add an allergy, if applicable. Refer to Activity 6-7 for help.

   - Enter past immunizations to the patient's chart. Refer to Activity 6-8 for help.

Table 6-8   James Smith: CC, Medications, Allergies, and Immunizations

CC for Visit	Follow-up exam/consultation; review lab and EKG
Medication	(1) Atorvastatin Calcium Oral Tablet 20 mg by mouth every night (2) Lasix Oral Tablet 20 mg by mouth every morning
Allergy	No known drug allergies
Past Immunization	Influenza vaccine October 1 of last year

5. Enter the patient's medical history using Source Document 6-1, located at the end of this case study. Refer to Activity 6-9 for help.

6. Record the patient's vital signs noted in **Table 6-9**. Refer to Activity 6-10 for help.

Table 6-9   James Smith: Vital Signs

Height	6 ft 2 in
Weight	201 lbs
BMI	(automatically calculates)
Blood Pressure	149/93
Pulse Rate	77
Temperature	98.6°F
Respiratory Rate	16
Pulse Oximetry	99%
Pain Level (0-10)	0/10

7. Create a progress note for Mr. Smith using the "IM OV Option 4 (v4) w/A&P" template. Complete the progress note using the information provided in Source Document 6-1, located at the end of this case study. Refer back to Activity 6-15 for guidance if needed.

After entering all of the information provided in the packet, print a chart summary (label it "Case Study 6-1A") and progress note (label it "Case Study 6-1B"), and place them in your assignment folder.

(continues)

CASE STUDIES (*continued*)

Source Document 6-1

James M. Smith DOB: 2/23/1965

Patient History

Reviewed

✔ Medication List Reviewed	✔ Past Medical History Reviewed
✔ Allergy List Reviewed	✔ Social History Reviewed
☐ Problem List Reviewed	✔ Family History Reviewed
☐ Denies significant past history.	☐ No recent change in medical history.

GENERAL MEDICAL HISTORY

☐ Alcoholism	☐ Depression	☐ Kidney Infections
☐ Allergies/Hayfever	☐ DM Type 1	☐ Kidney stone
☐ Anemia	✔ DM Type 2	☐ Migraine
☐ Anxiety	☐ Epilepsy	☐ Multiple Sclerosis
☐ Asthma	☐ Fracture	☐ Obesity
☐ Atrial Fibrillation	☐ Gastric ulcer	☐ Old MI
☐ Blood Transfusions	☐ Gastrointestinal Disease	☐ Osteoarthritis
☐ CAD	☐ GERD	☐ Osteoporosis
☐ Cancer	☐ Gestational Diabetes	☐ Pneumonia
☐ Cardiac Pacer	☐ Glaucoma	☐ Progressive Neurological Disorder
☐ Cardiovascular Disease	☐ Heart Murmur	☐ Pulmonary Disease
☐ CHF	☐ Hepatitis	☐ Rheumatic Fever
☐ Cirrhosis	☐ High Cholesterol	☐ Rheumatoid Arthritis
☐ Colitis	☐ Hyperlipidemia	☐ STD
☐ COPD	☐ Hypertension	☐ Terminal Illness
☐ CRF	☐ Hyperthyroidism	☐ Thyroid Disease
☐ Crohn's Disease	☐ Hypothyroidism	☐ TIA
☐ CVA	✔ Joint Pain	☐ Tuberculosis

HOSPITALIZATIONS

OTHER MEDICAL HISTORY

Tobacco Assessment

This section supports Stage 1 Meaningful Use
Smoking Status Current Everyday Smoker   ☒ Tobacco User
pack-years **25**   Date quit smoking
☐ Counseling on tobacco cessation
☐ Rx therapy for tobacco cessation
☒ Discussed Smoking/Tobacco Use Cessation Strategies

Social History

Alcohol Use Occasional	Educational level
Caffeine Use 2 servings per Day	Marital Status Single
☒ Drug Use	Exercise Habits moderate >3 x/wk
☒ sun protection	✔ seatbelts
☒ Tattoos	☐ Body piercings
☒ sexually active	birth control method
Race White	Birth Control Device insertion date
Native language	Birth Control Device removal date
☒ physical abuse	Religion
☒ domestic violence	Occupation **IT Support**
Other Social History	

Depression Screening

☐ Patient Refused
Little interest or pleasure in doing things At no time
Feeling down, depressed, or hopeless

Date of Last Depression Screening/PHQ-2
PHQ-2 Score **PHQ2 Score: 1**

OB/GYN HISTORY

LMP

Frequency of menstrual cycle   Days menstrual cycle
☐ Menopause has occurred
☐ History of abnormal pap smears
☐ Sexually Active   Birth Control
                                                                 Birth Control Device insertion date
☐ ectopic pregnancy   Birth Control Device removal date

PREGNANCY SUMMARY
Gravida
Term
Preterm
AB   Miscarriage
Live children   Elective Abortion
OTHER OB-GYN HISTORY ....   C-Section:

SURGICAL / PROCEDURAL

☐ No prior surgical history
☐ Appendectomy   ☐ Endometrial Ablation   ☐ Laparoscopy
☐ Breast Lumpectomy   ☐ Gall Bladder   Mastectomy
☐ Cataract Surgery   ☐ Heart Surgery   ☐ Myomectomy
Location:

Location:

☐ Colectomy   ☐ Hemorrhoids   ☐ Oophorectomy
☐ Cone Biopsy   ☐ Hernia   ☐ Tonsil/Adenoidectomy
☐ D&C   ☐ Hysterectomy   ☐ Tubal Ligation
OTHER SURGICAL
HISTORY

PREVENTIVE CARE

A1c %   HPV Test
Air Contrast Barium Enema   HPV Vaccine
Ankle Brachial Index   Last Complete Physical Exam
Blood Glucose   Lipids
Bone Density   Mammography
Chest X-Ray   Pap Smear
Chlamydia Screening   Pneumovax
Colonoscopy   10/14/2016   PSA   02/10/2017
Dilated Eye Exam   04/17/2017   Pulmonary Function Tests
DTaP Vaccine (90700)   Routine Eye Exam
Echocardiogram   Stool Occult Blood
Electrocardiogram   Stress Test
Flexible Sigmoidoscopy   Td
Flu Vaccine   10/09/2017   Tdap Vaccine, Adult
Foot Exam Date   Tuberculin PPD
HIV Test Date   Varicella
                                               Zoster Vaccine (90736)
Self-Management Goal

(continues)

CASE STUDIES *(continued)*

James M. Smith DOB: 2/23/1965

Sensitive Information

STD

☒ Vaginosis		☒ Gonorrhea	
☒ Trichomonas		☒ Chlamydia	
☒ Genital Warts		☒ Syphilis	
☒ PID		☒ HPV	

STD Info

SUBSTANCE ABUSE

☒ History of Substance Abuse

Abused Substances

MENTAL HEALTH

☒ Seeing mental health provider

Mental Health Provider Name
Mental Health Condition(s)

HIV Status

HIV Status
HIV Test Date
HIV Notes
Has never had an HIV test.

James M Smith DOB: 2/23/1965

Family History

GENERAL FAMILY HISTORY

☐ Adopted	☐ Denial of any knowledge of significant family history	
☐ Unknown Paternal Hx	☐ Unknown Maternal Hx	
☐ Alcoholism	☐ Congenital Anomaly	☑ Hypertension
☐ Anemia	☐ COPD	☐ Hypothyroidism
☐ Anxiety	☐ Crohn's Disease	☑ Kidney Disease
☐ Asthma	☐ Depression	☐ Liver Disease
☐ Birth Defects	☑ Diabetes	☐ Multiple Births
☐ CAD	☐ Epilepsy	☐ Osteoarthritis
☐ Cardiovascular Disease	☑ GERD	☐ Osteoporosis
☐ CHF	☐ Hypercholesterolemia	☐ Pulmonary Disease
Cancer	☑ Hyperlipidemia	☐ Stroke

Other
conditions ....

Case Study 6-2

Update Mr. Thompson's medical record and create a progress note. See the steps below for more information.

1. Click on *Clinical Today*.

2. In the *Appointments* screen within *Clinical Today*, bring up the date of Adam Thompson's appointment scheduled in Chapter 4. Be sure that *Resource* reflects "All." **Hint:** If you don't recall the date of the appointment, with the patient in context, click on the *History* tab in the *Scheduling* module to locate the patient's appointment. Do not create a new encounter for this activity, use only the appointment/encounter previously scheduled.

3. Click on Mr. Thompson's name. The patient's *Chart Summary* will open in a new window (refer to Figure 6-7).

4. Complete the following activities/entries using information from **Table 6-10**:

    *   Add medications. Refer to Activity 6-6 for help. **Note:** Select "Benefit outweighs risk" in the *Interaction Screening* dialog box when entering medication(s).

    *   Add an allergy. Refer to Activity 6-7 for help.

    *   Enter past immunizations to the patient's chart. Refer to Activity 6-8 for help.

Table 6-10　Adam Thompson: CC, Medications, Allergies, and Immunizations

CC for Visit	productive cough
Medication	(1) Atorvastatin Calcium Oral Tablet 20 mg by mouth every night (2) Micardis Oral Tablet 40 mg by mouth every night (3) Potassium Chloride Extended-Release Oral Capsules 10 mEq by mouth every morning (4) NEXIUM Delayed-Release Capsule 20 mg by mouth every morning one hour before food (5) Lasix Oral Tablet 20 mg by mouth every morning
Allergy	Penicillin V Potassium (reaction: anaphylaxis). Use date January 1, 1990
Past Immunization	(1) Influenza vaccine: September 1 of last year (2) Pneumococcal vaccine: September 1 of last year

5. Enter the patient's medical history using information from Source Document 6-2, located at the end of this case study. Refer to Activity 6-9 for help.

6. Record the patient's vital signs from **Table 6-11**. Refer to Activity 6-10 for help.

(continues)

CASE STUDIES *(continued)*

Table 6-11   Adam Thompson: Vital Signs

Height	5 ft 8 in
Weight	197
BMI	(automatically calculates)
Blood Pressure	151/87
Pulse Rate	62
Temperature	100.6°F
Respiratory Rate	19
Pulse Oximetry	95%
Pain Level (0-10)	4/10

7. Create a progress note for Mr. Thompson using the "IM OV Option 4 (v4) w/A&P" template. Complete the progress note using the information provided in Source Document 6-2 (located at the end of this case study). Refer back to Activity 6-15 for guidance if needed.

After entering all of the information provided in the packet, print a chart summary (label it "Case Study 6-2A") and progress note (label it "Case Study 6-2B"), and place them in your assignment folder.

Source Document 6-2

Adam Thompson DOB: 1/1/1942

Patient History

Reviewed

☑ Medication List Reviewed	☑ Past Medical History Reviewed
☑ Allergy List Reviewed	☑ Social History Reviewed
☐ Problem List Reviewed	☑ Family History Reviewed
☐ Denies significant past history.	☐ No recent change in medical history.

GENERAL MEDICAL HISTORY

☐ Alcoholism	☐ Depression	☐ Kidney Infections
☐ Allergies/Hayfever	☐ DM Type 1	☐ Kidney stone
☐ Anemia	☐ DM Type 2	☐ Migraine
☐ Anxiety	☐ Epilepsy	☐ Multiple Sclerosis
☐ Asthma	☐ Fracture	☐ Obesity
☐ Atrial Fibrillation	☑ Gastric ulcer	☐ Old MI
☐ Blood Transfusions	☐ Gastrointestinal Disease	☑ Osteoarthritis
☐ CAD	☑ GERD	☐ Osteoporosis
☐ Cancer	☐ Gestational Diabetes	☐ Pneumonia
☐ Cardiac Pacer	☐ Glaucoma	☐ Progressive Neurological Disorder
☑ Cardiovascular Disease	☐ Heart Murmur	☐ Pulmonary Disease
☐ CHF	☐ Hepatitis	☐ Rheumatic Fever
☐ Cirrhosis	☐ High Cholesterol	☐ Rheumatoid Arthritis
☐ Colitis	☐ Hyperlipidemia	☐ STD
☐ COPD	☑ Hypertension	☐ Terminal Illness
☐ CRF	☐ Hyperthyroidism	☐ Thyroid Disease
☐ Crohn's disease	☐ Hypothyroidism	☐ TIA
☐ CVA	☐ Joint Pain	☐ Tuberculosis

HOSPITALIZATIONS Cardiac Pacemaker Placement 02/15/2011. Overnight stay at Napa Valley Medical Center. No complications

OTHER MEDICAL HISTORY

Tobacco Assessment

This section supports Stage 1 Meaningful Use
Smoking Status Former smoker
\# pack-years **20**
☐ Counseling on tobacco cessation
☐ Rx therapy for tobacco cessation
☐ Discussed Smoking/Tobacco Use Cessation Strategies

☐ Tobacco User
Date quit smoking **03/14/1990**

Social History

Alcohol Use Occasional	Educational level
Caffeine Use 2 servings per Day	Marital Status
☒ Drug Use	Exercise Habits
☒ sun protection	☑ seatbelts
☒ Tattoos	☐ Body piercings
☒ sexually active	birth control method
Race	Birth Control Device insertion date
Native language	Birth Control Device removal date
☐ physical abuse	Religion
☐ domestic violence	Occupation
Other Social History	

Depression Screening

☐ Patient Refused
Little interest or pleasure in doing things
Feeling down, depressed, or hopeless

Date of Last Depression Screening/PHQ-2
PHQ-2 Score **PHQ2 Score: incomplete**

CASE STUDIES *(continued)*

OB/GYN HISTORY

LMP	Menarche Age
Frequency of menstrual cycle	Days menstrual cycle
☐ Menopause has occurred	
☐ History of abnormal pap smears	
☐ Sexually Active	Birth Control
	Birth Control Device insertion date
	Birth Control Device removal date
☐ ectopic pregnancy	

PREGNANCY SUMMARY

Gravida	
Term	
Preterm	Miscarriage
AB	Elective Abortion
Live children	C-Section:
OTHER OB-GYN HISTORY	

SURGICAL / PROCEDURAL

☐ No prior surgical history		
☐ Appendectomy	☐ Endometrial Ablation	☐ Laparoscopy
☐ Breast Lumpectomy	☐ Gall Bladder	Mastectomy
☐ Cataract Surgery	☐ Heart Surgery	☐ Myomectomy
☐ Colectomy	☐ Hemorrhoids	☐ Oophorectomy
☐ Cone Biopsy	☐ Hernia	☐ Tonsil/Adenoidectomy
☐ D&C	☐ Hysterectomy	☐ Tubal Ligation

OTHER SURGICAL HISTORY   Cardiac Pacemaker in 2011

PREVENTIVE CARE

A1c %	HPV Test
Air Contrast Barium Enema	HPV Vaccine
Ankle Brachial Index	Last Complete Physical Exam
Blood Glucose	Lipids
Bone Density	Mammography
Chest X-Ray	Pap Smear
Chlamydia Screening	Pneumovax
Colonoscopy 10/01/2008	PSA
Dilated Eye Exam	Pulmonary Function Tests
DTaP Vaccine (90700)	Routine Eye Exam
Echocardiogram	Stool Occult Blood 05/10/2010
Electrocardiogram	Stress Test 10/10/2013
Flexible Sigmoidoscopy	Td
Flu vaccine 09/15/2013	Tdap Vaccine, Adult
Foot Exam Date	Tuberculin PPD
HIV Test Date:	Varicella
	Zoster Vaccine (90736) 03/22/2007
Self-Management Goal	

Adam Thompson DOB: 1/1/1942

Sensitive Information

STD

☒ Vaginosis		☒ Gonorrhea	
☒ Trichomonas		☒ Chlamydia	
☒ Genital Warts		☒ Syphilis	
☒ PID		☒ HPV	

STD Info

SUBSTANCE ABUSE

☒ History of Substance Abuse

Abused Substances

MENTAL HEALTH

☒ Seeing mental health provider

Mental Health Provider Name

Mental Health Condition(s)

HIV Status

HIV Status

HIV Test Date

HIV Notes

Medicare High Risk Criteria

Age when became sexually active
☐ More than five sexual partners in lifetime
☐ DES history in mother
Pap Smear
☐ History of abnormal pap smears

Courtesy of Harris CareTracker PM and EMR

Adam Thompson DOB: 1/1/1942

Family History

GENERAL FAMILY HISTORY

☐ Adopted	☐ Denial of any knowledge of significant family history	
☐ Unknown Paternal Hx	☐ Unknown Maternal Hx	
☐ Alcoholism	☐ Congenital Anomaly	☑ Hypertension
☐ Anemia	☑ COPD	☐ Hypothyroidism
☐ Anxiety	☐ Crohn's Disease	☐ Kidney Disease
☑ Asthma	☐ Depression	☐ Liver Disease
☐ Birth Defects	☑ Diabetes	☐ Multiple Births
☐ CAD	☐ Epilepsy	☐ Osteoarthritis
☑ Cardiovascular Disease	☐ GERD	☐ Osteoporosis
☐ CHF	☐ Hypercholesterolemia	☐ Pulmonary Disease
Cancer lung	☐ Hyperlipidemia	☑ Stroke

Other
conditions

Completing the Visit

Learning Objectives

1. Complete requisitions for diagnostic orders: specialists, labs, and radiology.
2. Search for pharmacies, manage a list of favorites, and create and print prescriptions.
3. View, add, and create immunization records.
4. Search for, customize, and provide patient education materials for patients.
5. Access the Correspondence application to find, add, and print patient correspondence.
6. Create outgoing and incoming patient referrals.
7. View and resolve open encounters and unsigned notes by completing the visit and signing the Progress Note.

Real-World Connection

In this chapter, you will learn additional EMR functions, such as how to enter orders in the electronic medical record. You may be tempted to enter orders at the time you create a patient prevention or maintenance plan, but you should never enter any orders until the provider has reviewed and approved each order. Entering orders without the provider's approval is equivalent to practicing medicine without a license. You will also learn to capture a visit (selecting procedure and diagnosis codes for the patient's visit). The electronic health record makes orders and visit capture a seamless process. Your challenge is to learn the proper steps for entering orders into the patient's EMR, to avoid the temptation of entering orders without the provider's approval, and to select the proper codes for the patient's visit.

Before you begin the activities in this chapter, refresh your memory on working with Harris CareTracker by referring back to the Best Practices list on page xiv of this workbook. Following best practices will help you complete work quickly and accurately.

COMPLETING REQUISITIONS FOR DIAGNOSTIC ORDERS

Learning Objective 1: Complete requisitions for diagnostic orders: specialists, labs, and radiology.

To complete activities in this chapter, you will refer back to the patient's progress note *Assessment* and *Plan* (**Figure 7-1**).

ASSESSMENT:
(N39.0) - Urinary tract infection
(R30.0) - Dysuria
(I10) - Essential (primary) hypertension
(N02.9) - Recurrent and persistent hematuria

PLAN:
a. Stat lab test - "Urinalysis dipstick panel by Automated test strip
b. Send urine out for lab test "Urinalysis microscopic panel [#volume] in urine by automated count
c. Give patient educational handouts (1) Urinary Tract Infections in Women, and (2) What is Hematuria?
d. Bactrim DS Oral Tabs (80-160 mg), Sig 1 tab bid for 5 days, No refills
e. Enter Order for 3-phase CT cysturethrogram
f. Patient to return in 10 days for a Follow-Up UA
g. Set patient up for a referral with a urologist

PREVENTION GOALS
a. Patient to have her first Hepatitis B shot today
b. Set patient up for a mammogram

Courtesy of Harris CareTracker PM and EMR

Figure 7-1   *Assessment and Plan for Jane Morgan*

Activity 7-1

Access the *Orders* Application

The *Orders* application in Harris CareTracker EMR enables you to manage and track orders such as laboratory, radiology, pathology, and physical therapy directly from the patient's medical record. This ensures that all orders placed are followed up on by the office for patient compliancy. The *Orders* application works simultaneously with the *Results* application by providing quick access to test results of completed orders and enables entering manual results and linking to results received electronically.

The *Orders* application, accessed by clicking on *Orders* in the *Clinical Toolbar*, allows you to order tests directly from the *Medical Record* module.

TIP If you find that when you access a patient's medical record you receive a pop-up alert indicating some missing information (e.g., consent, PCP, NPP, etc.), it is best practice to update the patient's record in the demographics screen before moving forward.

Using patient Jane Morgan, complete the *Assessment* and *Plan* (A&P) *Orders* as outlined in the progress note from her encounter that you created in Chapter 6 (**Figure 7-2**). You will refer back to her *A&P* throughout this chapter's activities.

1. Access patient Jane Morgan's *Medical Record* module using one of the following methods:

   a. Pull patient Jane Morgan into context and click the *Medical Record* module.

   b. If the patient has an appointment, click the patient's name in the *Appointments* application of the *Clinical Today* module. (To find an appointment date with the patient in context, click on the *History* tab of the *Scheduling* module. It displays the most current appointment for the patient in context in either the *Pending Appointments* or *Rescheduled Appointments* sections in the center of the screen.)

2. In the *Patient Health History* pane of the *Medical Record* module, click *Orders/Referrals* (**Figure 7-2**). The *Orders* window displays with outstanding orders for the patient. You will see that there are no outstanding orders at this time. **(FYI)** If there were an open order, you would be able to see more details by clicking on the order number. You would be able to view the date and type of order, the test description, the ordering provider, encounter date, and associated diagnosis.

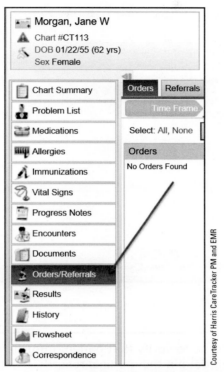

Figure 7-2   Orders/Referrals Application

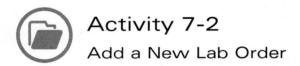

Activity 7-2
Add a New Lab Order

The *Orders* application, accessed by clicking *Order* 🔬 on the *Clinical Toolbar*, allows you to order tests directly from the *Medical Record* module.

Using patient Jane Morgan, complete the *Assessment* and *Plan* (A&P) *Orders* as outlined in the progress note from her encounter that you created in Chapter 6, Activity 6-15 (see **Figure 7-1**). You will refer back to her A&P throughout this chapter's activities. The first activity will be to add a new lab order (Activity 7-2).

1. Before beginning the steps in this activity, refer back and record patient Jane Morgan's appointment you scheduled in Chapter 4. Date/Time: _____.

2. Pull patient Jane Morgan into context, and then click the *Medical Record* module.

3. In the *Clinical Toolbar*, click *Order* 🔬

4. If an encounter is in context, Harris CareTracker EMR displays the *New Order* dialog box. If an encounter is not in context, Harris CareTracker EMR displays the *Select Encounter* dialog box. Click on the encounter you created with the appointment booked in Chapter 4, Activity 4-1 and the *Order* screen (**Figure 7-3**) will appear.

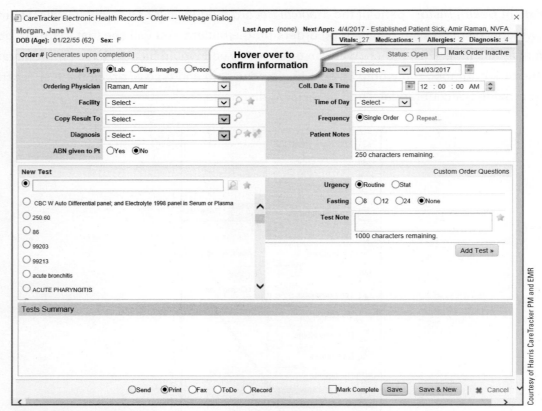

Figure 7-3   Order Screen

 TIP Best practice would be to verify that patient information such as medications, allergies, and diagnoses are up-to-date in the medical record. This is done by hovering over each category in the upper-right corner of the *Order* dialogbox (see **Figure 7-3**). This allows the opportunity for the medical assistant to add and update the information as necessary. For example, hover over the *Medications* category and the patient's medications will appear. This is informational only, and not a required step in this activity.

5. By default, the *Status* is set to "Open" in the *Order* dialog box (see **Figure 7-3**).

6. By default, the *Order Type* is set to "Lab." Leave this setting as is. The *Order Type* defaults to the option selected in the *Default Order Type*. **(FYI)** The order type can be changed by selecting *Lab, Diag. Imaging,* or *Procedure*. You can only select one order type per order and you must select the correct type to view pertinent tests.

7. By default, the *Ordering Physician* list displays the provider associated with the encounter. Confirm that the provider listed is Dr. Raman, Ms. Morgan's, PCP.

8. The *Facility* list displays the default facility set for the order type. Click the drop-down list. A list of favorite labs will appear. Select the first lab on the list. Because this is a live educational environment, you may see multiple entries for the same facility name. Only select the first lab on the list for this activity.

    (FYI) If you want to copy the result to another provider, in the *Copy Result To* list, click other providers to whom you wish to route results. If the provider is not on the list, click the *Search* 🔍 icon to search for the provider. (Skip this step.)

9. In the *Diagnosis* list, click *Search* icon. The *Diagnosis Search* dialog box will display (**Figure 7-4**). Type in the ICD-10 Diagnosis code associated with the order "R30.0" (Dysuria) and click *Search*. (**Note**: Do not select from the drop-down list for this activity. Because "favorites" may have been saved across the database it is important that you select the correct diagnosis using the *Search* feature only.)

Diagnosis Search

R30.0   Search

Diagnosis	ICD-9	ICD-10		
Dysuria				
Burning with urination	788.1	R30.0		
Difficult or painful urination	788.1	R30.0		
Dysuria after pancreas transplant using bladder drainage technique (BDT)	788.1	R30.0		
Painful urging to urinate	788.1	R30.0 S		
Scalding pain on urination	788.1	R30.0		
Spastic dysuria	788.1	R30.0		
Stranguria	788.1	R30.0		
Strangury	788.1	R30.0		

Courtesy of Harris CareTracker PM and EMR

Figure 7-4   *Diagnosis Search Dialog Box*

TIP   Steps to search for a diagnosis:

- Click the *Search* 🔍 icon next to the *Diagnosis* list. Harris CareTracker EMR displays the *Diagnosis Search* dialog box.

- In the *Search Text* box, enter the name, partial name, or diagnosis code.
  Note: If a partial name search does not return the result expected, enter the full name of the diagnosis or the code.

- Click *Search*. Harris CareTracker EMR displays a list of diagnoses that match the search criteria.

---

10. Click on the diagnosis you want (R30.0).

11. In the *ABN given to Pt* field, choose "Yes" or "No" to indicate if an advance beneficiary notice was given to the patient. This notifies the patient that Medicare can deny payment for that specific service and that the patient is responsible for payment if denied. Select "No" because this patient does not have Medicare as her insurance.

12. In the *Due Date* box, leave as -Select- and enter the date the order is due in MM/DD/YYYY format in the calendar field (Select the date of the patient's encounter and collection.) If you were to select the time period from the list, Harris CareTracker EMR would automatically calculate the due date. Because you may be working in the EMR on a date other than the current date, you will need to use the MM/DD/YYYY format for consistency; however, Harris CareTracker EMR will automatically date stamp your work with the day you perform the activity.

13. In the *Coll. Date & Time* box, enter the date and time for collecting the specimen. Use the date of the encounter and a time of 30 minutes past the patient's set appointment time (e.g., if Jane Morgan's visit was on July 30, 2018, at 9:00 a.m., the UA collection time would be 9:30 a.m.).

14. In the *Time of Day* list, use the drop-down and select the time of the day for completing the order, "Morning," "Afternoon," or "Evening" indicated by the appointment time/encounter.

15. In the *Frequency* field, select "Single Order" or "Repeat" to indicate if the order is a single order or must be repeated (select "Single Order"). (**Note**: If the *Frequency* is set to "Repeat," you can click the *Repeat* link to display the *Test Frequency* dialog box (**Figure 7-5**) and select from Daily, Weekly, Monthly, or Yearly, enabling you to record additional details about the tests that must be repeated.)

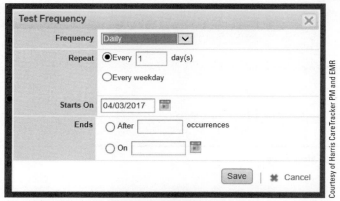

Figure 7-5   Test Frequency Dialog Box

16. *(Optional)* In the *Patient Notes* box, enter any notes about the order you want to display on the order form. Do not make any entries here.

17. The *New Test* section displays favorite tests for the order type, provider, and facility selected that had previously been entered.

18. You will search for the test by clicking on the *Search* icon. The *Search For* list defaults to the order type selected.

19. By default, the *Search Field* list displays "Description." Leave as "Description."

20. By default, the *Search Terms* list displays "Contains." However, you can change the option to "Begins with" if necessary. Leave as "Contains."

21. In the *Search Text* box, enter the keyword (enter "Urinalysis dipstick").

22. Click *Search*. Harris CareTracker EMR displays the *Orders Test Search* dialog box, which contains a list of tests that match the selected order type and the compendium associated with the facility (**Figure 7-6**).

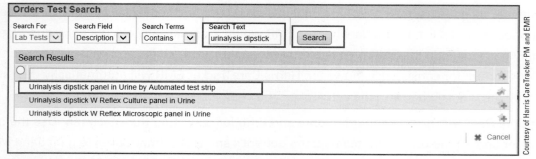

Figure 7-6   Orders Test Search Dialog Box

23. Select the tests indicated in the patient's A&P. Start by selecting "Urinalysis dipstick panel in Urine by Automated test strip" which is then pulled into the *New Test* section. (**Note:** You may see multiple entries in the *New Test* field. That is because each time an operator selected a test as a "favorite," it populates in the favorites field. Do NOT save as a favorite as part of this activity.)

24. In the *Urgency* field, select "Routine" or "Stat" based on the urgency level of the order. (Select "Stat" for this order.) **Note:** Select "Routine" for standard orders and "Stat" if results must be processed immediately.

25. In the *Fasting* field, select the option based on the fasting requirements for the test. (Select "None.") By default, a test that is a part of the Harris CareTracker PM and EMR compendium includes the fasting information as part of the AOE questions.

26. In the *Test Note* box, enter notes specific to the test to display on the order form. (Do not enter any additional notes in this field.)

27. Click *Add Test.* The test is added to the *Tests Summary* section. You can add multiple tests that are of the same order type, if necessary. You can also edit, view notes pertaining to the test, or remove a test from the *Test Summary* section.

28. Using the same settings (and steps 6 through 26 used to add the first test), add an additional *Stat* test named "Urinalysis microscopic panel [#/volume] in Urine by Automated count."

29. Click *Add Test.* In the *Tests Summary* section, both of the tests will now display.

30. At the bottom of the screen, select the appropriate option to process the order (select the *Print* radio dial button). Your screen of Ms. Morgan's *Order* should look like **Figure 7-7**.

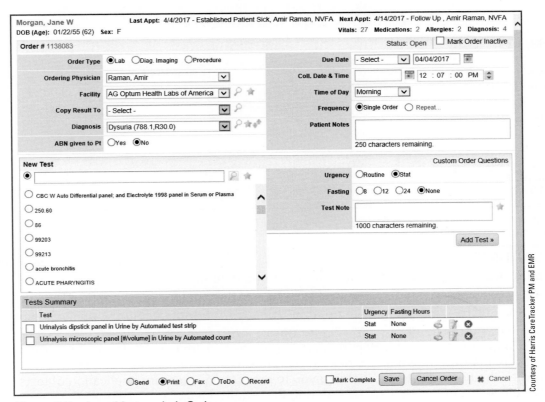

Figure 7-7   Jane Morgan Lab Order

31. Click *Save* to generate the order number and save the order. A copy of the order(s) is saved in the *Open Activities* section at the top of the patient's *Chart Summary*. Additionally, the open order displays in the *Today's Open Activities* dialog box when you access the patient's medical record from the *Clinical Today* module.

32. Once the order is saved, a pop-up box (**Figure 7-8**) will display the completed order. (**Note**: It may take a few moments for the completed order to display.) Print or save the order.

 Print the lab order. Label it "Activity 7-2" and place it in your assignment folder.

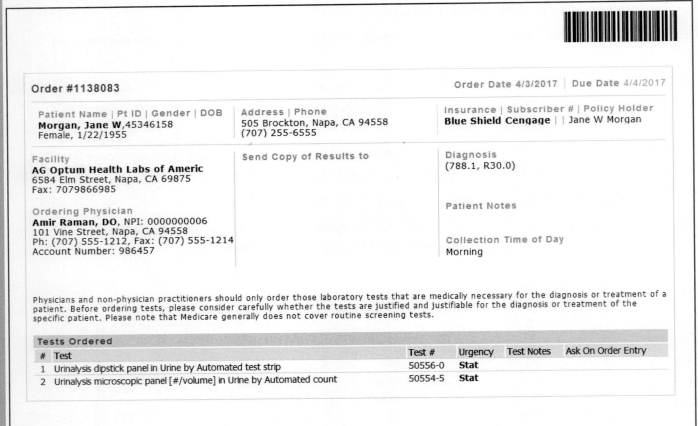

Order #1138083

Order Date 4/3/2017 | Due Date 4/4/2017

Patient Name | Pt ID | Gender | DOB	Address | Phone	Insurance | Subscriber # | Policy Holder
Morgan, Jane W,45346158 Female, 1/22/1955	505 Brockton, Napa, CA 94558 (707) 255-6555	**Blue Shield Cengage** | | Jane W Morgan

Facility	Send Copy of Results to	Diagnosis
AG Optum Health Labs of Americ 6584 Elm Street, Napa, CA 69875 Fax: 7079866985		(788.1, R30.0)

Ordering Physician
Amir Raman, DO, NPI: 0000000006
101 Vine Street, Napa, CA 94558
Ph: (707) 555-1212, Fax: (707) 555-1214
Account Number: 986457

Patient Notes

Collection Time of Day
Morning

Physicians and non-physician practitioners should only order those laboratory tests that are medically necessary for the diagnosis or treatment of a patient. Before ordering tests, please consider carefully whether the tests are justified and justifiable for the diagnosis or treatment of the specific patient. Please note that Medicare generally does not cover routine screening tests.

Tests Ordered

#	Test	Test #	Urgency	Test Notes	Ask On Order Entry
1	Urinalysis dipstick panel in Urine by Automated test strip	50556-0	**Stat**		
2	Urinalysis microscopic panel [#/volume] in Urine by Automated count	50554-5	**Stat**		

Amir Raman, DO
Ordering Physician

Figure 7-8   Order Completed Pop-Up Window

SPOTLIGHT The *Open Activities* section in the *Chart Summary* displays open orders that are overdue. Overdue tests display "Due" and the due date in red. An order with an urgency of "Stat" displays a bold "S" in parentheses (**S**) in the test description. For example: "Due 04/04/2017—Urinalysis microscopic panel [#volume] in Urine by Automated count; Urinalysis dipstick panel in Urine by Automated test strip" (**Figure 7-9**).

To print patient test orders to share with other health care professionals treating the patient, click on the drop-down arrow next to the order entry and select *Print* (**Figure 7-10**). This helps to review the history of tests, enabling you to prevent unnecessary duplication of tests and increase the efficiency of patient care by ordering the required tests.

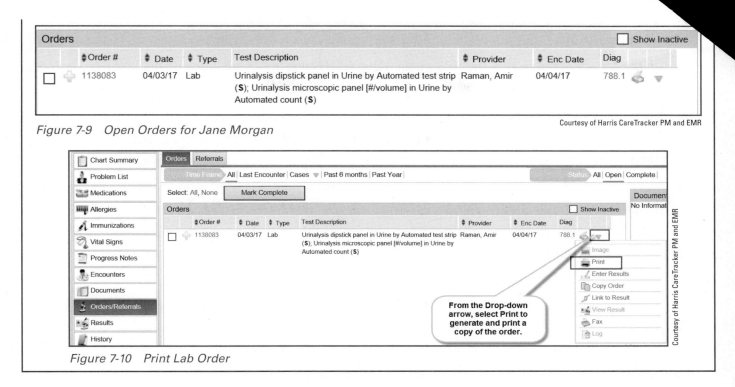

Figure 7-9   Open Orders for Jane Morgan

Figure 7-10   Print Lab Order

CREATING AND PRINTING PRESCRIPTIONS

Learning Objective 2: Search for pharmacies, manage a list of favorites, and create and print prescriptions.

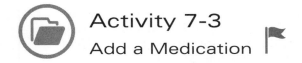

Activity 7-3
Add a Medication

The *Rx* application allows you to create prescriptions for both controlled (scheduled) and noncontrolled drugs. All prescriptions created through the *Rx Writer* application are recorded in the *Medications* application with the name, Rx Norm code, dosage, and other pertinent data.

Because your Harris CareTracker student version saves certain features across the database, you will not be saving a medication as a *Favorite*. In a live practice, the medical assistant would save medications as *Favorites* to streamline workflow. The medications saved as *Favorites* would be linked to the provider in the *Patient Medication* and *Prescription* dialog boxes.

You will now add a medication. It is important to know that you will need to click in the boxes of the dialog box vs. using the [Tab] key when adding medications/prescriptions. In addition, when you fill in the number of days in the quantity box, the SIG will pull the information into the screen.

1. Access the *Chart Summary* of Jane Morgan by clicking on her appointment in the *Clinical Today* module to add the medication noted in her progress note *A&P* (see **Figure 7-1**).If you are not in Jane Morgan's medical record, access it following the steps used below:

    *   Click on *Clinical Today*.
    *   In the *Appointments* screen within *Clinical Today*, bring up the date of Jane Morgan's appointment. Be sure that *Resources* reflect "All." **Hint:** If you don't recall the date of the appointment, click on the *History* tab in the *Scheduling* module to locate the patient's appointment. Do not create a new encounter for this activity, use only the appointment/encounter previously scheduled.

directly on the patient's name under *Appointments*, and the *Patient Health History* pane will ...ar (**Note**: Close out of the *Clinical Alerts* dialog box if displaying).

Clinical Toolbar, click the *Rx* icon. (This will launch the *Prescription* dialog box.)

...he *Pharmacy* field for now.

4. By default, the *Filling Provider* list displays the provider set in your batch. However, you can click another provider to add to your favorites. Confirm that the *Filling Provider* for patient Jane Morgan displays Dr. Raman.

5. Click on the *Search* 🔍 icon at the end of the *Medication* field. The *Medication Search* dialog box displays to search for a medication. By default, the *Search For* field displays "Medications." By default, the *Drug Type* list is set to "Dispensable."

6. By default, the *Search Terms* list is set to "Contains"; however, you can change the option to "Begins with" if necessary. (Leave as "Contains".)

7. Enter a keyword in the *Search Text* box. (Enter "Bactrim.")

8. Select the *Include Generics* checkbox to include generic versions of the medication in the search results. The generic version displays in *italics* for easy identification.

9. Click *Search*. Harris CareTracker EMR displays a list of medications matching the search criteria. (**Note:** By default, the search results do not show obsolete medications. To view medications that are obsolete, select the *Show Obsolete Drugs* checkbox. The obsolete medications appear dimmed in the search results. You cannot save obsolete medications.)

> **FYI** In your student environment, the *Drug Type* list is grayed out and automatically set to "Dispensable." In the real-world version of Harris CareTracker EMR, you can also select "Routed Drug" to record the medication without any dosage information. Routed refers to the way that a drug is introduced into the body, such as oral, enteral, mucosal, parenteral, or percutaneous.

10. Scroll down and click on the medication noted in the *A&P*: Bactrim DS Oral Tablet 800-160 MG (**Figure 7-11**). Click on the medication selected. (**Note:** If an *Interaction Screening* dialog box appears, select "Benefit outweighs risk" as the *Override Reason* and then click *Accept*.)

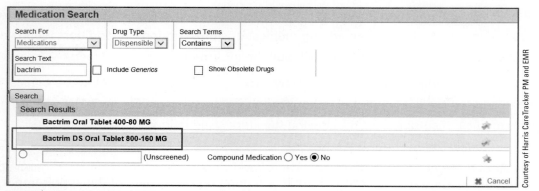

Figure 7-11   *Bactrim Search Results*

11. Continue completing the prescription by creating the SIG, as noted in the *Progress Note* in the *Dose* line of the *New Prescription* section ("SIG: 1 tab [tablet] bid [twice a day] for 5 days"). You can also click the *Dosing Calculator* icon, and the calculator will display the advised SIG. If the *Dosing Calculator* returned the SIG noted in the A&P, click on the radio dial, then scroll down and click *Select*. The SIG will populate in the *Prescription* dialog box. If the SIG returned by the *Dosing Calculator* is not the same as noted in the *Progress Note*, enter the SIG manually. In this case, the SIG will need to be entered manually.

    a. For *Amount*, enter "1."

    b. For *Unit,* select "Tablet."

    c. For *Frequency*, select "Twice a day."

    d. Enter a *Duration* of "5 Days."

12. In your student environment, you will need to change the *Start Date* and *Original Date* to reflect the date of the patient's encounter. However, the date stamp for audit purposes will reflect the actual date and time you recorded the information.

FYI When you click the *More Information* link next to the *Med Formulary* field, Harris CareTracker EMR displays the *Formulary-Additional Information* dialog box (**Figure 7-12**) with formulary, copay, coverage, and alternatives.

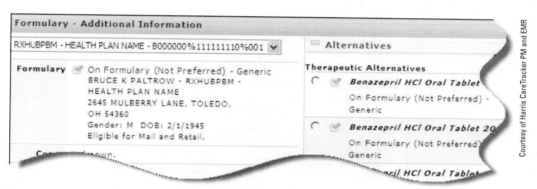

Figure 7-12   Formulary Information Dialog Box

You can select the original or an alternative medication and click *Select*. (**Note:** The selected medication is screened against the patient's active diagnoses, medications, and allergies. If the screening triggers an interaction that is higher than the severity settings set for the provider in the batch, the *Interaction Screening* dialog box displays for you to acknowledge the screening.)

---

13. Click *Add Rx* (**Figure 7-13**) and the prescription summary will display the newly added medication (**Figure 7-14**).

14. Click *Complete* to finish the prescription. The prescription will open in a new window (**Figure 7-15**). If you receive a prompt for a PIN to sign electronically, close out of the pop-up.

15. If your prescription did not print, follow the instructions in Activity 7-4 to reprint the prescription. Use reprint reason of "Printer Out Of Paper."

Courtesy of Harris CareTracker PM and EMR

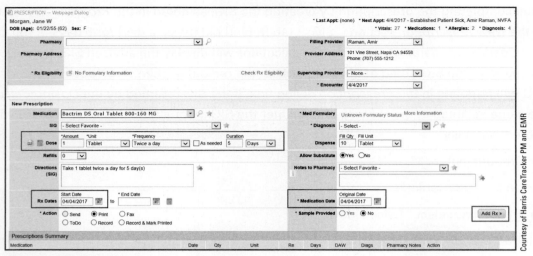

Figure 7-13 Add Rx

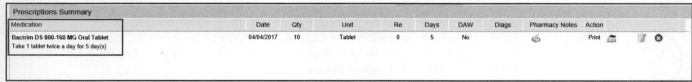

Figure 7-14 Rx Added to Prescription Summary

Courtesy of Harris CareTracker PM and EMR

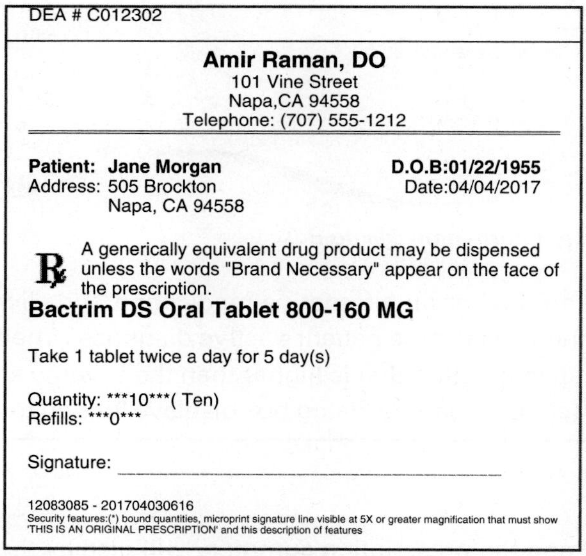

DEA # C012302

Amir Raman, DO
101 Vine Street
Napa,CA 94558
Telephone: (707) 555-1212

Patient: Jane Morgan **D.O.B:01/22/1955**
Address: 505 Brockton Date:04/04/2017
Napa, CA 94558

℞ A generically equivalent drug product may be dispensed unless the words "Brand Necessary" appear on the face of the prescription.

Bactrim DS Oral Tablet 800-160 MG

Take 1 tablet twice a day for 5 day(s)

Quantity: ***10***(Ten)
Refills: ***0***

Signature: ______________________________

12083085 - 201704030616
Security features:(*) bound quantities, microprint signature line visible at 5X or greater magnification that must show 'THIS IS AN ORIGINAL PRESCRIPTION' and this description of features

Courtesy of Harris CareTracker PM and EMR

Figure 7-15 Printed Bactrim Rx

Print the Bactrim prescription ordered for Jane Morgan. Label it "Activity 7-3" and place it in your assignment folder.

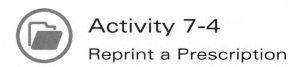

Activity 7-4
Reprint a Prescription

The *Medications* application helps review and print prescription information to give to a patient or fax to a pharmacy.

1. With patient Jane Morgan in context, click the *Medical Record* module.

2. In the *Patient Health History* pane, click *Medications*. Harris CareTracker EMR displays the *Medications* window.

3. Click on the checkbox next to the prescription you want to reprint. (Select *Bactrim*.)

4. In the *Actions* menu, click the *Arrow* icon for the prescription and click *Print* (**Figure 7-16**).

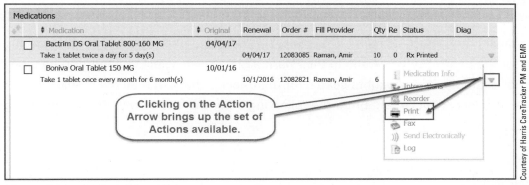

Figure 7-16   Actions Menu-Print

5. A *Reprint Prescription* dialog box will pop up. Select "Printer Out of Paper" as your *Reprint Reason* and click *Print*. The prescription displays in PDF format, enabling you to print. **Note:** If the prescription does not print, then print a screenshot of the *Reprint Prescription* dialog box with "Printer Out of Paper" selected instead. You can check your student companion website for more information.

   (FYI) If you had uploaded a digital signature, Harris CareTracker EMR would display the *Provider Signature* dialog box. Because no digital signature has been uploaded, print the prescription as is. In the *Medication* window, the *Status* of the medication changes to "Rx Printed."

 Print a copy of the prescription. Label it "Activity 7-4" and place it in your assignment folder.

Activity 7-5
Search for a Pharmacy

The *Rx Writer* application includes a *Pharmacy* list that includes the following two categories:

- Patient Pharmacies: Displays patient pharmacies listed under the *Relationships* application in the *Patient* module. By default, the *Pharmacy* list displays the patient's preferred pharmacy recorded for the patient in the *Relationships* application of the *Patient* module.

- Favorite Pharmacies: Displays pharmacies your practice most frequently uses. The favorite pharmacy list is set via the *Quick Picks* application of the *Administration* module. To access the application, click the *Administration* module, *Setup* tab, and then click the *Quick Picks* link under the *Financial* section. Click *Pharmacies* from the list to search and add favorite pharmacies for your practice. For more information on the *Quick Pick Setup* application, see *Administration Module > Setup > Financial > Quick Pick Setup* in the *Help* system.

You need to include the pharmacy information when sending a prescription electronically. Because you cannot send electronic prescriptions in your student version of Harris CareTracker EMR, you can only complete this function up to the point of searching for a pharmacy. Follow the instructions in this activity to familiarize yourself with this task.

1. With patient Jane Morgan in context, click the *Medical Record* module.

2. In the *Clinical Toolbar*, click the *Rx* icon.

3. If an encounter is in context, Harris CareTracker EMR displays the *Prescription* dialog box. (**Note:** If an encounter is not in context, the *Select Encounter* dialog box displays for you to select or create a new encounter. Click on the encounter you already created for this patient. The *Prescription* dialog box will display.)

4. If Ms. Morgan does not have any favorite pharmacies saved yet, you will need to click the *Search* icon next to the *Pharmacy* list. Harris CareTracker EMR displays the *Search Pharmacies* dialog box.

5. Enter search criteria such as name, city, state, zip code, and phone number in the specific boxes to search for the pharmacy you want. In the *Pharmacy Type* list, select the appropriate type of pharmacy. For example, if you want to search for pharmacies that can mail the medication to the patient, you would select "Mail Order." Enter the following criteria in the *Search Pharmacies* dialog box:

   a. *Name:* CVS

   b. *City:* Napa

   c. *State:* CA

   d. *Pharmacy Type:* Retail

   Note: The *State* list defaults to the patient's home address state and is a required field. In the *Name* box, enter the first few characters of the pharmacy name to display more results and prevent from eliminating results based on the way the name is spelled.

   Example: Entering *wal* will display all results with "wal" such as walmart, wal mart, and wal-mart, etc.

6. Click *Search*. Harris CareTracker EMR will return all pharmacies matching your criteria (**Figure 7-17**).

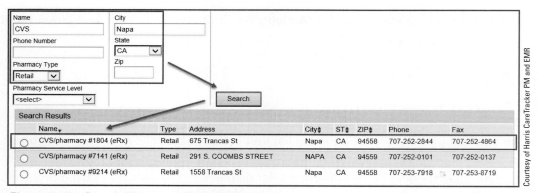

Figure 7-17   Search Pharmacy Criteria Results

📧 **Print a copy of the Search Pharmacy dialog box. Label it "Activity 7-5" and place it in your assignment folder.**

7. Select CVS # 1804. (**Note:** If you get an error message, close the dialog box and begin the search over.)

8. Do not add in the medication name or SIG at this time because this activity is only to learn to use the *Search* feature for pharmacies.

9. Click *Cancel* in the bottom right corner of the *Prescription* dialog box.

10. Click *OK* in the *Cancel Prescription* box.

PROFESSIONALISM CONNECTION

Health care professionals have access to stock medications, sample medications, and prescription tools. Providers must have absolute faith that they can trust the individuals they employ. This is why many health care workers are required to have a background check prior to employment. Never allow an individual, such as a family member or friend, pressure you into taking medication samples or creating prescriptions. It is vital that you behave in an ethical manner at all times. As a practical matter, your identification follows you everywhere you go in the electronic medical record, so even though your name may not be on the prescription anywhere, your identification is logged in as the individual who created the prescription.

ACCESSING THE IMMUNIZATION APPLICATION

Learning Objective 3: View, add, and create immunization records.

Activity 7-6
Access the Immunizations Application

The *Immunizations* application consists of a list of newly administered immunizations, immunizations administered in the past, and immunizations that the patient refused to have administered.

Additionally, the *Immunizations* application provides access to the Centers for Disease Control and Prevention (CDC) website. The website provides quick reference for recommended child and adolescent immunization schedules and a catch-up schedule for children who missed a scheduled immunization. You can review and print the immunization schedules from the CDC site.

1. Pull patient Jane Morgan into context and click the *Medical Record* module.

2. In the *Patient Health History* pane, click *Immunizations*. Harris CareTracker EMR displays the *Immunizations* window with a list of patient immunizations (**Figure 7-18**).

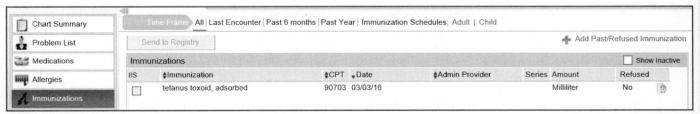

Figure 7-18   Immunizations Window

Courtesy of Harris CareTracker PM and EMR

💾 **Print a screen shot of the Immunizations window. Label it "Activity 7-6" and place it in your assignment folder.**

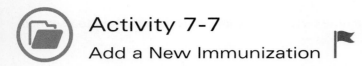

Activity 7-7
Add a New Immunization

The *Immunizations* application helps maintain a complete record of a patient's immunizations by adding past immunizations administered and immunizations that the patient refused to have administered in addition to new immunizations recorded. This helps store an up-to-date record of a patient's immunization history in one location and provides the ability to track immunizations that are due.

The *Immunization Writer* application, accessed by clicking the *Immunizations* icon on the *ClinicalToolbar,* allows you to maintain an up-to-date record of immunizations by recording information about immunizations administered. This helps your practice report accurate and complete patient immunization records to other entities, track inventory of immunizations, improve patient safety, and more.

Prior to adding a new immunization, you must set your *Administered By* list, which is defined through the *Immunization Administrator Maintenance* application accessed via the *Administration* module (**Figure 7-19**).

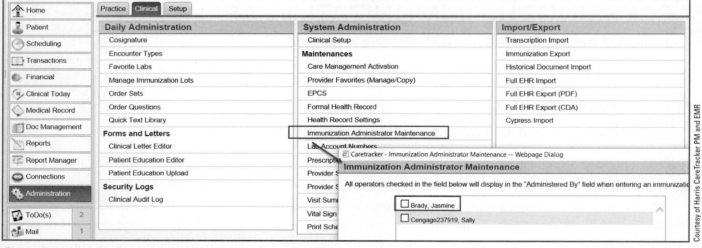

Figure 7-19   Immunization Administrator Maintenance

1. Go to the *Administration* module> *Clinical* tab and select the *Immunization Administrator Maintenance* link. Place a check mark next to your name (or if you didn't change your operator name in Activity 2-8, select your "Training Operator" number), then click *Save,* and then click on the red "X" (Close). You are now ready to add immunizations. (**Note:** You may receive an error message that the web page is trying to close; if so, click *Yes.* You can close out of the *Immunization Administrator Maintenance* dialog box by clicking the "X" in the upper-right corner. You have been added as an administrator to *ImmunizationMaintenance.*)

2. Pull patient Jane Morgan into context, and then click the *Medical Record* module.

3. In the *ClinicalToolbar*, click the *Immunizations* icon.

4. If an encounter is in context, Harris CareTracker EMR displays the *Immunization Writer* dialog box. If there was no encounter in context, the *Select Encounter* dialog box would display for you to select an

encounter. Select the appointment date/encounter you created for this patient in Chapter 4, which will launch the *Immunization Writer* dialog box.

5. The *Encounter* list defaults to the encounter date selected or created. (Leave as is.) If the encounter date is different, select the date of the encounter using the calendar icon.

6. The *Admin Date* defaults to today's date. To change the date of administration, enter the date or click the *Calendar* icon to select the date. (Change the *Admin Date* so that it matches the encounter date.) Select the time the immunization is administered. (Enter a time that is 15 minutes past the patient's appointment time.)

> **TIP** You can also click the *Reset* 🜲 icon to reset to the current date and time.

7. In the *Administered By* list, click the provider who administered the immunization. The screen should populate with your name or operator number. (Leave as is.)

8. In the *Ord Provider* list, click the provider who ordered the immunization. (Select "Dr. Raman.")

9. Click on the *Add Lot* ✚ icon in the *Immunization* section. Referring to the details in **Figure 7-20**, add immunization lot information and enter the following information in the *Lot Management* dialog box.

   a. Enter the *Lot Number* (enter "Hep" followed by your operator number as the lot number).

   b. Click the *Search* 🔍 icon next to *Immunization*.

       i. Enter "Hep B" in the *Search Text* field. Click *Search*.

       ii. Select "Hep B, adult" from the *Search Results* list.

   c. Click the *Search* 🔍 icon next to *Manufacturer*.

       i. Enter "me" in the *Search Text* field. Click *Search*.

       ii. Select the radio dial button next to "Merck & Co." under *Search Results*.

   d. Enter *Received Date* of January 1, 20XX (current year).

       (**Note:** Adjust the years in the *Received Date* and *Expiration Date* fields depending on the date of the encounter. For example, if your encounter takes place in 2018, the *Received Date* should occur in 2018, and the *Expiration Date* should be on the same month/day in 2019.)

   e. Enter *Expiration Date* of January 1, 20XX (following year). (See prior note on the *Expiration Date*.)

   f. Enter "20" in the *# Doses in Lot* field.

   g. Enter *Standard Dose* of "1.0" mL (note: the screen may reflect ml vs. mL).

   h. Select *StandardRoute* of "IM."

   i. *State Supplied* defaults to "No. "

   j. *Active* defaults to "Yes."

   k. Click *Save*.

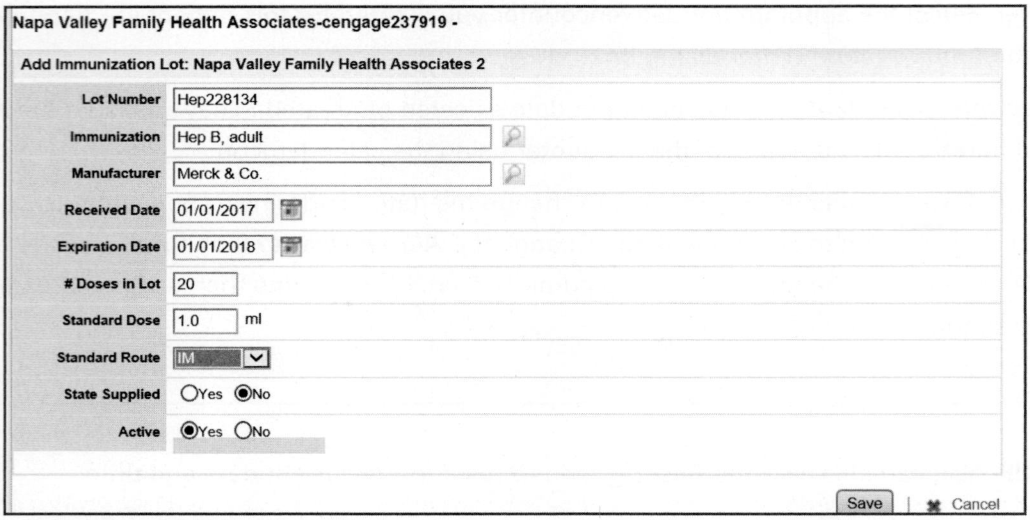

Napa Valley Family Health Associates-cengage237919 -

Add Immunization Lot: Napa Valley Family Health Associates 2

Lot Number	Hep228134
Immunization	Hep B, adult
Manufacturer	Merck & Co.
Received Date	01/01/2017
Expiration Date	01/01/2018
# Doses in Lot	20
Standard Dose	1.0 ml
Standard Route	IM
State Supplied	○Yes ●No
Active	●Yes ○No

Save | ✖ Cancel

Courtesy of Harris CareTracker PM and EMR

Figure 7-20   Add Immunization Lot

10. Select the lot you just created from the *Lot Number* drop-down list.

SPOTLIGHT Important!!

- If the lot number is not selected, a warning message displays, prompting you to select a lot number.

- All state departments of health require reporting the amount of an immunization administered in milliliters (mL).

11. By default, the *Dose Route* list displays the standard route information selected in the *Lot Management* dialog box. However, you can change the method by which the immunization is administered by making another selection from the *Dose Route* list. (Leave the *Dose Route* as "IM.")

12. By default, the *Amount* field displays the amount entered in the *Lot Management* dialog box. You can change this by manually entering another amount. (Leave the *Amount* as "1" Milliliter.)

13. In the *Series* list, select the appropriate sequence when the immunization administered is from a series of several shots (i.e., initial challenge and boosters). For example, if administering the patient with a series of hepatitis immunizations and it is the first immunization in the series, select "1" in the *Series* list. (Select "1.")

SPOTLIGHT **Three doses are generally required to complete the hepatitis B vaccine series for adults.**

- First injection—given at any time

- Second injection—at least one month after the first dose

- Third injection—six months after the first dose

When documenting a patient encounter, the series information displays in the narrative.

14. In the *Site* list, click the area of the patient's body where the immunization or drug is administered. (Select "Left Deltoid.")

15. In the *VIS Date* box, Harris CareTracker EMR automatically fills in the date from the *Support* database (leave as is). **Note:** If the date does not display, enter the date on the *Vaccine Information Statements* (VIS) handed out to the patient when the immunization was administered. (Enter date of the first day of the current year you are working in. For instance, if you are working in 2018, you would enter "01/01/2018.") **(FYI)** This feature only works on immunizations given via the *Immunization Writer*, and will not display for the information entered via the *Add Past/Refused Immunization* historical data.

16. In the *Date VIS given to Pt* box, enter the date the VIS was given to the patient. (Enter the date of the patient encounter.)

17. By default, the *Adverse Reactions* list is set to "Pt Tolerated Well." However, you can select one or more other reactions the patient had as a result of the immunization administered. (Leave the selection as is.)

18. In the *Administration Notes* box, enter additional comments about the immunization if necessary. (Enter: "Patient to return in 4–5 weeks for second injection, and return 6 months after the 1st dose for 3rd injection.") Your screen should look like **Figure 7-21**.

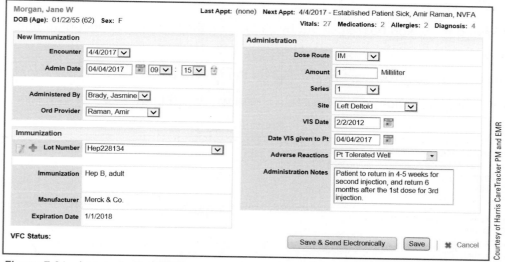

Figure 7-21   *Immunization Writer*

19. Click *Save* to save the administered immunization to the patient's medical record, *Chart Viewer,* and the narrative of the *Progress Note* template. (**Note:** To save and send the immunization information to the Department of Health in your state, you would click *Save & Send Electronically.*)

20. Refresh your *Immunizations* screen by clicking on the *Immunizations* application, and you will see the newly added Hep B immunization (**Figure 7-22**).

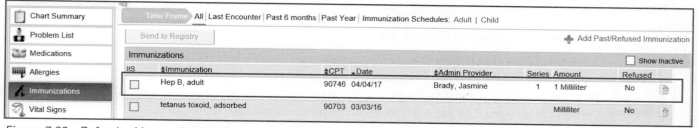

Figure 7-22   *Refreshed Immunization Screen*

Courtesy of Harris CareTracker PM and EMR

Print the updated Immunizations window. Label it "Activity 7-7" and place it in your assignment folder.

Activity 7-8
Print Immunization Records

The *Immunizations* application allows you to print immunization records to give to patients. This printed record helps to review the immunization history, provides the ability to know when an immunization is due, and prevents over-immunization. It also helps to share the patient immunization history with other entities such as clinics, schools, and camps, enabling compliance with safety and health regulations.

1. Pull patient Jane Morgan into context, and then click the *Medical Record* module.

2. In the *Patient Health History* pane, click *Immunizations*. Harris CareTracker EMR displays the *Immunizations* window with a list of immunizations administered to the patient.

3. Click on your name or operator number in the *Admin Provider* column. The information regarding the immunization displays.

4. After viewing the dialog box, close out by clicking on the "X" in the upper-right-hand corner of the dialog box.

5. Click the drop-down arrow next to *Print* on the *Patient Detail* bar, and click *Print Immunization*.

6. The patient immunization record opens in a new window (**Figure 7-23**).

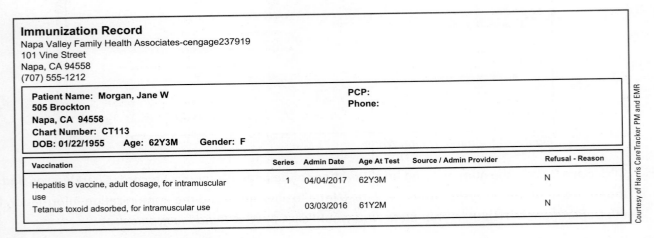

Figure 7-23   Print Immunization Record

 Print the Immunization Record. Label it "Activity 7-8" and place it in your assignment folder.

7. Close out of the *Immunization Record* tab.

> ✓ **TIP** The *Immunization Record* displays a detailed list of active immunizations for the patient. Immunizations marked as inactive do not display in the report.

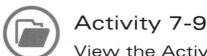

Activity 7-9
View the Activity Log of an Immunization

The *Activity Log* tracks all activity related to immunizations recorded in the patient's medical record. It is a helpful reference for audit purposes and displays information such as date, user responsible for the action, the action performed, and comments associated with an action. The log provides protection to patients, and helps providers demonstrate compliance with privacy laws and regulations such as HIPAA.

1. With patient Jane Morgan in context, click the *Medical Record* module.

2. In the *Patient Health History* pane, click on the *Immunizations* application. Harris CareTracker EMR displays the *Immunizations* window with a list of immunizations administered to the patient.

3. Now click the *Log* icon for the immunization you entered in Activity 7-8 and the *View Clinical Logs* dialog box displays each event based on the type of action performed. (**Note:** If the log is not displaying, you may need to adjust the date in the *From Date* [e.g., select "01/01/2018"] and *To Date* [use current date] boxes to include previously administered immunizations [**Figure 7-24**]).

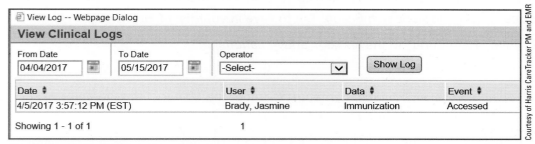

Figure 7-24   View Clinical Logs

 Print a screen shot of the Immunization Log. Label it "Activity 7-9" and place it in your assignment folder.

4. Close out of the *Log* by clicking the "X."

PULLING UP AND RECORDING PATIENT EDUCATION

Learning Objective 4: Search for, customize, and provide patient education materials for patients.

Activity 7-10
Access and Search for Patient Education

The *Patient Education* application provides a comprehensive library of patient education material available through Krames StayWell that covers the most common conditions. You can search for education material using keywords, ICD or CPT® codes, or search for material by navigating the tree structure. The content in this site is updated quarterly based on material received from Krames StayWell. You can also browse a list of favorite education materials via the *Favorites* tab. The material includes access to a database of health care advisories and clinical education handouts in different languages. You can give these materials to the patient based on the patient's condition and treatment options.

1. With patient Jane Morgan in context, click on the *Medical Record* module.

2. In the *Clinical Toolbar*, click the *Patient Education* (Edu) icon.

3. If an encounter is in context, the *Patient Education* dialog box displays and defaults to the tab set in the *Patient Education Default* list in the *Set Chart Summary Defaults* dialog box. If an encounter is not in context, Harris CareTracker EMR displays the *Select Encounter* dialog box. Select the appointment date/encounter you created for the patient in Chapter 4. This will launch the *Patient Education* dialog box.

4. By default, the *Search By* option is set to "Keywords." However, you can change the search option to CPT®, ICD-9, or ICD-10 code if necessary. (Leave as is.)

5. By default, the age and gender criteria default to the information saved for the patient in context. However, you can change the age and gender selections if necessary. (Change the *Age* selection to "All.")

6. In the *Language* list, click the language of the education material you want. (Select "English.")

7. In the blank box above *Language* type in the keywords "Urinary Tract Infection."

8. Click *Search*.

9. Under *Search Results* scroll down and select "Urinary Tract Infections in Women." Click on the *Favorite* ⭐ icon in the *Search Results* bar to save in your list of *Favorites*.

10. Now enter "Hematuria" in the text box above *Language*.

11. Click *Search*.

12. Scroll down and select "What Is Hematuria?" under the *Urinary Tract Problems* header. Click on the *Favorite* ⭐ icon to save in your list of *Favorites*.

13. To print the handouts for "Urinary Tract Infections in Women" and "What Is Hematuria":

    a. Click on the *Favorites* tab at the top of the *Patient Education* dialog box (**Figure 7-25**).

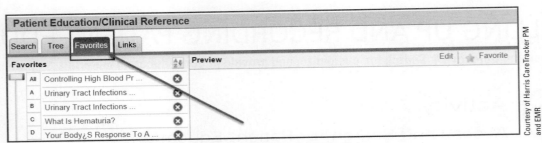

Figure 7-25   *Patient Education/Clinical Reference Favorites Tab*

    b. Select the required handout(s) from the *Favorites* list. The handout displays in the *Preview* section of the window.

    c. Click *Print* on the top right of the window to print the handout. **Hint:** You must actually print (or print to PDF) the handout for it to appear in the *Correspondence* section.

📧 **Label the printed Patient Education Sheet(s) "Activity 7-10a and 7-10b" and place them in your assignment folder.**

14. Close out of the *Patient Education/Clinical Reference* tab.

PROFESSIONALISM CONNECTION

At the beginning of any educational session, establish the patient's preferred learning style. Harris CareTracker PM and EMR provides an array of educational tools for patient education, but do not forget that the Internet has many tools that can be used when delivering patient education. Sometimes, a video or animation explains a disease or procedure much better than a handout. Make certain the provider approves all educational materials before use. Bookmark websites that have excellent educational tools so that you can bring these sites up quickly during future educational sessions.

CREATING CLINICAL LETTERS

Learning Objective 5: Access the Correspondence application to find, add, and print patient correspondence.

Activity 7-11
Create Clinical Letters

The *Letters* application provides the ability to use letter templates to create letters for patients. You can include the company logo; patient information, such as progress note data; lab reports; and more, in the letter. You can utilize the editor that is similar to other desktop editors like MS Word® to format and edit each letter. After creating the letter, you can save, print, or attach the letter to a *ToDo*, mail, or fax.

1. Pull patient Jane Morgan into context, and then click the *Medical Record* module.

2. In the *Clinical Toolbar*, click the *Letters* 🖊 icon.

3. If an encounter is in context, Harris CareTracker EMR displays the *Letter Manager* dialog box. (**Note:** If an encounter is not in context, Harris CareTracker EMR displays the *Select Encounter* dialog box. Select the appointment date/encounter you created for the patient in Chapter 4. This will launch the *Letter Manager* dialog box.)

4. To select the *Letter Template* you want to use ("NVFHA Consult Letter COPY"):

   a. Click the *Manage Favorites* ☆ icon to search for the required letter.

   b. In the *Manage Letter Favorites* dialog box, select "NVFHA Consult Letter COPY" under *ClinicalNote* (**Figure 7-26**). The selected letter template will now appear in the *Letter Manager* dialog box.

5. The Harris CareTracker EMR *Letters* application pulls in the referring provider (Dr. Richard Shinaman) and information from the patient encounter, creating the *Consult Letter* to send to Dr. Shinaman (**Figure 7-27**). **Note:** There must be a *Progress Note* associated with the encounter for the *Letter*(s) to pull in.

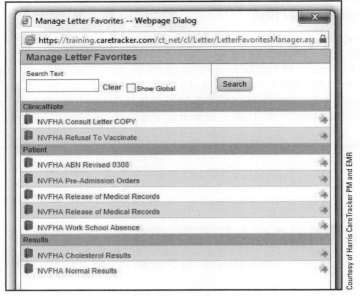

Figure 7-26   Manage Letter Favorites

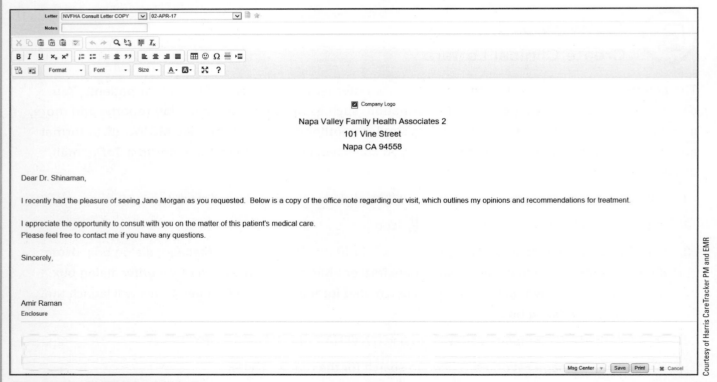

Figure 7-27   NVFHA Consult Letter

6.   In the bottom right corner of the screen, select *Print* to print a copy of the consult letter.

Label the printed consult letter "Activity 7-11" and place it in your assignment folder.

7.   Close out of the *Letter* screen.

TIP

- To save a letter as a favorite and add it to the *Letter* list, click the *Add as Favorite* ⚒ icon to the right of the letter name in the *Manage Letter Favorites* dialog box. You can check the box next to "Show Global" and the *Letters* available in the database will display. Any *Letter* previously added as a *Favorite* will have the *Saved as Favorite* ⚒ icon displayed.

- If printing a *Clinical Note* type letter, you must select the encounter. This allows you to generate a letter with information and progress note data from the encounter. If printing a *Results* letter type, you must select the specific result to include in the letter.

Activity 7-12
Add a Patient Correspondence

The *Correspondence* application displays any correspondence your practice has had with the patient in context and with another provider regarding the patient. This includes items such as *ToDo*(s), emails, phone calls, letters pertaining to the patient, patient education material given to the patient, and more. This helps keep track of all communications associated with the patient in a central location. The *Correspondence* application is accessible from the following locations:

- *Name Bar > Corr* icon 📇
- *Patient Info* 📇 icon on the *Name Bar>Documents* tab *>Correspondence* tab (**Figure 7-28**)
- *Home* module *>Practice* tab *>Unprinted Correspondence* link (*Front Office* section)
- *Financial* module *>Correspondence* tab
- *Medical Record* module *>Correspondence* pane

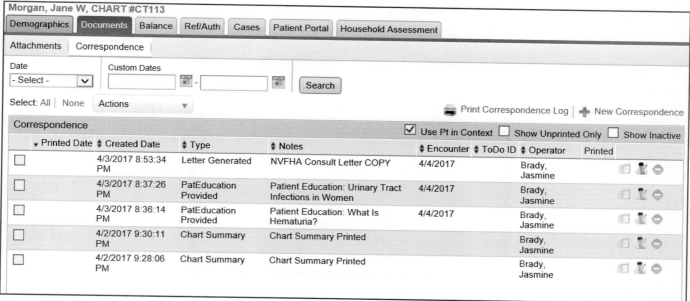

Figure 7-28   Patient Info - Correspondence Tab

Courtesy of Harris CareTracker PM and EMR

The *Correspondence* application allows you to add any correspondence, including medical record disclosures associated with a patient. When recording a medical record disclosure, a dialog box displays to enter additional details such as date and information disclosed. Additionally, you can link a correspondence to a specific encounter or to a document uploaded to the patient's medical record.

Patient Jane Morgan requested that a copy of her medical records be mailed to her home address because she is considering relocating to Colorado and wants to have all her records in her possession. She has completed the required authorization form.

1. Pull patient Jane Morgan into context, and then click the *Medical Record* module.

2. In the *Patient Health History* pane, click *Correspondence*. Harris CareTracker EMR displays the *Correspondence* window.

3. Click *+ New Correspondence* (**Figure 7-29**). Harris CareTracker EMR displays the *Add Correspondence* dialog box. The *Printed Date* box is grayed out, so no dates can be entered here.

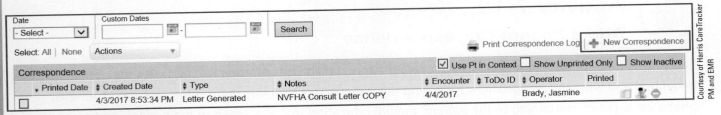

Figure 7-29   Add New Correspondence

4. In the *Type* field, scroll down to "Medical Record Disclosure" and select it.

5. In the pop-up *Correspondence Type*: *Medical Records* dialog box, enter the following details (**Figure 7-30**):

   a. *Date of Disclosure*: Enter today's date

   b. *Operator Name*: Enter your name or operator number

   c. *Reported to*: Enter "Patient, Jane Morgan"

   d. *Recipient's Address*: Leave blank

   e. *Information Disclosed*: Enter "Medical Record"

   f. *Purpose of Disclosure*: Enter "Pt requested copy of medical record"

   g. Click *Save*.

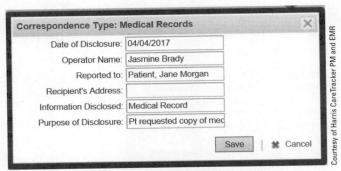

Figure 7-30   Correspondence Type: Medical Records

6. You will be taken back to the *Add Correspondence* dialog box. In the *Encounter ID* list, select the encounter to link to the correspondence. Use the last encounter you created for the patient.

7. In the *Document* list, you would click the attachment given to the patient. No document appears in the list.

8. By default, *Active* is set to "Yes." (Leave as is.)

9. In the *Notes* box, you can enter additional comments about the patient correspondence. Enter "Mailed copy to patient's home address on (use today's date)." Verify that the information entered in the *Correspondence Type* dialog box appears here (**Figure 7-31**).

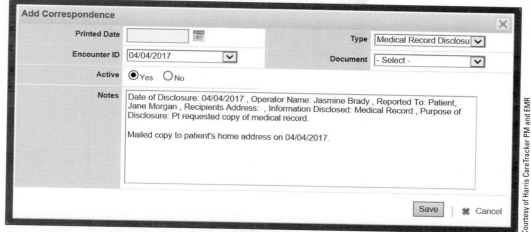

Figure 7-31   *Review Patient Correspondence Notes*

10. Click *Save* (**Figure 7-32**).

11. You will receive a *Success!* box. Close out of the *Success!* box. Close the *Add Correspondence* window if still displaying.

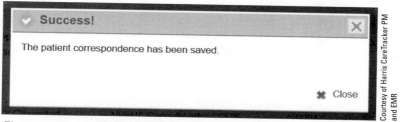

Figure 7-32   *Correspondence Saved*

The correspondence is saved in the *Correspondence* window of the *Correspondence* module (**Figure 7-33**).

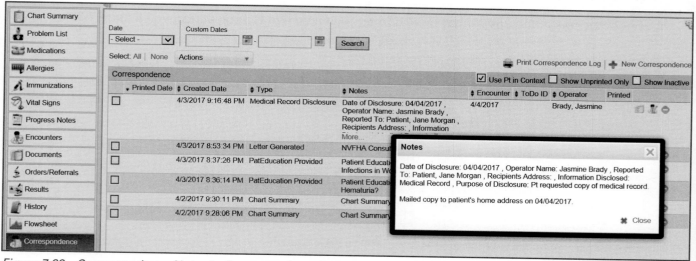

Figure 7-33   *Correspondence Notes in Correspondence Tab*

Courtesy of Harris CareTracker PM and EMR

📇 **Print a screenshot of the Patient Correspondence window. Label it "Activity 7-12" and place it in your assignment folder.**

Activity 7-13
Set an Item as Inactive or Active

The *Correspondence* application allows you to view correspondences and any attachments. You can view any documents or letters attached to patient correspondences in the *Correspondence* window.

You can set items as inactive in the *Correspondence* window. Inactive items display the *Set Active* icon. You can also change the status of an inactive item to active.

1. With patient Jane Morgan in context, click the *Medical Record* module.

2. In the *Patient Health History* pane, click *Correspondence*. Harris CareTracker EMR displays the *Correspondence* window.

3. First, mark the "Patient Education: What Is Hematuria?" document as inactive. Click the *Set Inactive* icon pertaining to this correspondence and then click *OK* to confirm the change (**Figure 7-34**).

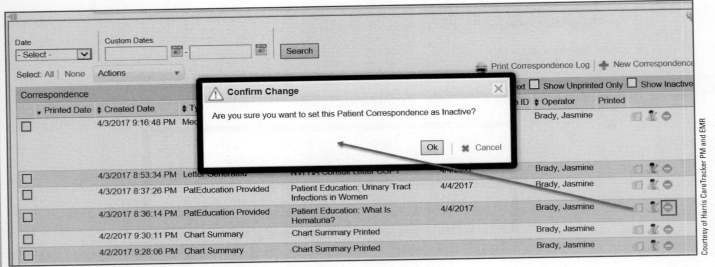

Figure 7-34   *Set as Inactive Confirmation Box*

4. Check the box in the upper-right-hand corner of your screen to "show inactive" (**Figure 7-35**).

Figure 7-35   *Show Inactive Box*

Courtesy of Harris CareTracker PM and EMR

📧 Print the screen of the Inactive Patient Correspondence, label it "Activity 7-13a," and place it in your assignment folder.

5. Now, mark the inactive document "Patient Education: What is Hematuria?" as active by clicking the *Set Active* icon pertaining to the inactive correspondence.

6. Click *OK* to confirm the change.

Print the screen of the Activated Patient Correspondence, label it "Activity 7-13b," and place it in your assignment folder.

> **FYI** In a live environment, to view and print correspondence attachments, follow the instructions below:
> 1. With patient Jane Morgan in context, click the *Medical Record* module.
> 2. In the *Patient Health History* pane, click *Correspondence*. Harris CareTracker EMR displays the *Correspondence* window.
> 3. If the *Letters* icon is grayed out, you cannot view the actual correspondence in this tab. To view a letter in a live environment, click the *Letters* icon on the right-hand side of your screen. For example, click the *Letters* icon next to "NVFHA Consult Letter COPY" to open the letter in a new window. It may take a few moments for the *Letter* to pull up.
> 4. Click *Print* to print the selected letter(s).

Activity 7-14
Print the Correspondence Log

The *Correspondence Log* is a summary of all patient correspondences.

1. Pull patient Jane Morgan into context, and then click the *Medical Record* module.

2. In the *Patient Health History* pane, click *Correspondence*. Harris CareTracker EMR displays the *Correspondence* window.

3. Uncheck *Show Inactive*.

4. Click the *Print Correspondence Log* (**Figure 7-36**) link at the top right of the screen. The application displays the log in a new window (**Figure 7-37**). (**Note:** If the log does not appear within a few seconds, go on to step 5.)

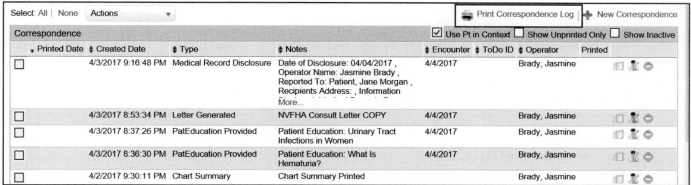

Figure 7-36   Print Correspondence Log

Courtesy of Harris CareTracker PM and EMR

5. Click back on the home screen (first tab in your browser), where you will see the PDF report on the lower part of your screen (**Figure 7-38**). You will be asked if you want to *Open* or *Save* the PDF. Click *Open* and then *Print* by right-clicking your mouse in the screen and selecting *Print* from the *Menu*. **Note**: If you still don't see the report, follow the steps in the Tip Box at the end of this activity.

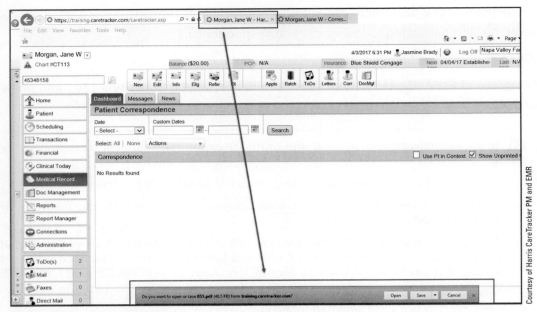

Figure 7-37   Correspondence Log

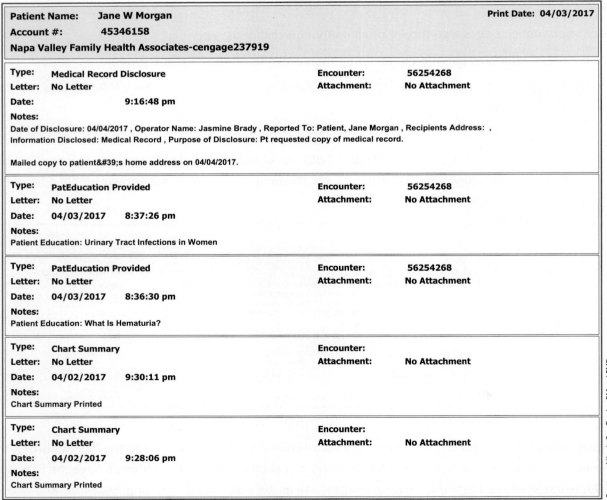

Figure 7-38   Correspondence Log PDF

TIP Depending on the version of Internet Explorer you are working in, you may have some difficulty loading the *Correspondence Log*. If you are experiencing difficulty, you can try to troubleshoot as follows:

Click back on the home screen, where you will see a message at the top of the screen indicating that Internet Explorer has blocked the correspondence file from downloading. Click on the message and select "Download file" from the drop-down menu (see **Figure 7-39**). The home page will reload.

a. Go back into the patient's medical record, and in the *Correspondence* module click on the *Print Correspondence Log* link.

b. A *Generating Report* window will pop up, telling you that the log is processing. (**Note:** If the correspondence log is taking too long to load, you can close out of the *Generating Report* window and the patient's medical record. Go back to the home screen and click the *Medical Record* module. Click the *Correspondence* tab and select the *Print Correspondence Log* link again. The correspondence log PDF should now load quickly.)

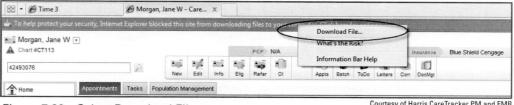

Figure 7-39   Select Download File   Courtesy of Harris CareTracker PM and EMR

 Print the Correspondence Log. Label it "Activity 7-14" and place it in your assignment folder.

CREATING REFERRALS

Learning Objective 6: Create outgoing and incoming patient referrals.

 ## Activity 7-15
Create an Outgoing Referral

The *Referrals and Authorizations* application enables providers to create inbound and outbound referrals and associated authorizations directly via the patient's medical record. You can provide data about the patient's condition and needs, referring and referred-to provider details, treatment authorization data, and referral dates and ranges. Referrals enable you to track patient compliance with the referral instructions, eliminating the need for paperwork.

There are several ways to access the *Referrals and Authorizations* application:

- Click the *Patient* module and then click the *Referrals & Authorizations* tab.
- Click the *Refer* icon on the *Name Bar*.
- Click the *Medical Record* module and then click the *Refer* icon on the *Clinical Toolbar*.

The *Referral To* list displays the providers in your *Refer Provider To* quick picks list. The *Referral From* list displays the providers in your *Refer Provider From* quick picks list. The quick picks list is set up via the *Quick Picks* application. The *Quick Picks* application is accessible by clicking the *Administration* module, *Setup* tab, and then clicking the *Quick Picks* link under the *Financial* section.

1. Pull patient Harriet Oshea into context.

2. With the patient in context, click on the *Medical Record* module. Harriet had been seen by
    Dr. Brockton on March 20, 2017, and complained of hip and back pain. She was to follow up with
    Dr. Brockton in one month. However, Harriet called the office on today (use today's date) complaining
    that the pain had increased and requested a referral to an orthopedic specialist.

3. In the *Clinical Toolbar*, click the *Refer* 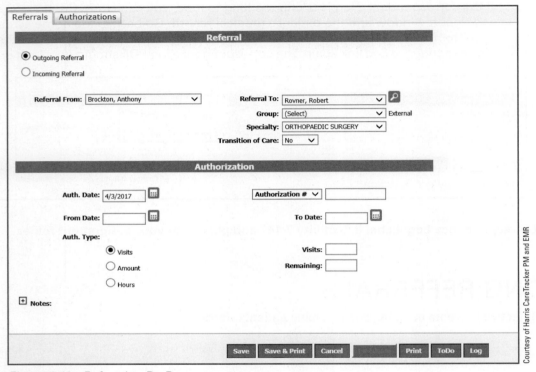 icon. A *Select Encounter* dialog box will pop up. Select the
    encounter dated March 20, 2017. Harris CareTracker EMR displays the *Referrals and Authorizations*
    dialog box (**Figure 7-40**).

Figure 7-40   Referral to Dr. Rovner

4. If the default selection is set to *Outgoing Referral* in your batch, leave as is. If not, change the field to
    Outgoing Referral for this activity.

5. If the *Default Referral to Billing Provider* list is set to "Yes" in your batch, then the *Referral From* list defaults
    to the billing provider set in the batch. However, you can select a different provider if needed. Confirm that
    Dr. Brockton is listed as the referring provider. If not, use the drop-down and select Dr. Brockton.

6. From the *Referral To* list, select the provider to whom you want to refer the patient. Click the
    Search icon to search for a provider.

    a. In the *Provider Search* dialog box, enter the *Name* and *State* information for Dr. Robert Rovner in
        San Ramon, California. Click *Search*.

    b. Click on Robert Rovner's name under the *Provider Name* heading and Harris CareTracker EMR will
        pull his information into the referral dialog box.

        (FYI): If the provider you are referring to is within the same practice as the referring from provider
        (internal), Harris CareTracker EMR automatically populates the information in the *Group* and
        Specialty lists.

7. If the provider is outside the practice (external), you must select the provider's group and specialty. (Select "Orthopaedic Surgery" in the *Specialty* field.)

8. By default, the *Transition of Care* list is set to "Yes" to indicate that the outgoing referral is a transition of care to another provider. However, you can change the option if necessary. (Select "No.")

9. Change the *Auth. Date* to today (use today's date / the date Harriet called, requesting a referral).

10. *(Optional—Authorization)* Harriet's insurance does not require an authorization. Leave blank.

11. Click *Save & Print* (see **Figure 7-40**) at the bottom of the screen. Harris CareTracker EMR saves the referral (**Figure 7-41**). (**Note:** Once you have saved the referral, you may have to close out of the *Referral* and *Authorization* dialog box to see the *Referral Print* screen.)

Referral

Referred From:	Anthony Brockton 101 Vine Street Napa, CA 94558 (Phone):(707)555-1212 (Fax):(707)555-1214	Referred To:	Robert Rovner ORTHOPAEDIC SURGERY 5801 Norris Canyon Rd Ste 210 San Ramon, CA 945835440 (Phone):(925)355-7350 (Fax):(925)244-1457
Chart #:	CT151		
Patient Name:	HARRIET OSHEA	**DOB:** 11/22/1972 **Age:** 45	
Address:	5545 Wilson Way Sonoma, CA 95476	**Sex:** F	
Phone:	(Home): (707)222-5707 (Work): (800)967-4663		
PCP:	No Provider Found		
Primary Insurance Plan:	Proplan	**Subscriber #:**	
Auth Date:	4/3/2017	**Authorization:**	PENDING
From Date:	1/1/1900	**To Date:**	1/1/1900
Notes:			

Courtesy of Harris CareTracker PM and EMR

Figure 7-41   Referral Form for Harriet Oshea

Print the Outgoing Referral by clicking on the Print button, or by right-clicking your mouse and selecting Print from the menu. Label it "Activity 7-15" and place it in your assignment folder.

12. Close out of the *Referral* print dialog box.

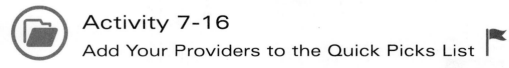

Activity 7-16
Add Your Providers to the Quick Picks List

Incoming referrals are generally received by specialty physicians and must be processed during check-in or on a pre-visit basis. The referral is necessary for the specialty provider to receive appropriate payment. For example, if a women's health care specialist receives a referral from an outside practice to treat a patient for polycystic ovarian syndrome, this is referred to as an incoming referral.

Prior to creating incoming *Referrals*, you must set up your providers in the "Refer Provider To" list via the *Quick Picks* link. In previous chapters, you learned how to create *Quick Picks*. Follow the steps below to add your providers to the *Quick Picks* list.

1. Click on the *Administration* module >*Setup* tab >*Financial* header >*Quick Picks* link.

2. In the *Screen Type* drop-down, scroll down and select *Refer Provider To*.

3. Your screen will display either (a) "Paul T Endo" in the *Refer To Providers* box (if you completed Case Study 2-1) who is not a NVFHA provider, or (b) "There are no quick picks" (if you did not complete Case Study 2-1).

4. Click the *Search* 🔍 icon and enter the providers of NVFHA (Rebecca Ayerick, Anthony Brockton, Gabriella Torres, and Amir Raman).

   a. In the *Provider Search* dialog box, enter the provider's last name (Ayerick) and state (California) to narrow your search (**Figure 7-42**). Click *Search*.

   b. Click on Rebecca Ayerick's name.

   c. You will receive a *Success* box stating "Quick Pick information has been updated."

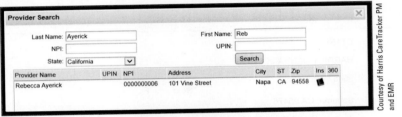

Figure 7-42   Quick Pick-Refer Providers To

5. Repeat step 4 for each of the remaining providers in the NVFHA group (Anthony Brockton, Amir Raman, and Gabriella Torres).

6. Click *Close* to exit out of the *Success* box after each provider has been added. When you have completed each entry, your screen should look like **Figure 7-43**.

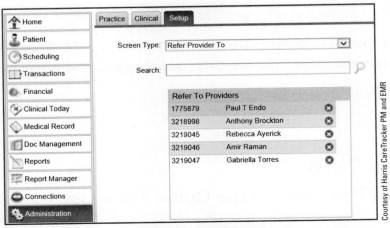

Figure 7-43   Refer Provider To Quick Pick List

💾 **Print the Refer Provider To Quick Picks screen, label it "Activity 7-16" and place it in your assignment folder.**

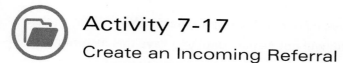

Activity 7-17

Create an Incoming Referral

Now that your referring provider *Quick Picks* have been set up, you will be able to create an incoming referral.

1. Pull patient Edith Robinson into context and then click on the *Medical Record* module. Ms. Robinson was referred to Dr. Raman of NVFHA as her new PCP by orthopedic specialist Dr. David Dodgin.

2. In the *Clinical Toolbar*, click the *Refer* icon.

   a. If you are taken to a *Select an Encounter* dialog box, select the most recent encounter for the patient. If no encounter is available to select, then follow the Tip box steps below.

   b. If the *Referral and Authorization* dialog box displays, you can proceed with Step 3.

3. (FYI) Only if the patient does not have a previous encounter listed, select the *Create a New Encounter* link and enter the following information in the *Create a New Encounter* dialog box:

   a. *Type*: Select "Other"

   b. *Service Date*: Enter the date of the appointment you scheduled for Ms. Robinson in Chapter 4.

   c. *Responsible Provider*: Select "Dr. Raman"

   d. *Patient Case*: Leave as "Default"

   e. *Location*: Leave as "NVFA"

   f. *Transition of Care*: Leave as "No"

   g. Click *Ok*.

4. In the *Referrals* dialog box, select *Incoming Referral* if not already selected (**Figure 7-44**). (The default selection for this field is set in your batch.)

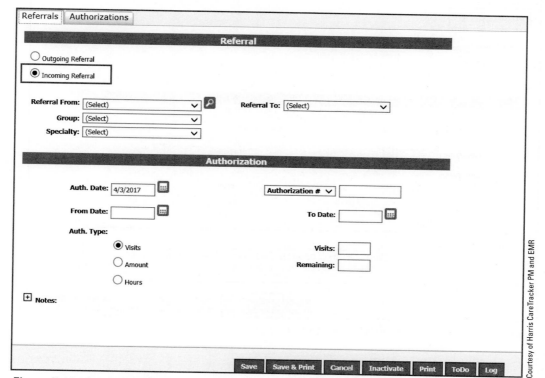

Figure 7-44   Incoming Referral

Courtesy of Harris CareTracker PM and EMR

5. Click *New*. Harris CareTracker PM and EMR displays the incoming referral fields. (**Note:** If the patient did not have a previous encounter, the *New* button will not display until you save this incoming referral, allowing you to create another. Skip this instruction and continue with the rest of the activity if the *New* button is not displayed.)

6. In the *Referral From* list, select the provider referring the patient. (Select "David Dodgin.") Alternatively, click the *Search* 🔍 icon to search for a provider. If you use the search feature to select a provider, Harris CareTracker EMR automatically adds the provider to the *Providers* (tab) application of the *Patient* module.

7. Leave the *Group* field as "(Select)."

8. In the *Specialty* field, select "Orthopaedic Surgery" from the drop-down list.

9. The *Referral To* list defaults to the billing provider set in your batch (if the batch setting of *Default Referral* to Billing provider is listed as "Yes"), but you can select a different provider if needed using the drop-down arrow. Select "Dr. Raman."

10. No authorization is required; however, change the *Auth. Date* to your encounter date (the first appointment date that the patient has/had with Dr. Raman).

11. Click + *Notes* to enter comments related to the authorization. Enter notes: "Edith Robinson is a patient of Dr. Dodgin and has recently moved to Napa and would like to establish with Dr. Raman as her PCP" (**Figure 7-45**).

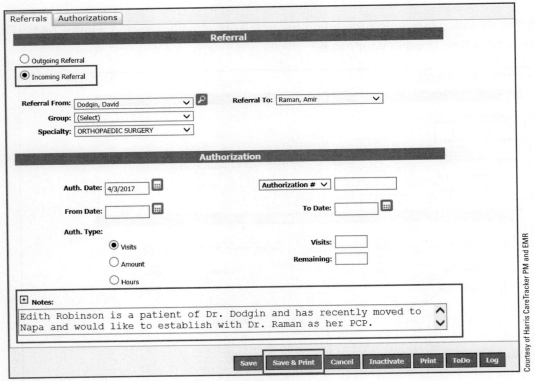

Figure 7-45   *Incoming Referral for Edith Robinson*

12. Click *Save & Print.* Harris CareTracker EMR saves the referral and the *Print* dialog box will appear (**Figure 7-46**). (**Note**: You may need to close out of the *Referral and Authorization* dialog box to see the *Referral Print* box.)

```
Print
```

Referral

Referred From:	David Dodgin	Referred To:	Amir Raman
	5201 Norris Canyon Rd		101 Vine Street
	Ste 300		Napa, CA 94558
	San Ramon, CA 945835405		(Phone):(707)555-1212
	(Phone):(925)820-6720		(Fax):(707)555-1214

Chart #:	CT143		
Patient Name:	EDITH ROBINSON		
Address:	3072 Sacramento St	DOB: 1/1/1948	Age: 69
	Sonoma, CA 95476	Sex: F	
Phone:	(Home): (707)245-9898		
	(Work): (800)941-7044		
PCP:	No Provider Found		

Primary Insurance Plan:	Medicare Cengage	Subscriber #:	
Auth Date:	4/3/2017	Authorization:	PENDING
From Date:	1/1/1900	To Date:	1/1/1900

Notes:	Edith Robinson is a patient of Dr. Dodgin and has recently moved to Napa and would like to establish with Dr. Raman as her PCP.

Courtesy of Harris CareTracker PM and EMR

Figure 7-46   Incoming Referral Print Box

🖫 **Print the Incoming Referral by clicking the Print button in the Referral Print dialog box, or by right-clicking your mouse and selecting Print from the menu. Label it "Activity 7-17" and place it in your assignment folder.**

13. Close out of the *Referral* print screen.

COMPLETING A VISIT FOR BILLING PURPOSES

Learning Objective 7: View and resolve open encounters and unsigned notes by completing the visit and signing the Progress Note.

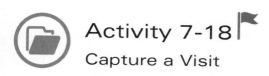 Activity 7-18 🚩

Capture a Visit

In Chapter 6, you completed much of the patient work-up to the point of completing and printing the progress note. In order for a patient visit to be billable, any open encounters must be resolved and the visit must be completed and the note signed. The provider is the person who is responsible for signing the progress note; however, to enhance your understanding of workflows in the EMR, you will be completing the visit, resolving open encounters, and electronically signing the note.

To generate claims, charges must be captured for the patient's appointment. The *Visit* application allows you to capture charges and enter procedure, NDC, and diagnosis codes for a patient's appointment.

Visits can be entered into Harris CareTracker PM and EMR via several applications. Access the *Visits* application by one of the following methods:

- Left-click on a patient's appointment in the *Book* application and select *Visit* from the pop-up mini-menu.

- Pull a patient into context, click the *Appts* button in the *Name Bar,* pull the appointment into context, and select *Visit* from the *Actions* menu.

- Click the *Appointments* link under the *Appointments* section of the *Dashboard* tab in the *Home* module, pull the patient appointment into context, and then select *Visit* from the *Actions* menu.

- Click the *Visits* link from the *Actions* drop-down list for a patient listed in the *Appointments* application of the *Clinical Today* module.

- Click the *Visit* icon on the *Clinical Toolbar* within the *Medical Record* module.

The *Visit* window contains a number of applications, but to save a visit you only need to enter the procedure and diagnosis code(s). Please note that a visit can only be edited prior to becoming a charge. For our first *Visit* activity, refer to patient Harriet Oshea's appointment on March 20, 2017, with Dr. Brockton. Best practice would be to access the *Assessment* tab in the *Progress Note* (**Figure 7-47**) and review the problem list to determine which diagnoses were selected for this visit. You would then capture the *Visit* following the instructions in this activity.

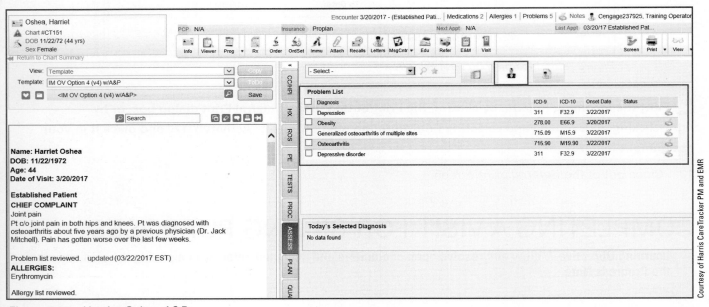

Figure 7-47   Harriet Oshea A&P

1. Click the *Scheduling* module. Harris CareTracker PM and EMR opens the *Book* application by default.

2. Move the schedule to display the date of service for which you want to confirm an appointment. This can be done by manually entering in the date in the *Date* box, by clicking the *Calendar* icon, or by selecting a time period from the *Move* list. (Enter "March 20, 2017" in the *Date* box.)

3. You will need to set the *Resources* field (just to the right of the calendar) to "All Resources" using the drop-down to select "All Resources" in order for the full schedule and all providers to display.

4. Click *Go.*

5. Left-click the appointment for which you want to enter visit information and select *Visit* from the mini-menu (select Harriet Oshea's appointment). The application displays the *Visit* window (**Figure 7-48**). When you first bring up the *Visit* window, it automatically displays the procedures section (*Procedures* tab located at the top left of the window).

| Procedures | Diagnosis | Visit Summary | | | | | | | EncoderPro.com |

Pt Name Oshea, Harriet (F)		PCP		Admit Date N/A		Notes		
DOB 11/22/1972 (44 yrs)		Ref Provider Brockton, Anthony		Last Surgery Date N/A				
Primary Ins Proplan		Case Ins Proplan		Next Appointment None		Complaint Joint Pain		

Procedure Search: _____ 🔍

OFFICE VISIT EST PTS	Mod	Units	OFFICE PROCEDURES	Mod	Units	PREVENTIVE MEDICINE EST	Mod	Units
☐ 99212 Office Outpatient Visit 10 Min		1	☐ 93000 Ecg Routine Ecg W/Least 12 Lds		1	☐ 99395 Periodic Preventive Med Est Pa		1
☐ 99213 Office Outpatient Visit 15 Min		1	☐ G0102 Pros Cancer Screening; Digtl R		1	☐ 99396 Periodic Preventive Med Est Pa		1
☐ 99214 Office Outpatient Visit 25 Min		1	☐ 94760 Noninvasive Ear/Pulse Oximetry		1	☐ 99397 Periodic Preventive Med Est Pa		1
☐ 99215 Office Outpatient Visit 40 Min		1	☐ J7650 Isoetharine Hci Inhal Thru Dme		0	**PREVENTIVE MEDICINE NEW**	**Mod**	**Units**
OFFICE VISIT NEW PTS	**Mod**	**Units**	☐ 94620 Pulmonary Stress Testing Simpl		1	☐ 99384 Initial Preventive Medicine Ne		1
☐ 99201 Office Outpatient New 10 Minut		1	☐ D7911 Complicated Suture-Up To 5 Cm		1	☐ 99385 Initial Preventive Medicine Ne		1
☐ 99202 Office Outpatient New 20 Minut		1	☐ 93225 Xtrnl Ecg < 48 Hr Recording		1	☐ 99386 Initial Preventive Medicine Ne		1
☐ 99203 Office Outpatient New 30 Minut		1	☐ V5008 Hearing Screening		1	☐ 99387 Initial Preventive Medicine Ne		1
☐ 99204 Office Outpatient New 45 Minut		1	☐ 3210F Group A Strep Test Performed		1	**INJECTIONS**	**Mod**	**Units**
RADIOLOGY	**Mod**	**Units**	**OTHER SERVICES**	**Mod**	**Units**	☐ 90471 Imadm Prq Id Subq/Im Njxs 1 Va		1
☐ 71020 Radiologic Exam Chest 2 Views		1	☐ Q0091 Screen Pap Smear; Obtain Prep		1	☐ 90658 Influenza Virus Vaccine Split		1
☐ 72100 Radex Spine Lumbosacral 2/3 Vi		1	☐ 88143 Cytp C/V Flu Auto Thin Mnl Scr		1	☐ G0008 Administration Of Influenza Vi		1
☐ 73100 Radex Wrist 2 Views		1	☐ 99051 Svc Prv Office Reg Schedd Evn		1	☐ G0009 Administration Of Pneumococcal		1
☐ 73500 Radex Hip Unilateral			☐ 00000 Handle&/Or Conveu					

Figure 7-48   Harriet Oshea Visit Window

Courtesy of Harris CareTracker PM and EMR

6. The *Procedures* screen contains a list of procedure codes that mirror the CPT® codes on the encounter form. Place and verify that the checkboxes next to each code associated with the patient's appointment are selected. SelectCPT® codes 99213, 73565, 73520, and 36415 for this visit. (**Note:** If no *Visit* had yet been entered for the patient, the encounter form would display with no checkboxes next to procedure or diagnosis codes. If you see the code you want to select for the *Visit*, you can select the checkbox next to the code. Alternatively, you could enter either a code or key term in the *Procedure Search* box and click *Search* to locate the desired code.)

Source: Current Procedural Terminology © 2017 American Medical Association.

TIP   If you need to search for a CPT® code:

- Enter a partial code, complete code, or a keyword in the *Procedure Search* field, and then click the *Search* icon. The application opens the *Procedure Search* window.

- *(Optional)*To search for an NDC Code, select *NDC Code* from the *Search Type* list and then click *Search*.

- Click on the desired procedure to select it. The codes selected from the search are added to the patient's *Visit* window, and there is no limit to the number of codes you can select.

---

7. Enter any modifiers in the *Mod* field next to each selected procedure code, if applicable. (No modifier is required.)

8. If needed, enter the number of units in the *Units* field for each selected procedure code. (Number of units is "1" per CPT® code for this activity [as noted in **Figure 7-48**].)

9. Click the *Diagnosis* tab in the *Visit* window. The application displays the *Diagnosis* application.

10. The *Diagnosis* screen displays a list of codes that mirror the ICD codes on the encounter form. Select the checkbox next to each code associated with the patient's appointment. (Select ICD-10 code M15.0 as in **Figure 7-49**.)

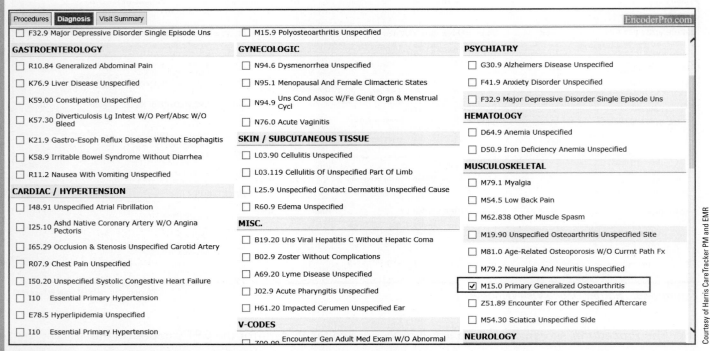

Procedures	**Diagnosis**	Visit Summary		EncoderPro.com

☐ F32.9 Major Depressive Disorder Single Episode Uns   ☐ M15.9 Polyosteoarthritis Unspecified

GASTROENTEROLOGY
☐ R10.84 Generalized Abdominal Pain
☐ K76.9 Liver Disease Unspecified
☐ K59.00 Constipation Unspecified
☐ K57.30 Diverticulosis Lg Intest W/O Perf/Absc W/O Bleed
☐ K21.9 Gastro-Esoph Reflux Disease Without Esophagitis
☐ K58.9 Irritable Bowel Syndrome Without Diarrhea
☐ R11.2 Nausea With Vomiting Unspecified

CARDIAC / HYPERTENSION
☐ I48.91 Unspecified Atrial Fibrillation
☐ I25.10 Ashd Native Coronary Artery W/O Angina Pectoris
☐ I65.29 Occlusion & Stenosis Unspecified Carotid Artery
☐ R07.9 Chest Pain Unspecified
☐ I50.20 Unspecified Systolic Congestive Heart Failure
☐ I10 Essential Primary Hypertension
☐ E78.5 Hyperlipidemia Unspecified
☐ I10 Essential Primary Hypertension

GYNECOLOGIC
☐ N94.6 Dysmenorrhea Unspecified
☐ N95.1 Menopausal And Female Climacteric States
☐ N94.9 Uns Cond Assoc W/Fe Genit Orgn & Menstrual Cycl
☐ N76.0 Acute Vaginitis

SKIN / SUBCUTANEOUS TISSUE
☐ L03.90 Cellulitis Unspecified
☐ L03.119 Cellulitis Of Unspecified Part Of Limb
☐ L25.9 Unspecified Contact Dermatitis Unspecified Cause
☐ R60.9 Edema Unspecified

MISC.
☐ B19.20 Uns Viral Hepatitis C Without Hepatic Coma
☐ B02.9 Zoster Without Complications
☐ A69.20 Lyme Disease Unspecified
☐ J02.9 Acute Pharyngitis Unspecified
☐ H61.20 Impacted Cerumen Unspecified Ear

V-CODES
☐ Z00.00 Encounter Gen Adult Med Exam W/O Abnormal

PSYCHIATRY
☐ G30.9 Alzheimers Disease Unspecified
☐ F41.9 Anxiety Disorder Unspecified
☐ F32.9 Major Depressive Disorder Single Episode Uns

HEMATOLOGY
☐ D64.9 Anemia Unspecified
☐ D50.9 Iron Deficiency Anemia Unspecified

MUSCULOSKELETAL
☐ M79.1 Myalgia
☐ M54.5 Low Back Pain
☐ M62.838 Other Muscle Spasm
☐ M19.90 Unspecified Osteoarthritis Unspecified Site
☐ M81.0 Age-Related Osteoporosis W/O Currnt Path Fx
☐ M79.2 Neuralgia And Neuritis Unspecified
☑ M15.0 Primary Generalized Osteoarthritis
☐ Z51.89 Encounter For Other Specified Aftercare
☐ M54.30 Sciatica Unspecified Side

NEUROLOGY

Courtesy of Harris CareTracker PM and EMR

Figure 7-49   Harriet Oshea Diagnosis Codes

> **TIP** If you need to search for a diagnosis code:
> - Enter a partial code, a complete code, or a keyword in the *Diagnosis Search* field, and then click the *Search* icon. The application opens the *Diagnosis Search* window.
> - Click on the desired ICD-10 code to select it. The codes selected from the search are added to the patient's *Visit* window.

11. Click the *Visit Summary* tab in the top left corner of the *Visit* window. Harris CareTracker PM displays a summary of the visit information.

12. To check out the patient directly from the *Visit* application, select the *Check out Patient?* checkbox (**Figure 7-50**) at the bottom of the screen.

13. Review the screen (see Figure 7-50) and verify the accuracy of the information including the *Location*, *Place of Service (POS)*, *Referring Provider*, *Insurance*, *Billing*, and *Servicing Provider*.

14. (If applicable) To link the visit to a case, you would select a case from the *Case* list. (No *Case* number is associated with this visit.)

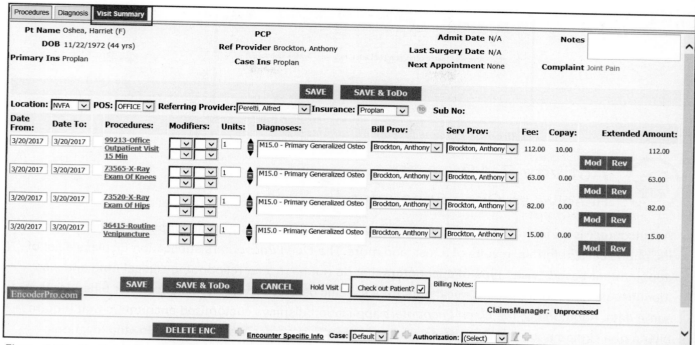

Figure 7-50   *Harriet Oshea Visit-Summary Window*   Courtesy of Harris CareTracker PM and EMR

15. Select an authorization number from the *Authorization* list, if applicable (not applicable in this activity).

16. From the *Billing Type* list, select the billing type "Professional" at the bottom of the *Visit* screen (**Figure 7-51**).

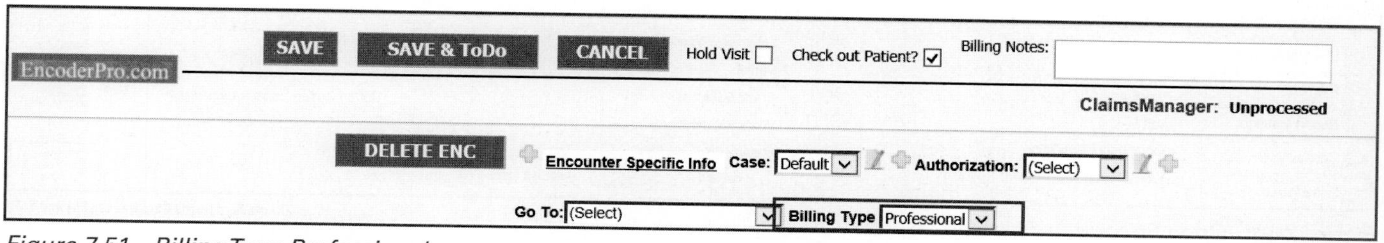

Figure 7-51   *Billing Type-Professional*   Courtesy of Harris CareTracker PM and EMR

17. *(Optional)* Click *EncoderPro.com* to obtain coding information from *EncoderPro*. This information can be used as a guide to correct the visit information.

🖫 **Print the Visit Summary screen. Label it "Activity 7-18," and place it in your assignment folder.**

18. Click *Save* at the top or bottom of the screen. Once you hit *Save*, you will receive a pop-up message (**Figure 7-52**) stating "An error occurred connecting to Claims manager. Transaction saved." You must <u>wait</u> for this error message before continuing with the activity. Once you receive the error message, <u>click</u> *OK* on the pop-up. When the visit is saved, the coding information is sent to *ClaimsManager* for screening. In addition, Harris CareTracker PM and EMR automatically checks out the patient on the schedule and a check mark appears next to the patient's name confirming that the visit has been captured. Your *ClaimsManager* feature is not active in your student version of Harris CareTracker which is why you receive the error message, but the visit is saved for this activity and future billing activities.

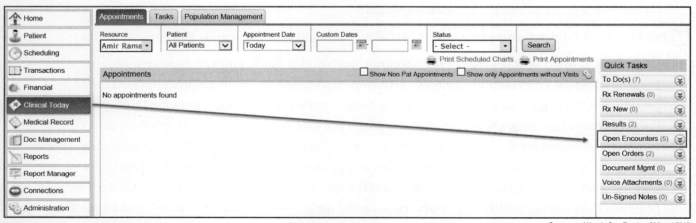

Figure 7-52   Claims Manager Error Message

Activity 7-19
Resolve an Open Encounter

An encounter is an interaction with a patient on a specific date and time. Encounter types include visits, phone calls, referrals, results of a test, and more. The *Open Encounters* application displays a list of appointment-based "visit" type of encounters that do not have a corresponding clinical note and also identifies patients who have a clinical note for a specific date of service but no encounter billed for that same date. Additionally, the *Open Encounters* application displays customized encounters that require billing or a signed note. The *Open Encounters* application is accessible from the following locations:

- *Home* module > *Dashboard* tab > *Open Encounters* link (*Clinical* section) (**Figure 7-53**)

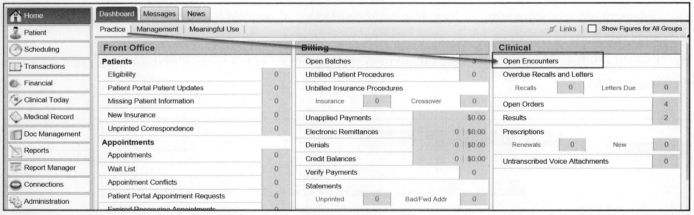

Figure 7-53   Open Encounters Link on Dashboard Tab

Courtesy of Harris CareTracker PM and EMR

- *Clinical Today* module > *Tasks* tab > *Open Encounters* (from the *Tasks* menu on the right side of the window) (**Figure 7-54**)

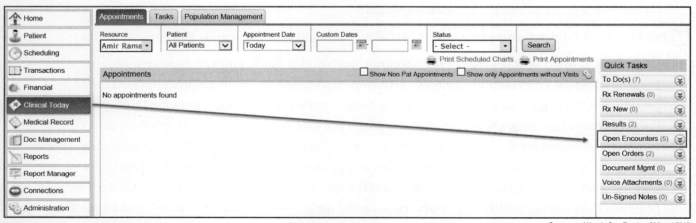

Figure 7-54   Open Encounters from the Clinical Today module

Courtesy of Harris CareTracker PM and EMR

Access the list of *Open Encounters* by going to your *Home* module >*Dashboard* tab >*Open Encounters* link (*Clinical* section). You may need to change the *Provider* to "All" using the drop-down arrow; otherwise the encounters might not display (**Figure 7-55**).

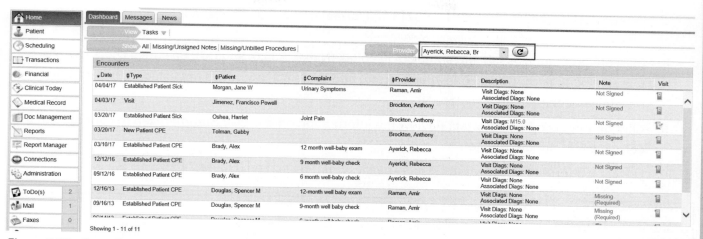

Figure 7-55   *Open Encounters-Select All Providers*

Courtesy of Harris CareTracker PM and EMR

The *Open Encounters* application helps resolve appointment-based "visit" type of encounters by entering the visit information, reviewing, transcribing (if the note contains an untranscribed file), signing the note, and then billing. All tasks related to the note can be completed via the *Progress Note* application in the *Medical Record* module. *Visit* information is captured by entering the appropriate CPT® and ICD codes using the *Visit* application. For this activity, you will want to view the *Progress Note* and confirm (resolve) that all items in the A&P for the encounter have been completed. If there are any outstanding items, complete them before you sign the note.

1. Access the *Open Encounters* application from the *Home* module >*Dashboard* tab >*Open Encounters* link (*Clinical* section). If the encounter you are looking for does not display, use the drop-down feature next to *Provider*, select *All*, and then click the *Change Resource* (search) 🔍 icon.

2. Find the encounter you want to resolve (**Figure 7-56**). (Locate the encounter you created for Jane Morgan.)

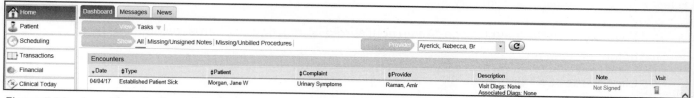

Figure 7-56   *Jane Morgan Open Encounter*

Courtesy of Harris CareTracker PM and EMR

3. Under the *Note* column, click the *Not Signed* link. The *Progress Note* application displays, enabling you to complete and sign the note if instructed.

4. As Best Practice, you would confirm (resolve) that all items in the *A&P* for the encounter have been completed. This is the opportunity for the medical assistant to complete any orders, education materials, future appointments, etc.

5. Do <u>not</u> sign the note at this time.

6. Click on the *Visit* 🗔 icon in the *Clinical Toolbar*. The *Visit* application will display.

(**Note:** If you completed the Billing Module Quick Start prior to completing this activity, you will get a message that says, "There are already Financial Records written associated with this Encounter." <u>If you get this message, click *OK* and skip steps 7 through 13 of this activity.</u>)

7. Enter/select the appropriate CPT® (99213 and 90746) in the *Procedures* tab.

    Source: Current Procedural Terminology © 2017 American Medical Association.

8. Click on the *Diagnosis* tab and enterICD-10 codes (N39.0, R30.0, and I10). Be sure a check mark is placed next to each ICD-10 code you selected, and de-select any codes not listed in this activity that may have been previously entered.

9. Click on the *Visit Summary* tab. Review the information on the *Visit Summary* tab to confirm that the correct codes are displaying.

10. Once the information is confirmed in the *Visit Summary* screen (**Figure 7-57**), click *Save.*

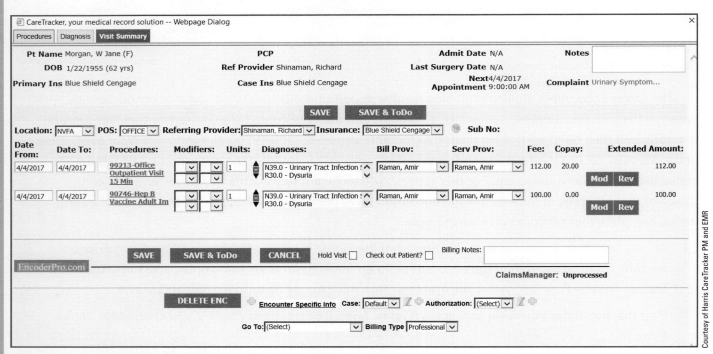

Figure 7-57   *Jane Morgan Visit Summary Screen*

11. You must wait for the message "An error occurred connecting to Claims manager. Transaction saved" before moving on.

12. Click on the "OK" button.

13. When the visit information is saved, the icon in the *Visit* column changes to "Visit Complete." (**Note:** If you don't see the change, "Refresh" the *Open Encounters* screen to see the updated *Visit* column entry. You can refresh clicking on the *Refresh* icon located next to the Provider name field.)

🖥 **Print a screenshot of the updated Open Encounters window, label it "Activity 7-19," and place it in your assignment folder.**

14. Now that you have completed the tasks assigned, click back on Ms. Morgan's medical record, and review the *Progress Note* for the appointment date/encounter you scheduled for her in Chapter 4. Scroll down to the bottom and confirm that all orders, immunizations, referrals, and educational materials ordered in the A&P have been completed (**Figure 7-58**).

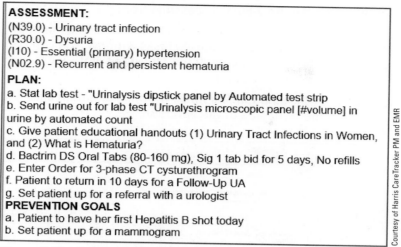

ASSESSMENT:
(N39.0) - Urinary tract infection
(R30.0) - Dysuria
(I10) - Essential (primary) hypertension
(N02.9) - Recurrent and persistent hematuria

PLAN:
a. Stat lab test - "Urinalysis dipstick panel by Automated test strip
b. Send urine out for lab test "Urinalysis microscopic panel [#volume] in urine by automated count
c. Give patient educational handouts (1) Urinary Tract Infections in Women, and (2) What is Hematuria?
d. Bactrim DS Oral Tabs (80-160 mg), Sig 1 tab bid for 5 days, No refills
e. Enter Order for 3-phase CT cysturethrogram
f. Patient to return in 10 days for a Follow-Up UA
g. Set patient up for a referral with a urologist

PREVENTION GOALS
a. Patient to have her first Hepatitis B shot today
b. Set patient up for a mammogram

Figure 7-58   Completed A&P for Jane Morgan

15. You note that the patient is to return in 10 days for a follow-up UA.

    a. Schedule a Follow-Up Appointment for Jane Morgan with Dr. Raman for 10 days from her original encounter (**Figure 7-59**). Write "10-day follow up for UA" in the chief complaint. (Refer to Chapter 4, Activity 4-1, if you need to review the instructions for making an appointment.)

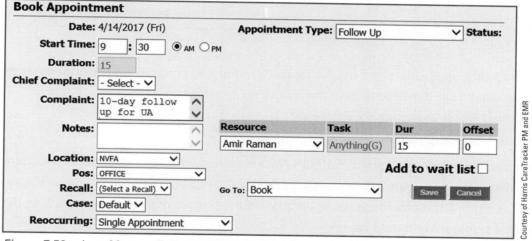

Figure 7-59   Jane Morgan Follow-Up Appointment

16. You will sign the note in Activity 7-20. After both the progress note and billing process are complete, the encounter is deleted from the *Open Encounters* application and is saved under the *Encounter* section of the patient's medical record for reference. Harris CareTracker PM and EMR updates the status of the *Note* and *Visit* columns to "Complete," and "Visit Complete."

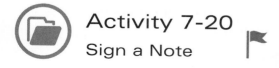

Activity 7-20
Sign a Note

The *Unsigned Notes* application displays a list of progress notes that are not signed or require a co-signature by the provider set in the batch. A co-signature is required when a progress note is documented by a nonphysician provider such as a physician assistant (PA) or a nurse practitioner (NP).

The *Unsigned Notes* application (**Figure 7-60**) is accessible from the following locations:

- *Clinical Today* module >*Tasks* tab >*Unsigned Notes* (from the *Tasks* menu on the right side of the window) or click an unsigned notes task in the *All Tasks* window. You can sort on the *Tasks* column to easily identify unsigned note tasks. (**Note:** If the *Unsigned Note* is not displaying, change the provider to "All" and click the refresh icon.)

- An alternative method is to click the *Clinical Today* module, and then click *Unsigned Notes* from the *Quick Tasks* menu (on the right side of the window).

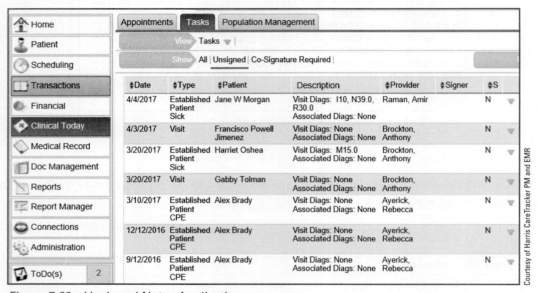

Figure 7-60 Unsigned Notes Application

The *Unsigned Notes* application lists notes that the treating and supervising provider must review and sign. The note can be signed directly from the following locations:

- *Unsigned Notes* application
- *Progress Note* application

It is important to know that once a *Progress Note* is signed, you can no longer make changes to it, and any open items/orders that were not completed prior to signing the note will not display within the A&P. When a note is signed, the provider's name displays at the bottom of the progress note as the treating provider with a signature and date stamp.

To Sign a Note:

Once you have confirmed that all tasks outlined in the *A&P* are completed:

1. Access the *Unsigned Notes* application by clicking on the *Home* module, *Open Encounters* under the *Clinical* column.

2. In the *Encounters* screen, *Note* column you will find Ms. Morgan's note, stating "Not Signed."

3. Click on "Not Signed" in the *Note* column and the progress note launches. **Hint:** If you do not see the note, remember to change the "Resource" (Provider) to *All* and then search.

4. Review the progress note for accuracy then click the *Sign* 🖉 icon.

5. A message prompts to confirm the action (**Figure 7-61**). Click *OK*. (**Note:** Alternatively, you could point to the *Arrow* icon in the *Action* menu and click *Edit Note* to open the note in a new window, review, make changes, and sign or co-sign the note.)

6. Once the *Progress Note* is signed, it will disappear from the *Unsigned Notes* application. **Note:** You may need to click the *Refresh* icon first.

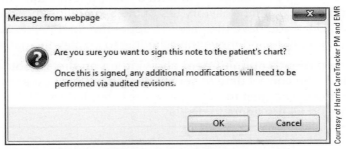

Figure 7-61   Sign Note Pop-Up Window

7. With patient Jane Morgan in context, click on the *Medical Record* module.

8. Click on *Progress Notes* from the *Patient Health History* pane, and select the progress note you created for Jane Morgan. The note launches on the right side of the pane.

9. Click the *Print* 🖪 icon on the *Progress Note* (**Figure 7-62**) tab that you just signed. A dialog box will display where you can select *Print* or *PDF*. Select *Print*.

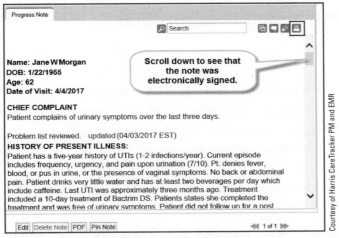

Figure 7-62   Progress Note with Print Icon

🖪 **Print the signed Progress Note. Label it "Activity 7-20," and place it in your assignment folder.**

10. Close the dialog box when you have finished printing.

11. Now access the *Open Encounters* application again from the *Home* module >*Dashboard* tab >*Open Encounters* link (*Clinical* section). Using the drop-down feature next to *Provider*, select *All*, and then click the *Change Resource* icon to refresh the screen. You will note that Jane Morgan's encounter is no longer listed in the *Open Encounters* link.

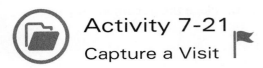

Activity 7-21 ⚑
Capture a Visit

Using what you learned in Activity 7-18, capture the visit for the following patients. This activity is required in order to create the data needed to complete billing and collections activities in Chapters 9 and 10.

TIP Before you begin work, review these helpful hints for capturing visits.

- **What do I do if I can't remember the date of the patient's appointment?** With the patient in context, look in the History tab of the Scheduling module to locate the patient's appointment. Once you have the patient's appointment date, go back to the Book tab of the Scheduling module and move the schedule to display the patient's date of service.
- **Why isn't the patient's appointment showing up on the schedule?** Be sure you moved the schedule to the correct date of service for the patient you are working with. Be sure to set the Resources field (just to the right of the calendar) to "All Resources" in order for the full schedule and all providers to display.

A—Ellen Ristino

1. Using steps you learned throughout this chapter (refer to Activity 7-18), and using the information below, capture the visit for Ellen Ristino for the appointment/encounter you created in Chapter 4.
   - *CPT® Codes*: 99213; 3210F; 36415; 94760; 86308
   - *ICD-10 Codes*: J06.9; J20.9

   Source: Current Procedural Terminology © 2017 American Medical Association.

2. Remember to wait for the pop-up error message to appear before moving on.

Print a screenshot of the completed visit and label it "Activity 7-21A." Place the document in your assignment folder.

B—Craig X. Smith

3. Referring to Activity 7-18, and using the information that follows, capture the visit for patient Craig X. Smith. Refer to the appointment/encounter you created for Mr. Smith in Chapter 4.
   - *CPT® Codes:* 99213; J7650; 71020 (**Note:** for CPT® code J7650 you will need to enter "1" in the *Units* field of the *Visit Summary* screen.)
   - *ICD-10 Code:* R06.2

   Source: Current Procedural Terminology © 2017 American Medical Association.

4. Remember to wait for the pop-up error message to appear before moving on.

Print a screenshot of the completed visit and label it "Activity 7-21B" and place in your assignment folder.

C—Barbara Watson

5. Referring to Activity 7-18, and using the information that follows, capture the visit for patient Barbara Watson. Refer to the appointment/encounter you created for Ms. Watson in Chapter 4.
   - *CPT® Codes:* 99213; 94760
   - *ICD-10 Code:* R50.9

   Source: Current Procedural Terminology © 2017 American Medical Association.

6. Remember to wait for the pop-up error message to appear before moving on.

Print a screenshot of the completed visit and label it "Activity 7-21C." Place the document in your assignment folder.

D—Edith Robinson

7. Referring to Activity 7-18, and using the information that follows, capture the visit for patient Edith Robinson. Refer to the appointment/encounter you created for Ms. Robinson in Chapter 4.

- *CPT ® Code:* 99203
- *ICD-10 Codes:* M54.5; M99.03; M99.05; I10; E11.9

    Source: Current Procedural Terminology © 2017 American Medical Association.

8.   Remember to wait for the pop-up error message to appear before moving on.

💾 **Print a screenshot of the completed visit and label it "Case Study 7-21D." Place the document in your assignment folder.**

E—Alex Brady

9.   Referring to Activity 7-18, and using the information that follows, capture the three visits for patient Alex Brady's encounters. Refer to the *History* tab in the *Scheduling* module to obtain the date/time/provider for Alex's appointments. Use the CPT and ICD-10 codes noted below for the visit dated 09/12/2016:

- *CPT® Code:* 99391
- *ICD-10 Code:* Z00.129

    Source: Current Procedural Terminology © 2016 American Medical Association.

10.   Remember to wait for the pop-up error message to appear before moving on.

11.   Once the visit has been captured, sign the *Progress Note* for Alex Brady's 09/12/2016, encounter. Refer to Activity 7-20 if you need a refresher of the instructions.

💾 **Print screenshots of the completed visits and label them "Activity 7-21E1." Print the signed** *Progress Note* **and label it "Activity 7-21E2." Place all the documents in your assignment folder.**

12.   Now capture the visit for Alex Brady for his encounter dated 12/12/2016. (**Note:** Do <u>not</u> sign the Progress Note for this encounter at this time.)

- *CPT® Code:* 99391
- *ICD-10 Code:* Z00.121

    Source: Current Procedural Terminology © 2017 American Medical Association.

13.   Remember to wait for the pop-up error message to appear before moving on.

💾 **Print a screenshot of the completed visits and label it "Activity 7-21E3." Place the document in your assignment folder.**

14.   Now capture the visit for Alex Brady for his encounter dated 03/10/2017. (**Note:** Do <u>not</u> sign the *Progress Note* for this encounter at this time.)

- *CPT ® Code:* 99391
- *ICD-10 Code:* Z00.121

    Source: Current Procedural Terminology © 2017 American Medical Association.

15.   Remember to wait for the pop-up error message to appear before moving on.

💾 **Print screenshots of the completed visits and label them "Activity 7-21E4." Place the document in your assignment folder.**

F—Francisco Powell Jimenez

16. Referring to Activity 7-18, and using the information that follows, capture the visit for patient Francisco Powell Jimenez. Refer to the appointment/encounter you created for Francisco in Chapter 4.

    - *CPT® Code:* 99214
    - *ICD-10Code:* Z00.129

    Source: Current Procedural Terminology © 2017 American Medical Association.

17. Remember to wait for the pop-up error message to appear before moving on.

💾 **Print screenshots of the completed visit and label it "Activity 7-21F." Place the document in your assignment folder.**

G—Gabby Tolman

You can also capture the visit through the *Clinical Today* module. For Gabby's visit, you will need to access her appointment through the *Clinical Today* module / *Appointments* application.

18. Pull Gabby Tolman into context. Click on the *Clinical Today* module (on the left side of your screen) and set the following search criteria;

    a. Change *Resource* to "All".

    b. Change *Patient* to "All Patients".

    c. Enter "03/20/17" in the *Custom Dates* fields.

    Then click Search.

19. In the row for Gabby Tolman, click on the drop-down arrow next to *Actions*, and select *Visit*.

    - *CPT ® Codes*: 99202
    - *ICD-10Codes*: K59.00 and R39.15

    Source: Current Procedural Terminology © 2017 American Medical Association.

20. Remember to wait for the pop-up error message to appear before moving on.

💾 **Print a screenshot of the completed visit and label it "Activity 7-21G." Place the document in your assignment folder.**

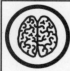 **CRITICAL THINKING** At the beginning of this chapter, you were challenged to learn the proper steps for entering orders into the patient's EMR, to avoid the temptation of entering orders without the provider's approval, and to select the proper codes for the patient's visit. Having completed the activities, what do you rate your level of understanding and proficiency for entering orders and capturing visits with the appropriate codes? Were there any activities that seemed difficult? If yes, what steps did you take to resolve the issue? Did you remember to read through the entire activity first before beginning to enter data? Would you have entered a lab order before the patient was seen by the provider if the reason for the visit was burning and urgent urinary symptoms? Explain your decision.

CASE STUDIES

If the demographic pop-up alerts you to missing information when you pull a patient into context, it is best practice to update as necessary. Update patients' PCP, subscriber numbers, and confirm (Y) to Consent, HIE, and NPP as needed throughout the remainder of your activities and case studies.

Case Study 7-1

Complete an *Order* for a mammogram referral for patient Jane Morgan. Refer to Activity 7-2 for help.

- *Order Type:* Diag. Imaging
- *Ordering Physician*: Dr. Raman
- *Due Date*: The date of the encounter
- *Diagnosis*: Select "Encounter for screening mammogram for malignant neoplasm of breast (Z12.31)" (**Note:** Search under "Mammogram" to locate the diagnosis).
- *New Test*: Search for and select this test from the database "Mammography; bilateral." Do <u>not</u> free text and add your own entry. Patient information is entered into a reminder system with a target due date for the next mammogram (RAD).
- Scroll down under *New Test* and select the type of test ordered (see above "Mammography; bilateral").
- Click *"Add Test."*
- Scroll to the bottom of the *Order* screen. With "Print" selected, click "Save."

📠 **Print the mammogram order for Ms. Morgan. Label it "Case Study 7-1" and place it in your assignment folder.**

Case Study 7-2

To complete Case Study 7-2, you must have completed the case studies from the previous chapters for patient James Smith. If you did not complete the previous case studies for James Smith, skip Case Study 7-2 and complete Case Study 7-3.

Patient James Smith was seen by Dr. Ayerick to review lab and EKG results. Based on the findings in the lab and EKG reports, Dr. Ayerick would like Mr. Smith to see a cardiologist and recommends Dr. Mark Nathan in Walnut Creek, California.

a. Refer patient to Dr. Mark Nathan in Walnut Creek, California, a well-respected Cardiologist (**Note:** you will not select a "Specialty" for this *Referral* and this is not a transition of care). Follow the steps in Activity 7-15 for help.

b. Schedule a follow up appointment for repeat lab work and visit with Dr. Ayerick. Schedule the appointment four weeks from today (refer to Activity 4-1 for help).

c. Now that the visit is complete, capture the visit for James Smith. Use steps you learned in Activity 7-18, and the procedure and diagnosis codes that follow.

- *CPT® Codes:* 99213 and 93000
- *ICD-10 Code:* I48.91; R00.2; and I10

Source: Current Procedural Terminology © 2017 American Medical Association.

d. Once the visit has been captured, sign the *Progress Note* for James Smith. Refer to Activity 7-20 for help if needed.

📠 **Print a screenshot of the Referral, Visit Capture, and signed Progress Note, and label them "Case Study 7-2." Place the documents in your assignment folder.**

(continues)

CASE STUDIES *(continued)*

Case Study 7-3

To complete Case study 7-3 in its entirety, you must have completed Case Study 6-3 for patient Adam Thompson. If you did not complete Case Study 6-3 for Adam Thompson, skip Part A and complete only Part B of Case Study 7-3 (Capture the Visit).

a. Complete the outstanding orders for patient Adam Thompson. Use the steps you learned throughout this chapter and in Activity 7-2 for help. To accurately complete the order, refer to the information contained in the A&P of the *Progress Note* you created for Mr. Thompson in Case Study 6-3 and the information that follows:

 • *Order Type*: Lab

 • *Due Date:* The date of the encounter

 • *Ordering Physician* (select Mr. Thompson's PCP)

 • *Facility*: Select the first facility noted in the drop-down list

 • *Frequency*: Select "Single Order"

 • *Diagnosis*: Select ICD-10 code "Z00.00"

 • *ABN given to Pt:* Yes

 • *Due Date:* The date of the encounter

 • *New Tests*: Add the following tests:

  1) CBC W Auto Differential panel in Blood

  2) Electrolytes 1998 panel in Serum or Plasma

 • *Urgency*: Routine

 • *Fasting*: 12

When the order information has been entered, select "Print" and then click *Save*.

b. Using the information that follows, capture the visit for Adam Thompson. Refer to Activity 7-18 for help if needed.

 • *CPT® Codes*: 99213; 71020; 94760; 93000

 • *ICD-10 Codes:* J18.9; K21.9; I10; M19.90

 Source: Current Procedural Terminology © 2017 American Medical Association.

c. Once the visit has been captured, sign the *Progress Note* for Adam Thompson following the steps in Activity 7-20.

🖫 **Print a copy of the order and label it "Case Study 7-3." Place the document in your assignment folder.**

Other Clinical Documentation

8

Learning Objectives

1. Edit, add an addendum to, sign, and print a *Progress Note*.
2. Manually enter *Results* into the patient's medical record.
3. Record messages in Harris CareTracker PM and EMR.
4. Create and update patient *Recall Letters*.
5. Run an immunization report using the *Clinical Export* feature.

Real-World Connection

In the past, medical assistants have often had the responsibility of retrieving faxed or printed lab results for the provider to review; however, with electronic connectivity, this task will diminish over time. Whether lab results are automatically uploaded to the provider's portal or scanned into the EMR, the medical assistant should always consider the patient's peace of mind. Unfortunately, health care workers often view the retrieval of lab results as secondary to other tasks, but to an anxious patient, the wait can be agonizing. When you have a patient who is anxious about a result, watch for the result and alert the provider once it is available. This will reduce the patient's wait time. You will learn how to enter lab results into the patient's EMR in this chapter, but I urge you to think about the flip side of the result—the patient's peace of mind. Another very important consideration is that as you input data into the *Results* application; think about the integrity of the data entered. Imagine what would happen if you made an entry error that would adversely affect the results and the effect it would have on the patient and patient care.

Before you begin the activities in this chapter, refresh your memory on working with Harris CareTracker by referring back to the Best Practices list on page xiv of this workbook. Following best practices will help you complete work quickly and accurately.

THE *PROGRESS NOTES* APPLICATION

Learning Objective 1: Edit, add an addendum to, sign, and print a Progress Note.

Activity 8-1

Access the *Progress Notes* Application

The *Progress Notes* application allows you to navigate the list of notes saved for the patient and click a note to view and manage from the right pane. A progress note is a document, written by the clinician or provider that describes the details of a patient's encounter and is sometimes referred to as a chart note.

TIP **Important!!** Complete and sign all progress notes before any billing information is submitted to the payers.

The *Progress Notes* application displays a list of notes recorded during each patient visit and progress note–type documents that are uploaded. Progress notes include information such as the patient's history, medications, allergies, as well as a complete record of all that happened during the visit. This information is required for medical, legal, and billing purposes.

You can use the application to browse through all the patient notes, including uploaded notes, on the right pane of the window. When viewing uploaded notes, the right pane displays the document in the *Document Viewer* and fits the width of the pane. However, you can click the *Expand/Collapse* 🔲 icon to control the view.

There are several ways to access the *Progress Notes* application. Use the following method for this activity.

1. Pull patient Alex Brady into context.

2. Click the *Medical Record* module.

3. Click on the *Progress Notes* application in the *Health History* pane. (**Note:** This patient has three visits that were scheduled on 09/12/2016, 12/12/2016, and 03/10/2017.)

4. The *Progress Notes* window displays a list of signed and unsigned notes for the patient (**Figure 8-1**).

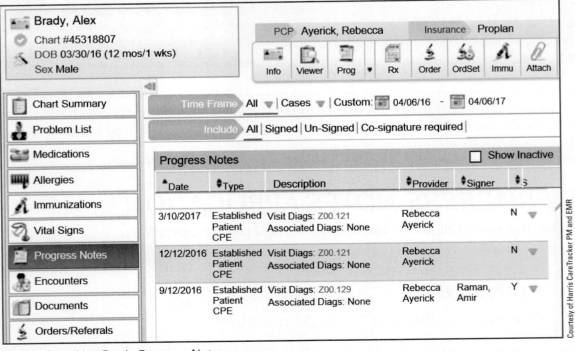

Figure 8-1   Alex Brady Progress Notes

5. On a blank sheet of paper (or new document), write down (or type) the list of the signed and unsigned progress notes for the patient. Label the page "Activity 8-1" and place it in your assignment folder.

Activity 8-2

Access *Progress Notes* from the *Clinical Toolbar*

In addition to the *Progress Notes* application, Harris CareTracker EMR provides quick access to progress notes via two other locations:

- *Progress Note* icon on the *Clinical Toolbar*
- *Select Encounter* dialog box

> **TIP** You can also access the *Progress Note* application by clicking the *Encounters & Progress Notes* section (**Figure 8-2**) title in the *Chart Summary*.

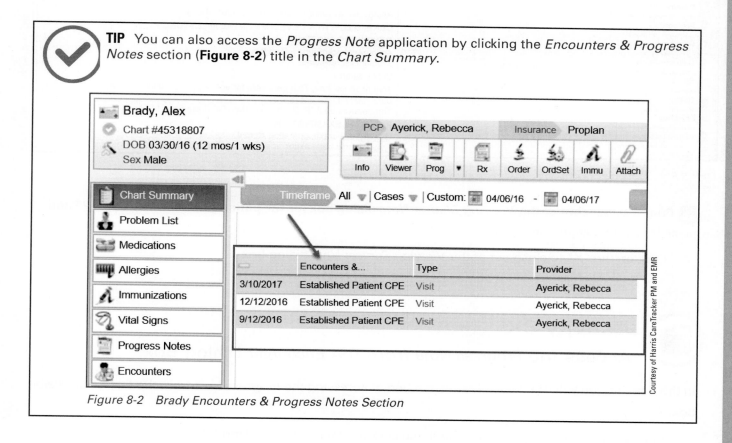

Figure 8-2   Brady Encounters & Progress Notes Section

1. Pull patient Alex Brady into context and click the *Medical Record* module.

2. In the *Clinical Toolbar*, click the *Arrow* ▼ icon next to the *Progress Notes* icon. Harris CareTracker EMR displays the *Note* icon next to the encounters that have a progress note. A pop-up with the *Progress Note* summary will appear.

3. Click the *Note* icon next to the encounter dated September 12, 2016. Harris CareTracker EMR displays the *Viewing Clinical Note* dialog box with the selected progress note to the right of the date (see **Figure 8-3**).

> **ALERT!** You must actually click on the *Note* icon, not just on the encounter date (Figure 8-3) to receive the pop-up summary. If you click on the encounter date, the entire progress note application will pull in to context.

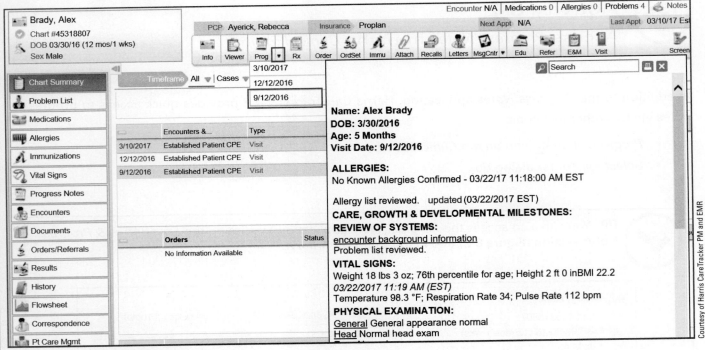

Figure 8-3   *Alex Brady Progress Note*

 Print a screenshot of the *Viewing Clinical Note* dialog box for the patient. Label it "Activity 8-2" and place it in your assignment folder.

4.   Click on the "X" to close out of the *Viewing Clinical Note* dialog box.

Activity 8-3

Access the *Progress Note* from the *Encounter* Dialog Box

In this activity, you will use the alternative method of accessing the *Progress Note* from the *Encounter dialog box.*

1.   Pull patient Jane Morgan into context and click the *Medical Record* module.

2.   In the *Patient Detail* bar, click the *Encounter* link (**Figure 8-4**).

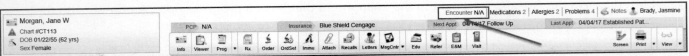

Figure 8-4   *Encounter Link*

Courtesy of Harris CareTracker PM and EMR

3.   Harris CareTracker EMR displays the *Select Encounter* dialog box (**Figure 8-5**). Encounters with progress notes display the *Note* 📝 icon next to the encounter.

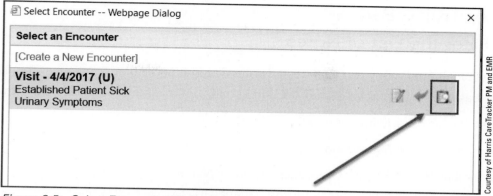

Figure 8-5   Select Encounter Dialog Box

4. Click the *Note* 📋 icon next to the encounter you created for the patient in Chapter 6. Harris CareTracker EMR displays the *View Clinical Note* dialog box with the selected progress note (**Figure 8-6**).

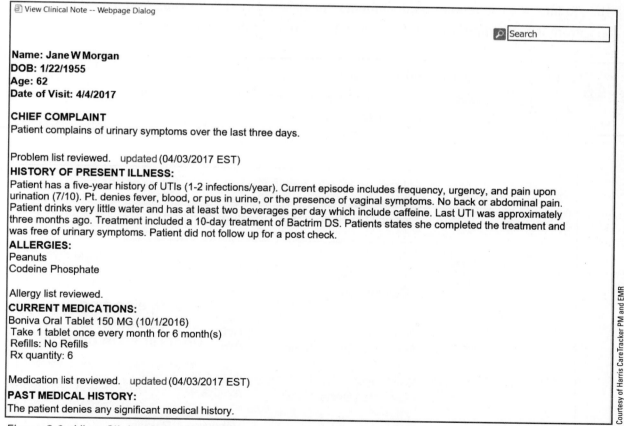

Figure 8-6   View Clinical Note Dialog Box

💾 **Print a screenshot of the *View Clinical Note* dialog box for the patient. Label it "Activity 8-3" and place it in your assignment folder.**

5. Click on the "X" to close the *View Clinical Note* dialog box.

6. Click on the "X" to close the *Select Encounter* dialog box.

Activity 8-4
Filter the List of Notes

The *Progress Notes* application can filter a list of notes documented during a patient encounter. You can filter the list of notes based on the approval status, document date, or the diagnoses associated with the note.

1. Pull patient Alex Brady into context.

2. Click on the *Medical Record* module.

3. In the *Patient Health History* pane, click *Progress Notes.* The *Progress Notes* window displays with a list of signed and unsigned notes for the patient.

4. Practice filtering by doing each of the following (**Figure 8-7**), and then take a screenshot of each for your Activities folder:

   a. To filter the list of notes by approval status, click the *Signed, Un-Signed*, or *Co-signature required* in the *Include* tab just below the *Time Frame* tab

   b. To filter the list of notes by documented date, select *Last Encounter, Past 6 months*, or *Past Year* from the *All* drop-down menu directly to the right of the *Time Frame* tab.

FYI To filter the list of notes by case:

- Click the *second drop-down menu to the right of the Time Frame tab.*
- Select *Cases, All Cases*, or *Default.*

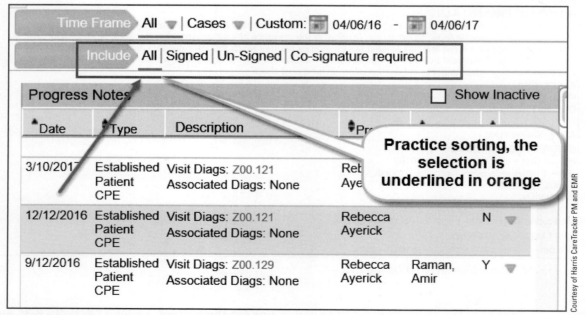

Figure 8-7   Filter the List of Progress Notes

---

   c. To filter the list of notes by diagnoses selected in the *A&P* (Assessment) tab of a progress note:

   i. Select *Diag. Filter* from the *All* drop-down menu to the right of the *Time Frame* tab. Harris CareTracker EMR displays the *Select Diagnosis* dialog box (**Figure 8-8**). (**Note:** If no diagnoses have been entered in the *A&P* (*Assessment* tab) of the *Progress Note*, the dialog box will be blank. If a diagnosis appears, you would select the checkbox pertaining to the diagnosis you want.)

ii. Click *Select*. Harris CareTracker EMR displays the notes associated with the selected diagnoses.

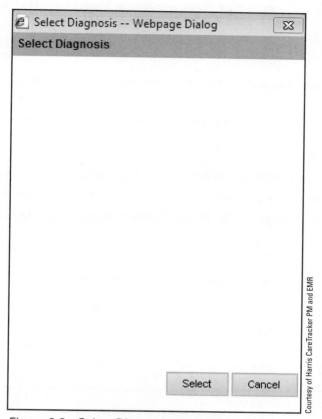

Figure 8-8   Select Diagnosis Dialog Box

 SPOTLIGHT The *Diag. Filter* tab displays all diagnoses selected in the *A&P* (*Assessment*) tab of a progress note when documenting a patient encounter. It does not display the primary diagnosis selected via the *Visit* application.

💾 **Print a screenshot of the filtering methods that displays the Time Frame of "All" and Include Unsigned only. Label it "Activity 8-4" and place it in your assignment folder.**

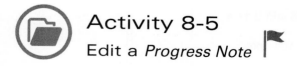 **Activity 8-5**
Edit a *Progress Note* 🚩

Edits can be made to a progress note until it is signed by the provider. If the note requires a co-signature, it can be edited until the supervising provider signs the note. If a note is signed, the template is unavailable to prevent any changes being made to the note. However, the signing provider (you, in this case of student training) can unsign a note to make changes if necessary.

1. In the *Clinical Today* module, set the calendar to December 12, 2016, and click on Alex Brady's name in the *Appointments* window. This will launch his medical record. **Hint:** If you do not see the appointment, you will need to set the *Resources* field (just to the right of the calendar) to "All Resources" using the drop-down to select "All Resources" in order for the full schedule and all providers to display, then click *Search*, and then click on Alex Brady's name in the *Appointments* window.

2. In the *Patient Health History* pane, click *Progress Notes*. Harris CareTracker EMR displays the *Progress Notes* window.

 TIP If you had previously signed the progress note, unsign it so that you can make edits (see Activity 8-9).

3. To edit from the *Actions* menu:

    a. Click the *Arrow* ▼ icon next to the note dated December 12, 2016, and then click *Edit Note*. If the *Copy prior note* dialog box appears, click *Cancel*. Harris CareTracker EMR displays the *Progress Note Template* window (**Figure 8-9**). In the *Template* field, select "9 Month Well Child Visit" if not already displaying.

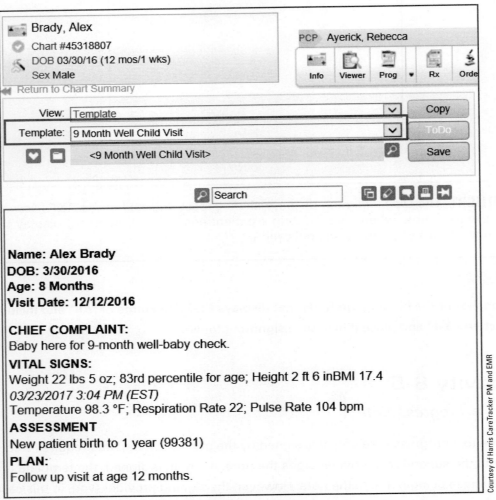

Figure 8-9 Progress Note Template Window

b. Notice that there is only a small amount of information recorded in the *Progress Note*. Refer back to Chapter 6 and, using the steps outlined in Activity 6-16, edit and update the progress note using the information packet for Alex Brady's 9-month exam (see Source Document 8-1, found at the end of this activity).

c. When you have finished entering the data from Source Document 8-1 into the progress note, click *Save*. **Note:** If your screen turns gray, close out of the *Progress Note* window, click back on the patient's medical record and open the *Progress Note*. You will see the information entered has been saved.

d. Sign the note (refer to Activity 7-20 if you need to review the steps). Recall that although your name/operator will display as the signer on the note, in the *Progress Notes* module, the signer will be noted as the provider set in your batch.

4. Using an alternate method (steps a–f following), edit the progress note dated March 10, 2017 from the preview in the *Progress Notes* screen. Repeat steps 1 and 2 of this activity but set the calendar to March 10, 2017 if needed.

a. Click on the progress note (<u>not</u> the *Actions Arrow* icon) you want to edit. Select the progress note dated March 10, 2017. The progress note displays on the right pane of the window.

b. Click *Edit* at the bottom of the screen (**Figure 8-10**).

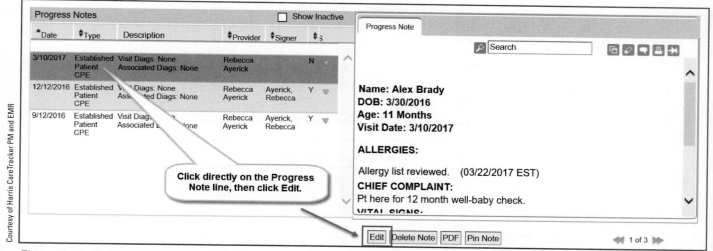

Courtesy of Harris CareTracker PM and EMR

Figure 8-10   Edit Button on Progress Note

c. If the *Copy prior note* dialog box displays, click *Cancel*. The *Progress Note* window launches, enabling you to edit the unsigned note. **Note:** If this *Progress Note* has already been signed, first *Unsign* it and then make your edits.

d. Using the steps outlined in Activity 6-16, edit the note using the information packet for Alex Brady's 12-month exam (see Source Document 8-2, found at the end of this activity).

e. When you have finished entering the data from Source Document 8-2, click *Save*.

f. Now sign the note.

📇 **Print the edited progress notes. Label the December 12, 2016 progress note "Activity 8-5a" and the March 10, 2017, progress note "Activity 8-5b," and then place them in your assignment folder.**

Source Document 8-1

PATIENT'S NAME: Alex Brady

DATE OF BIRTH: 03/30/2016 (**Note:** Since patient Alex Brady's date of birth is fixed in the database, his age may show as older than 9 months when you are completing this activity. However, he was 9 months old at the time of his December 2016 appointment.)

PROVIDER: Dr. Ayerick

PROGRESS NOTE

Template: Pediatric: 9-month well-child visit (You may need to search for this template)

Tab	Entry
Interval History	*Accompanied by:* Mother *Concerns and Questions:* Mother has no questions or concerns at this time. *Interval History:* Pt. is here a bit early for son's 9-month visit. Family will be out of the country for the next two months so mother wanted to bring Alex in before leaving for their trip.
ROS	**Nutrition** Select "Y" for *breast fed* *Times per day:* 3 *Minutes per side:* 10 Check the following boxes: *Drinks from cup, source of water, solid foods, juice* Add comment to the *solid foods* note box: "Eats approximately 3 jars of baby food/day. Solid foods include cereal with applesauce, peas, squash, and bananas." **Elimination** *Wet diapers per day:* 6 *Bowel movements per day:* 1 **Sleep** Select "Y" for *sleeping through the night* **Development** *Gross Motor:* Select "Y" for *sits well*, and *crawls*; Select "N" for *pulls to feel with support* *Fine motor:* Select "Y" for *Feeds self, bangs objects together*, and *pincer grasp* *Communication:* Select "Y" for *Responds to name, waves bye-bye*, and *imitates sound* *Social:* Select "Y" for *Peekaboo, Patty-cake*, and *Stranger anxiety*
PE	**Vital Signs** *Weight:* 22 lbs 05 oz *Height:* 30 in 76.2 cm *Temperature:* 98.3 F *Heart Rate:* 104 bpm *Respiration Rate:* 22 **Physical Examination** Select "N" for normal for all categories except female genitalia (leave that blank)
Anticipatory Guidance	*Nutrition:* Select "avoid choke foods" *Injury Prevention:* Select "crib safety," "choking hazards," "First Aid, CPR," and "sun exposure"
Assess & Plan	Assessment: Click on the box beside "established patient birth to 1 year (99391)" Immunizations: Click on the box beside "DTap-HepB-IPV (90723)" *Plan:* Click on the drop-down box beside *Follow-up/Next Visit* and select "3 months"

Source Document 8-2

PATIENT'S NAME: Alex Brady

DATE OF BIRTH: 03/30/2016 (**Note:** Since patient Alex Brady's date of birth is fixed in the database, his age may show as older than 12 months when you are completing this activity. However, he was 12 months old at the time of his March 2017 appointment.)

PROVIDER: Dr. Ayerick

PROGRESS NOTE

Template: Pediatric: 12-month well-child visit (You will need to search for this template.)

Tab	Entry
Interval History	*Accompanied by:* Father *Concerns and Questions:* Father has no questions or concerns at this time.
ROS	***Nutrition*** Select "N" for *breast fed.* Add comment to the *breast fed* note box: "Mom stopped breast feeding last month. Patient has adjusted well according to dad." Select "Y" for the following: *Drinks from cup, table foods, finger foods* ***Elimination*** *Wet diapers per day:* 6 *Bowel movements per day:* 2 ***Sleep*** Select "Y" for *sleeping through the night* ***Development*** *Gross Motor:* Select "Y" for *walks without assistance,* and *stands well alone* *Fine motor:* Select "Y" for *has a pincer grasp, bangs objects together, scribbles spontaneously* *Communication:* Select "Y" for *says mama/dada specifically, imitates simple daily tasks, language at 12 months* *Social:* Select "Y" for *plays pat-a-cake, waves bye-bye*
PE	***Vital Signs*** *Weight:* 21 lbs *Length 33 in / 83.8 cm* *Temperature:* 98.2 F *Heart Rate:* 100 bpm *Respiration Rate:* 22 ***Physical Examination*** Select "N" for normal for all categories except female genitalia (leave that blank)
Anticipatory Guidance	*Nutrition:* Select "whole milk," "healthy food choices," and "nutritious snacks, limit sweets" *Social competence:* Select "toilet training" *Injury Prevention:* Select "electrical outlets"
Assess & Plan	Click on the box beside "established patient birth to 1 year (99391)" *Immunizations:* Select "DTAP/HIB/IPV (90698)," "Polio Virus Vaccine (90713)," and "Measles, Mumps, Rubella Vaccine (90707)." Click on the drop-down box beside *Follow-up/Next Visit* and select "1 Month." *Plan:* Enter "Will bring patient back in for a weight check in 30 days."

Activity 8-6

Delete a *Progress Note*

You can only delete unsigned notes. When a note is signed, *Delete Notes* appears dimmed.

In a recent audit, you discovered a progress note from the year 2013 that was entered in error. To correct the error, you will delete the progress note.

1. Pull patient Donald Schwartz into context.

2. Click on the *Medical Record* module.

3. In the *Patient Health History* pane, click *Progress Notes*. Harris CareTracker EMR displays the *Progress Notes* window.

4. Click the progress note you want to delete. Select the note dated May 14, 2013. The progress note displays on the right pane of the window.

5. Click *Delete Note* (**Figure 8-11**). Harris CareTracker EMR displays the *Void* dialog box.

6. Select *Delete Reason*: "Other" (**Figure 8-12**).

7. You will be prompted to enter a reason. Enter "Test Activity 8-6."

8. Click *Save*. (**Note:** It may take a few moments for the note to be deleted.)

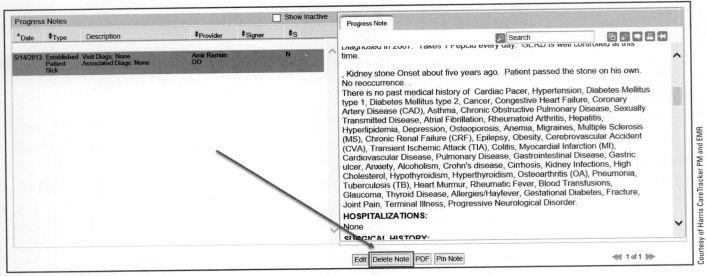

Figure 8-11   Delete Note Tab

Figure 8-12   Delete Reason Dialog Box

TIP A record of the deleted note is maintained in the *Clinical Log*. To access the *Clinical Log*, click the drop-down arrow next to the *View* 👓 icon at the top right of the *Chart Summary* screen, and then select *View Clinical Log*. The *View Log* dialog box will display (**Figure 8-13**). **Note:** You may need to adjust the *Time Frame* parameters to include the date of the *Progress Note* you deleted.

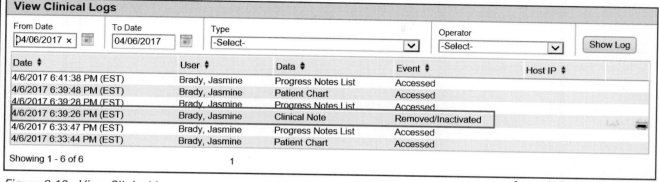

View Clinical Logs

Date ⬍	User ⬍	Data ⬍	Event ⬍	Host IP ⬍
4/6/2017 6:41:38 PM (EST)	Brady, Jasmine	Progress Notes List	Accessed	
4/6/2017 6:39:48 PM (EST)	Brady, Jasmine	Patient Chart	Accessed	
4/6/2017 6:39:28 PM (EST)	Brady, Jasmine	Progress Notes List	Accessed	
4/6/2017 6:39:26 PM (EST)	Brady, Jasmine	Clinical Note	Removed/Inactivated	
4/6/2017 6:33:47 PM (EST)	Brady, Jasmine	Progress Notes List	Accessed	
4/6/2017 6:33:44 PM (EST)	Brady, Jasmine	Patient Chart	Accessed	

Showing 1 - 6 of 6   1

Figure 8-13   View Clinical Logs   Courtesy of Harris CareTracker PM and EMR

📠 **Print a screenshot of the *Clinical Log*, which shows the deleted progress note (see Tip box above). Label it "Activity 8-6" and place it in your assignment folder.**

9. Close out of the *View Clinical Logs* dialog box by clicking on the "X" in the upper-right-hand corner.

 # Activity 8-7
Add an Addendum to a *Progress Note*

You can add an addendum to both a signed and an unsigned note to accommodate any clinical workflow your practice follows. An addendum is text that is added to a progress note after it is signed. The addendum displays at the end of the original progress note and helps track updates made to the note. Additionally, the "Addended By" label displays with the operator's name and the date and time of the addendum. This tracks changes made to the note and the person responsible for the change.

1. Pull patient Harriet Oshea into context.

2. Click on the *Medical Record* module.

3. In the *Patient Health History* pane, click *Progress Notes*. Harris CareTracker EMR displays the *Progress Notes* window.

4. Click the progress note to which you want to add an addendum. Select the note dated March 20, 2017. The progress note displays on the right pane of the window.

5. Click the *Add Addendum* 💬 icon. Harris CareTracker EMR displays the *Add Clinical Note Addendum* dialog box. (**Note:** If you receive an error message, close the dialog box and click on the *Add Addendum* icon again until the prompt displays.)

6. Enter additional note: "Pt requests referral to Dr. Robert Rovner for Orthopedic evaluation" (**Figure 8-14**).

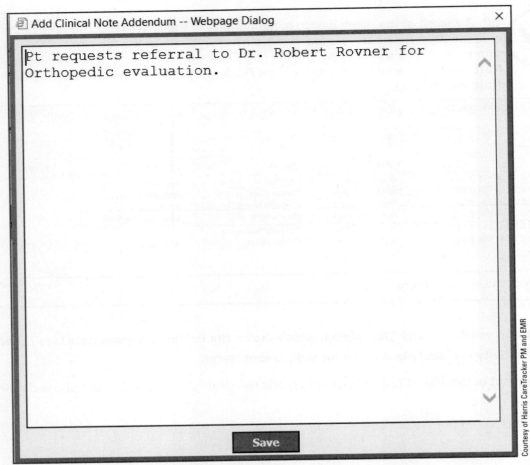

Figure 8-14   *Harriet Oshea Addendum Text*

7. Click *Save*.

 SPOTLIGHT   You can also choose to dictate the addendum or use the quick text feature to enter additional notes.

8. In the right pane, scroll to the bottom of the progress note where the *Addendum* has been added (**Figure 8-15**).

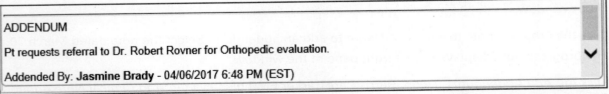

ADDENDUM

Pt requests referral to Dr. Robert Rovner for Orthopedic evaluation.

Addended By: **Jasmine Brady** - 04/06/2017 6:48 PM (EST)

Figure 8-15   *Harriet Oshea Addendum Added to Note*   Courtesy of Harris CareTracker PM and EMR

Print the progress note that now reflects the Addendum. Label it "Activity 8-7" and place it in your assignment folder.

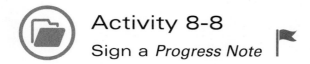

Activity 8-8
Sign a *Progress Note* ⚑

Having previously learned to sign the progress note in Chapter 7 (Activity 7-20), you will now sign the progress note(s) you have worked on in this chapter. (**Note**: Before you sign a progress note, be sure the visit has been captured with CPT® and ICD codes entered. Refer to Activity 7-18 if you need to review these steps.)

Before signing the progress note, with the encounter in context, first confirm that there is a captured *Visit* with the CPT® and ICD codes already entered (following instructions from Activity 7-18).

1. Pull patient Harriet Oshea into context.

2. Click on the *Medical Record* module.

3. In the *Patient Health History* pane, click *Progress Notes*. Harris CareTracker EMR displays the *Progress Notes* window.

4. Click the progress note you want to sign. Select the note dated March 20, 2017.

5. (Optional) Click on the *Expand* 🔲 icon to maximize the readability of the progress note you are viewing. You can click the icon again to collapse the narrative.

6. (Optional) As Best Practice, you would confirm that the addendum to the note has been added as instructed in Activity 8-7.

7. Click the *Sign* ✎ icon on the right pane of the window to sign the note.

8. Harris CareTracker EMR will display a pop-up window asking "Are you sure you want to sign this note to the patient's chart?" Click *OK*.

9. Harris CareTracker EMR will update the status of the note. When complete, you will note the electronic signature stamp at the bottom of the progress note (**Figure 8-16**).

Electronically Signed By: Jasmine Brady
Electronically signed: 4/6/2017 6:55:44 PM

Figure 8-16   Electronically Signed Progress Note

💾 **Print the signed progress note. Label it "Activity 8-8" and place it in your assignment folder.**

Activity 8-9
Unsign a *Progress Note*

You can unsign a signed note, if necessary. However, only the operator who signed the note is allowed to unsign a note based on the operator's role. Enter a reason for unsigning the note if required to complete the action. For audit purposes, a copy of the original note is maintained in the patient's clinical log.

1. After signing Ms. Oshea's progress note in the previous activity, you realize that Dr. Brockton is the provider who needs to sign the note, not you.

2. To unsign the note, with patient Harriet Oshea in context, click the *Medical Record* module.

3. In the *Patient Health History* pane, click *Progress Notes*. Harris CareTracker EMR displays the *Progress Notes* window.

4. Click the progress note you want to unsign. Select the note dated March 20, 2017. The progress note displays on the right pane of the window.

5. Click the *Unsign* 🖉 icon. Harris CareTracker EMR displays a confirmation message.

6. Click *OK* to unsign the note.

7. In the *Progress Notes* window, the note will now be listed as unsigned (**Figure 8-17**).

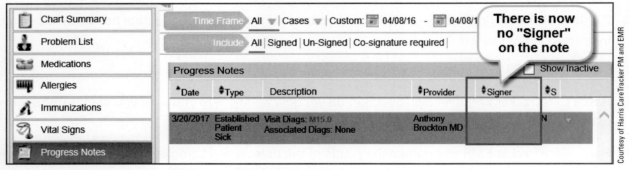

Figure 8-17   *Progress Note Window—Unsigned Note*

 Print a screenshot of the unsigned progress note. Label it "Activity 8-9" and place it in your assignment folder.

8. Now sign the progress note once again and save it so you can use this encounter in later activities.

Activity 8-10
Print the *Progress Note*

To print the progress note, follow the instructions:

1. With patient Harriet Oshea in context, click the *Medical Record* module.

2. In the *Patient Health History* pane, click *Progress Notes*. Harris CareTracker EMR displays the *Progress Notes* window.

3. With the March 20, 2017 progress note in context, use each of the following three print functions:

    a. Print from the *Actions* menu:

- Click the *Arrow* ▼ icon and click *Print*. Harris CareTracker EMR displays the *Clinical Note* dialog box.
- Click *Print*. A copy of the notes prints to the printer attached to your computer.
- Close out of the print dialog box when finished.

    b. Print from the preview in the right pane:

- Click the progress note you want to print. The progress note displays on the right pane of the window.
- Click the *Print* 🖫 icon. Harris CareTracker EMR displays the *Clinical Note* dialog box.
- Click *Print*. A copy of the note prints to the printer attached to your computer.
- Close out of the print dialog box when finished.

    c. Create a PDF of the progress note:

- Click the progress note you want to convert to PDF. The progress note displays on the right pane of the window.
- Click *PDF* at the bottom of the screen. Harris CareTracker EMR creates a PDF version of the documented progress note. You can print or save a copy.
- Close out of the print dialog box when finished.

🖫 **Print the progress note using each of the methods in the activity. Label the pages "Activity 8-10a," "Activity 8-10b," and "Activity 8-10c" and place them in your assignment folder.**

ACCESS AND RECORD RESULTS

Learning Objective 2: Manually enter *Results* into the patient's medical record.

Activity 8-11
Enter Results Manually

The *Open Orders* application enables you to manually enter the results of lab tests into the system or automatically download them from the facility. If the delivery method of results includes fax, phone, paper, or download, you must manually enter the results for the specific order. This automatically updates the order status and the results in the patient's medical record. When the result is entered, both the order and the result are removed from the *Open Orders* application under *Quick Tasks* and the *Open Activities* section of the *Chart Summary* in the *Medical Record* module.

    The *Results* application is where lab and radiology results are displayed. The medical assistant should monitor results on a continuous basis, determining that results are received, reviewed, and handled in an efficient manner. Be certain to reset the *Provider* field to *All* and then click *Search*. Results received electronically are saved in the following locations:

- *Home* module > *Dashboard* tab > *Clinical* section > *Results* link
- *Clinical Today* module > *Tasks* tab > *Results* (from the *Tasks* menu on the right side of the window) (**Figure 8-18**)

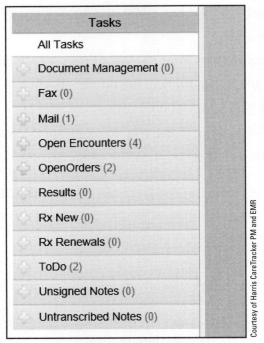

Tasks
All Tasks
Document Management (0)
Fax (0)
Mail (1)
Open Encounters (4)
OpenOrders (2)
Results (0)
Rx New (0)
Rx Renewals (0)
ToDo (2)
Unsigned Notes (0)
Untranscribed Notes (0)

Courtesy of Harris CareTracker PM and EMR

Figure 8-18   Results in Tasks Pane

- *Open Activities* section of the *Chart Summary*
- *Results* section of the *Chart Summary.*

In this activity, you will perform only an abbreviated results entry in the *Office Tests* section of the *Tests* tab in the *Progress Note.*

1. Pull patient Jane Morgan into context.

2. Click on the *Medical Record* module.

3. Access the *Progress Note* for the appointment/encounter you created for Ms. Morgan in Chapter 4.

4. If you had previously signed Ms. Morgan's *Progress Note*, unsign the note, following the steps in Activity 8-9, then click *Edit.*

5. Select the *TESTS* tab of the *Progress Note.*

6. In the *Office Tests* field enter "Negative" into the *Rapid Streptococcus Group Identification (Kit)* field drop-down at the top of the *Tests* tab of the *Progress Note.*

7. Click on *Save.*

8. Sign the *Progress Note.*

Print the Progress Note that displays the Rapid Strep Test result, and label it "Activity 8-11", and place it in your assignment folder.

RECORDING MESSAGES

Learning Objective 3: Record messages in Harris CareTracker PM and EMR.

In Chapter 2, you were introduced to the *Message Center* where you created *ToDos* and *Mail* messages and viewed *Queues* and *Fax* options. In this chapter, we expand on your previous activities: simulate the office environment and workflows, and record patient messages in Harris CareTracker PM and EMR.

Activity 8-12
Access the *Messages* Application

The *Messages* application is a communication tool accessed via the patient's medical record that allows you to manage customer, staff, and patient communications.

Use the steps outlined in this activity to access the *Messages* application each time you are instructed to create a *ToDo* or *Mail* message. The *ToDo* application is also accessible by clicking the *ToDo* 🗹 icon or the *ToDo* button in other applications accessed via the patient's medical record.

1. Pull patient Jane Morgan into context and click the *Medical Record* module.

2. In the *Clinical Toolbar*, click the drop-down arrow next to *Msg Cntr* 🗹 and select *New ToDo*. Harris CareTracker EMR displays the *New ToDo* dialog box.

📇 Print a screenshot of the *ToDos* screen, label it "Activity 8-12", and place it in your assignment folder.

3. Click "X" in the top right corner of the window to close it.

SPOTLIGHT You can use templates to create preformatted content for *ToDos*, faxes, and mail messages. For example, you can create a standard mail message used for outgoing referrals. Anytime that template is selected, the mail message is automatically populated with the text in the template. Templates help improve workflow, and are discussed in detail in Chapter 2.

Activity 8-13
Create a *ToDo*

ToDos are Harris CareTracker PM and EMR's internal messaging system that serves two primary functions: assigning a co-worker a task and communicating with the Harris CareTracker PM and EMR support team. You can also view *ToDos* for a patient if the *Messages* application is accessed when a patient is in context.

In Chapter 2, you created a "test" *ToDo* (see Activity 2-14). Now you will create a clinical *ToDo* related to EMR.

1. Pull patient Harriet Oshea into context.

2. Click on the *Medical Record* module.

3. Click on the *Msg Center* 🗹 icon in the *Clinical Toolbar*. This will launch the *New ToDo* window.

4. By default, the *From* list displays your operator name/number.

5. Of the options available in the *To* list, select "Operator."

6. If a patient is in context when sending a *ToDo*, the patient's name displays in the *Patient* box. If no patient is in context, click the *Search* 🔍 icon next to the *Patient* list. The *Patient Search* dialog box displays, enabling you to enter the required parameters to search for the patient. Patient Harriet Oshea should be in context.

7. By default, the *Subject* box displays information based on the selection in the *Type* and *Reason* lists. However, you can change the subject if necessary. Leave as is.

8. In the *Due Date* and *Due Time* boxes, enter the date and time by which the *ToDo* must be completed. This is important to track overdue items. Change to the date Ms. Oshea called the office requesting the referral (use today's date). Leave *Due Time* box blank.

9. From the *Template* list, select the template you want to use. Leave this blank.

10. From the *Category* list, select the appropriate *ToDo* category. (For example, if the *ToDo* created is for the Harris CareTracker PM and EMR *Support* entity, select "Support Center" from the *Category* list.) Select "Interoffice" for this activity.

11. By default, the *Type* list displays "EHR." Leave as is.

12. In the *Reason* field, use the drop-down and select "Phone Call (Patient)."

13. In the *Severity* list, click the priority of the *ToDo*. Select "Medium." Click the *Info* i icon to view a description of each severity level.

14. By default, the *Status* list is set to "Open." Leave as is.

15. Leave the *Duration* box blank.

16. In the *Notes* box, enter additional notes pertaining to the *ToDo*. You can format the note and spell-check the note entered. This is similar to the formatting toolbar in MS Word®. Enter the following text regarding referral to Dr. Rovner. "Patient called saying that her hip and back pain has increased and is requesting referral to Orthopedic Specialist. She has a friend that sees Dr. Robert Rovner in San Ramon and is very happy with him. Can you arrange a referral to Dr. Rovner? Her insurance does not require authorization." (**Figure 8-19**)

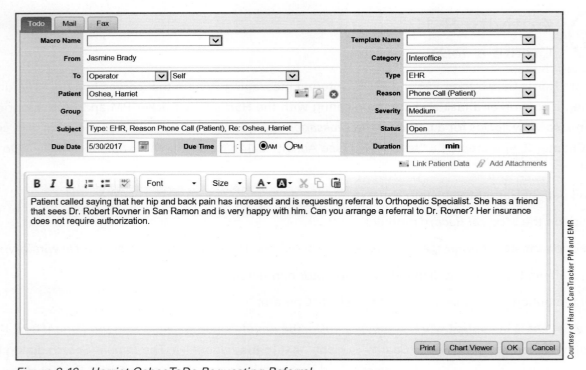

Figure 8-19   Harriet Oshea ToDo Requesting Referral

17. Click *OK*.

18. Refresh your *Home* module screen. The *ToDo* will be listed in the bottom left corner of the screen. Click on the *ToDo* link to view the *ToDo List* window (**Figure 8-20**).

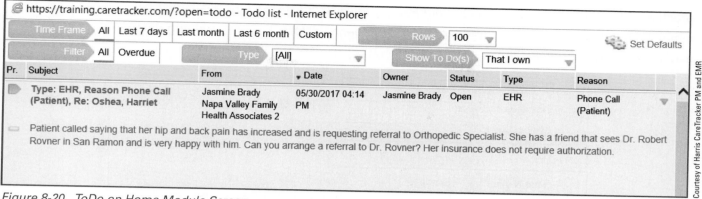

Figure 8-20   ToDo on Home Module Screen

19. Now repeat the activity and create *ToDo* as listed in **Table 8-1**. For the *ToDo* in **Table 8-1** use the *Category* "Interoffice," *Type* "EHR," and *Reason* "Phone Call (Patient)."

Table 8-1   New *ToDo* Messages

FROM	TO	SUBJECT	REASON/SEVERITY	NOTES (MESSAGE)	PATIENT
You	You *(in an actual practice, you would send this message to the provider)*	Fall/Refer to X-ray	Phone Call (Patient)/ High	Patient fell at home and hand is in extreme pain. He wants to know if he can get an X-ray in the office today, or if he should go to Urgent Care. Please call on cell phone ASAP. OK to leave message.	Domenic Scott

Courtesy of Harris CareTracker PM and EMR

 Print a screenshot of the contents of the *ToDo* you created. Label it "Activity 8-13," and place it in your assignment folder.

Activity 8-14
Create a Mail Message

The *Mail* application is similar to any standard email application and allows you to send, receive, organize, and reply to mail messages. In Chapter 2, Activity 2-15, you created a "Test Mail Message". This chapter expands by creating new *Mail* messages that mimic clinical workflows.

The *Mail* application allows you to communicate electronically with staff members, providers in your *Provider Portal,* and patients activated in the *Patient Portal.* The mail feature works similarly to other email applications, enabling you to open, view, create, send and receive, and delete messages. In Harris CareTracker PM and EMR, the mail application is a secure messaging system that users can participate in by invitation only and allows a user to send secure messages outside of the Harris CareTracker system to patients through the patient portal or to referring doctors who are part of the referral network. This is different from email because it is on a secure server, but the use and functions within the mail system are similar to standard email. In addition, you can link attachments such as patient encounter notes, documents, results, referrals, and authorization forms and set priorities and more. As a general rule, the *Mail* feature should only be used when sending a message to someone outside the practice, for example, to refer to providers (outside the practice), or to patients active in the *Patient Portal.* **Figure 8-21** lists the tabs available to use when selecting a mail recipient (*My Company, Provider Portal,* or *Patients*). (**Note:** For your training environment, you will use only the *My Company* tab.)

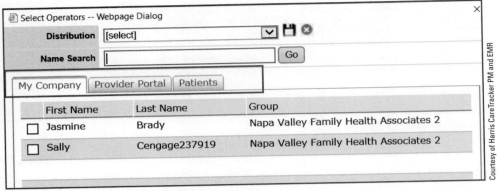

Figure 8-21   *Select Mail Recipients*

TIP   Important!! If you want a task to be completed by a specific person within the practice, send a *ToDo* and not a *Mail* message.

SPOTLIGHT   If sending *Mail* messages to a patient, be sure to follow HIPAA policy and protocol.

This will be a simulated activity because your student version of Harris CareTracker does not include an active *Patient Portal* or *Provider Portal*. For this activity, you will remain in the *My Company* tab.

1. With no patient in context, click the *Home* module.

2. Click on the *Messages* tab. The *Messages Center* opens and displays all of your open *ToDos*.

3. Click *Send Mail* in the bottom right corner of the screen (**Figure 8-22**), which opens the *New Mail* dialog box.

FYI   The *From* list defaults to the operator creating the mail message (you) and cannot be edited.

---

4. In the *To* field, click the *Search* 🔍 icon. Harris CareTracker PM and EMR opens the *Select Operators* dialog box. You will be the only operator available to select (along with any operators you have created). In a live environment, you would select the most appropriate person (this could also be a provider or a patient). Check the box next to your operator name or number, and click *Select* at the bottom of the screen.

5. If a patient is in context, the patient's name displays in the *Patient* box. However, you can also send a mail message about a different patient by clicking on the *Search* 🔍 icon. You can delete a patient from the list by clicking the *Remove Patient* ⊗ icon. There should be no patient in context, so leave the *Patient* field blank.

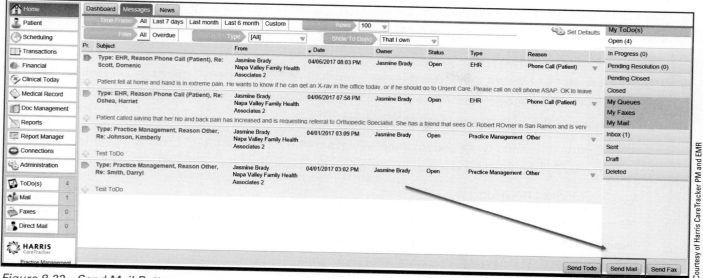

Figure 8-22   Send Mail Button

6. In the *Subject* box, enter "Cardiology Group Presentation." If the subject is patient related, be sure the correct patient's name displays in the *Subject* box. If the message does not relate to a patient, be sure to remove the patient's name. Remove any patient from the *Subject* box.

7. By default, the *Severity* list displays "Medium." However, you can change the priority of the mail message if necessary. Leave as is.

8. In the *Notes* box, enter the message and format the information as directed in **Figure 8-23**. "Hello Dr. Raman, the Napa Valley Cardiology Group would like to make a presentation at your next providers meeting. Would you like me to arrange it? Thanks." (Sign the note with your operator name/number.)

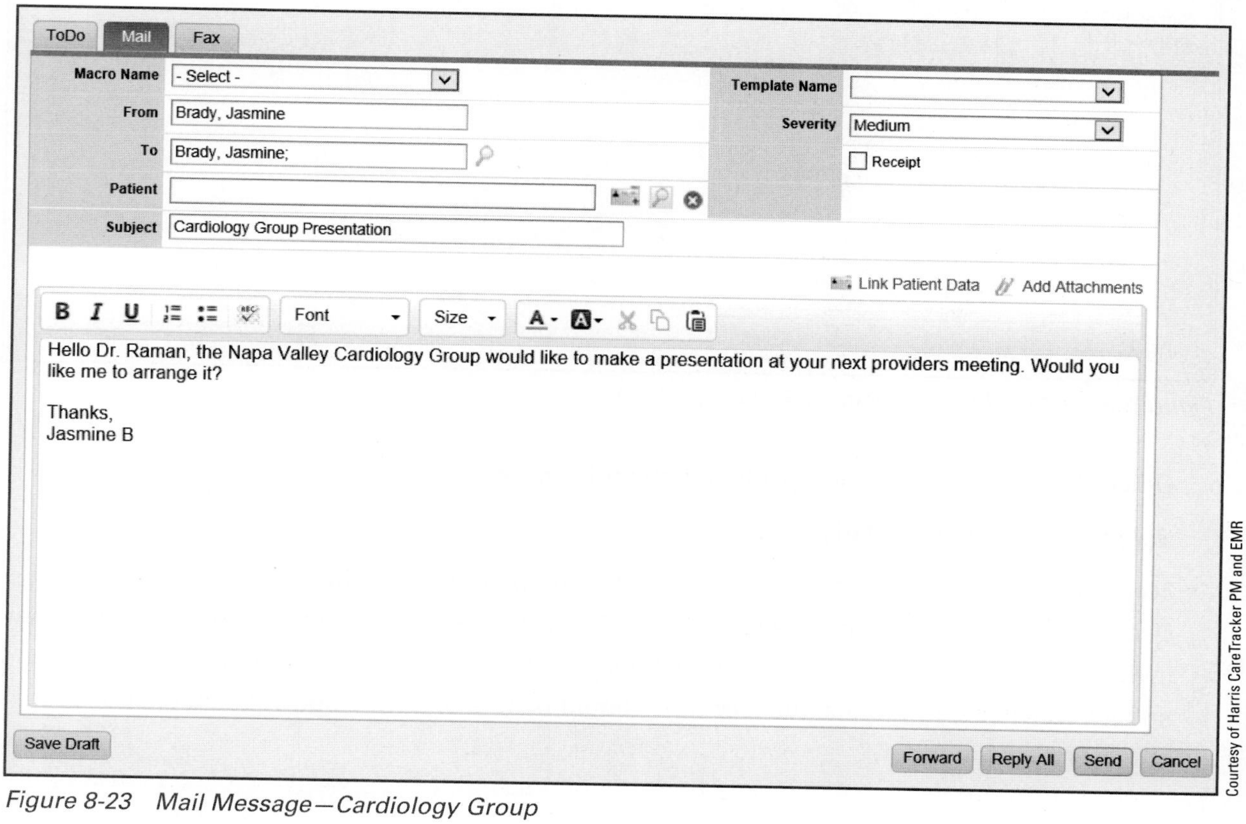

Figure 8-23   Mail Message—Cardiology Group

9. Click *Send* to send the mail message to the selected operators. The message(s) you created will now appear in your *Inbox* (see **Figure 8-26**) listed under *My ToDo(s)* on the right-hand side of the screen.

10. Repeat these steps to create the "Patient Portal" and "Office Holiday Party" messages in **Figures 8-24 and 8-25**. Figure 8-26 shows your *Inbox* with all these messages. You would click the + sign to expand the message and the–sign to collapse the message.

a. Patient Portal message (with patient Jane Morgan in the *Patient* field): ***This is a simulated mail message as Patient Portal is not active in the student version of Harris CareTracker***

Subject: Medical Records

Message Text: "Hello Ms. Morgan, your medical records have been copied and mailed per your request. If there is anything else I can do for you, please let me know. Sincerely, (your operator name/number)"

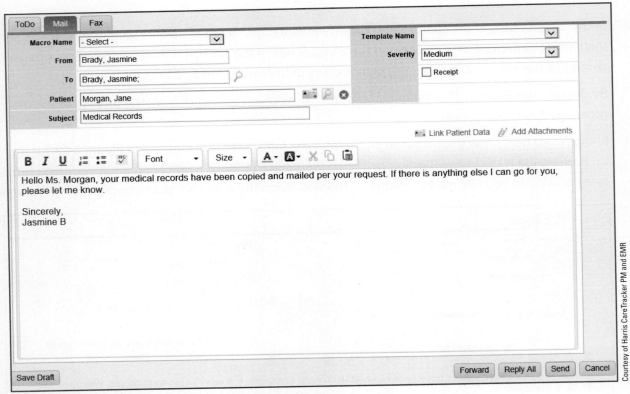

Figure 8-24   *Mail Message—Patient Portal Simulation*

b. Office Holiday Party message (with no patient in context):

Subject: Office Holiday Party

Message Text: "Hello all Providers and Staff. We are planning an Office Holiday Party on December 15th. Reservations have been made at Vic Stuart's Restaurant for 6:30 p.m. You may invite a guest as well. Please respond no later than December 1st if you are planning to attend and if you will be bringing a guest or not. Should be lots of fun!! Hope you can attend. Best, (your operator name/number)"

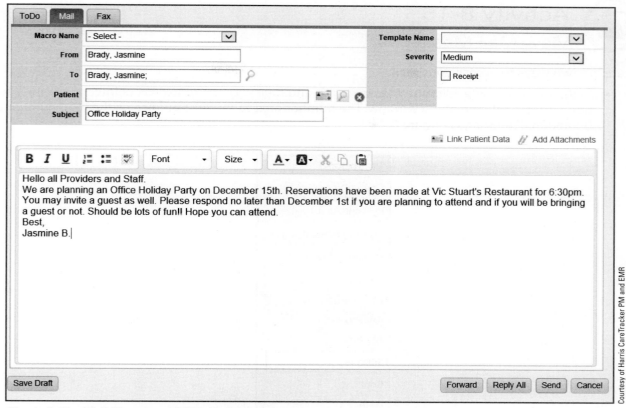

Figure 8-25   Mail Message—Office Holiday Party

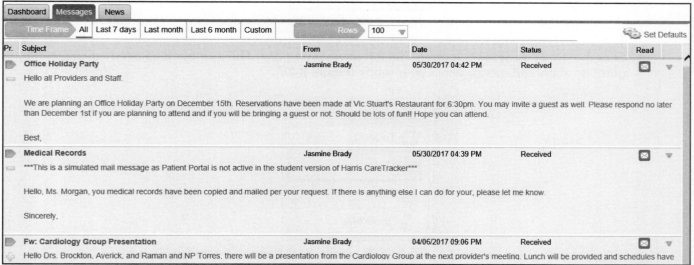

Figure 8-26   Mail Messages in Inbox

 Print the screen that displays the contents of each mail message by clicking on the *Inbox* under *My ToDo(s)* on the right-hand side of the screen. Label it "Activity 8-14" and place it in your assignment folder.

PROFESSIONALISM CONNECTION

When a patient sends you an electronic mail message, always respond as quickly as possible, even if you do not have an answer. This demonstrates that the patient's question is important and that you are handling it. Follow through with what you conveyed in the return email so that the patient does not lose trust in your word.

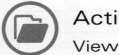

Activity 8-15
View Mail Messages

There are two ways to access your mail:

- In the *Home* module, click the *Messages* tab and then click the *Inbox* link below the *My Mail* section on the right side of the window. The number next to the *Inbox* indicates the total number of unread mail messages (**Figure 8-27**).

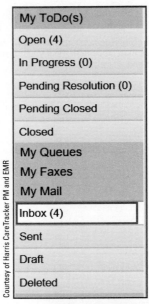

Figure 8-27   Access Mail Messages from the Inbox Link

- Click the *Mail* link at the bottom of the left navigation pane. The number displayed indicates the number of unread messages in your inbox (**Figure 8-28**).

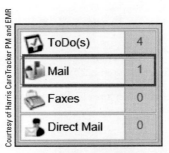

Figure 8-28   Access Mail Messages from the Mail Link

To View Mail Messages:

1. Access your mail messages from the *Home* module.

2. Click the *Messages* tab.

3. Click on the *Inbox* link below the *My Mail* section on the right side of the window. (**Note:** You may have to refresh your screen for the recent activity to display.)

4. Click on the plus sign [+] next to the messages to quickly review the message thread without opening the message.

5. Now click the minus sign [–] to close the thread (**Figure 8-29**).

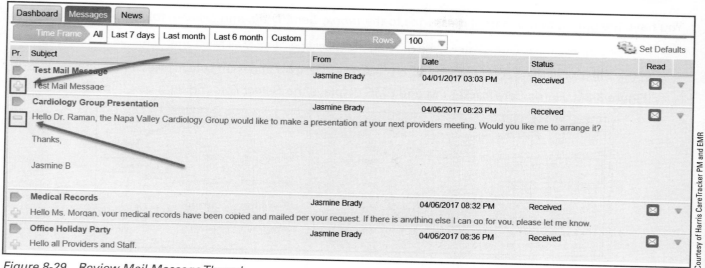

Figure 8-29   *Review Mail Message Thread*

6. To open the mail message, either click on the *Subject* line or point to the *Arrow* ▼ icon at the far right end of the row, and then select "Open." Harris CareTracker PM and EMR opens the message.

7. From the *Actions* column you can choose to move to folder, open, delete, reply, reply all, or forward (**Figure 8-30**). (You will move, reply, forward, and delete messages in later activities.)

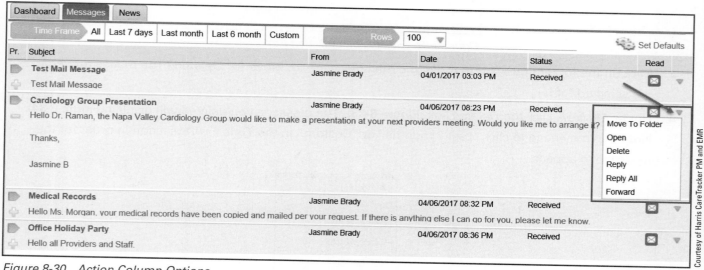

Figure 8-30   *Action Column Options*

🖷 **Print the screen that displays the contents of the Mail Messages Inbox. Label it "Activity 8-15" and place it in your assignment folder.**

Activity 8-16
Move a Mail Message

You have the option to move mail messages to the *Inbox, Sent, Draft*, and *Deleted* folders.

1. Access your mail messages. You will be moving the message "Test Mail Message" (created in Activity 2-15).

2. In the "Test Mail Message" row, point to the *Arrow* ▼ icon and then select "Move To Folder" (**Figure 8-31**). Harris CareTracker PM and EMR displays the *Select Folder* dialog box (**Figure 8-32**).

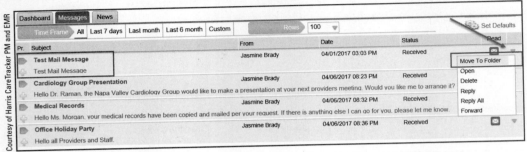

Figure 8-31   Move to Folder

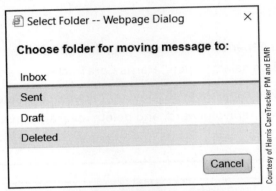

Figure 8-32   Select Folder Dialog Box

3. Click on the folder you want to move the mail message to: Move to "Deleted." The mail is moved to the selected folder.

4. Under *My Mail,* click the *Deleted* link (**Figure 8-33**). The message you deleted will display (**Figure 8-34**). **Note:** You may need to click "Last 6 months" or "Custom" in the *Time Frame* section in order for the message to appear.

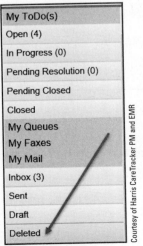

Figure 8-33   Deleted Link

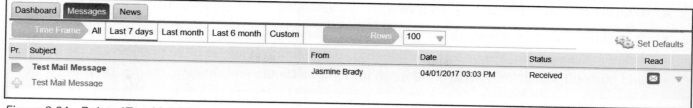

Figure 8-34   Deleted Test Mail Message   Courtesy of Harris CareTracker PM and EMR

Print the Deleted message screen. Label it "Activity 8-16" and place it in your assignment folder.

Activity 8-17
Reply to a Mail Message

1.   Access the mail messages in your *Inbox*. You will reply to the mail message "Office Holiday Party."

2.   To reply to only the sender, point to the *Arrow* ▼ icon in the *Actions* column and then click "Reply."
     Note: If there were multiple recipients on a mail message, you could reply to all of the recipients by pointing the *Arrow* ▼ icon in the *Actions* column and clicking *Reply All*.

3.   Type the reply message as noted in **Figure 8-35**: "Count me in for 2!! Thank you."

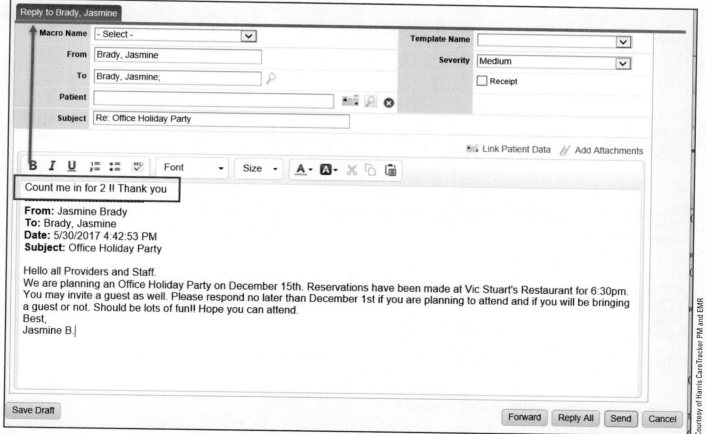

Figure 8-35   Holiday Party Reply Mail Message

4. Click *Send*. You may need to refresh your screen before the message appears in your *Inbox*.

5. Repeat the activity and reply to the "Cardiology Group Presentation." Type the reply message as noted in **Figure 8-36**: "Yes, please arrange the presentation and advise other providers in the group and block off schedules. Please order lunch from Tulio's for the presentation. Thanks, Dr. R."

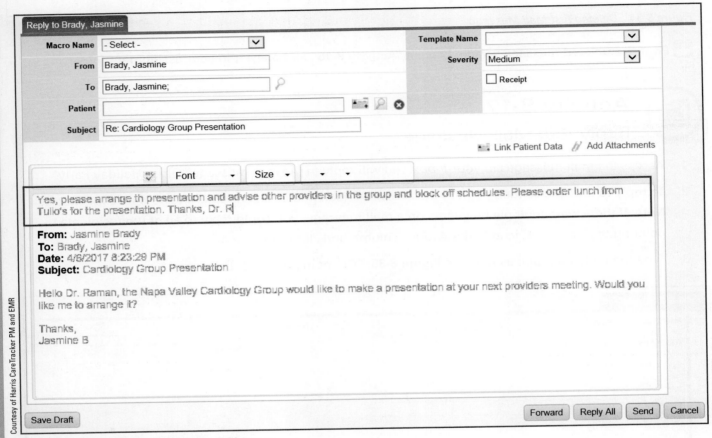

Figure 8-36   Cardiology Reply Mail Message

6. Click *Send*.

Print the screen that displays the mail message replies. Label it "Activity 8-17" and place it in your assignment folder.

Activity 8-18
Forward a Mail Message

Forwarding allows you to send the original mail message to a new recipient.

1. Access your *Inbox*. You will forward the mail message "Cardiology Group Presentation" (forward the message reply, not the original message).

2. In the *Actions* column, point to the *Arrow* ▼ icon and then select "Forward." Harris CareTracker PM and EMR displays the *Forward Message* window.

3. In the *To* field, click the *Search* 🔍 icon. The *Select Operators* dialog box displays. In this training environment, you will be the only operator listed (along with any operators you have created).

4. Select the checkbox next to the person (you) to whom you want to forward the message.

5. Click *Select.* Harris CareTracker PM and EMR closes the *Select Operators* dialog box. Free text the following message to forward: "Hello Drs. Brockton, Ayerick, and Raman and NP Torres, there will be a presentation from the Cardiology Group at the next provider's meeting. Lunch will be provided and schedules have been blocked. Thank you, (your name/operator number)" (**Figure 8-37**).

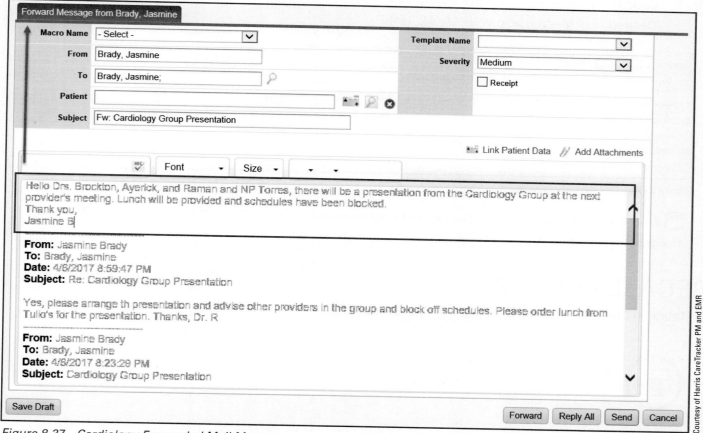

Figure 8-37   Cardiology Forwarded Mail Message

6. Click *Send.* The message is forwarded to the selected recipients.

📇 **Print the screen that displays the forwarded mail message. Label it "Activity 8-18" and place it in your assignment folder.**

Activity 8-19
Delete a Mail Message

Once you finish with a mail message, it is best practice to clean up your mail box. This means you should delete messages that no longer require attention or a response.

1. Access your *Inbox*. You will delete the original "Office Holiday Party" and "Cardiology Group Presentation" messages.

2. In the *Actions* column for each message, point to the *Arrow* ▼ icon and then select "Delete." Harris CareTracker PM and EMR deletes the message from the list.

3. Click the *Deleted* link under *My Mail* to view your deleted message. **Figure 8-38** represents the *Deleted Mail Messages* in your *My Mail* tab.

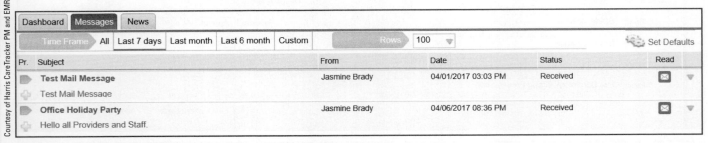

Figure 8-38   *Deleted Messages*

🖳 **Print the screen that displays the deleted mail messages. Label it "Activity 8-19" and place it in your assignment folder.**

RECALL LETTERS

Learning Objective 4: Create and update patient Recall Letters.

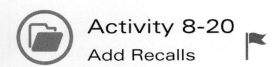

Activity 8-20
Add Recalls

Recalls are reminders to patients that an appointment needs to be booked. Rather than scheduling a future appointment, a recall date is set for the appointment in the *Scheduling* module. Harris CareTracker PM and EMR tracks all recalls, enabling you to generate recall letters at the appropriate time intervals. The *Recalls/Letters Due* application allows you to generate and print letters and labels.

1. Pull patient Gabby Tolman into context.

2. The *Patient Alerts* pop-up alert will note any missing information (**Figure 8-39**).

3. As best practice, update Ms. Tolman's demographics screen as noted below.

   a. Click on the *Patient* module

   b. Click on *Edit*

   c. Change her *Group Provider*, *Referred By*, and her *PCP* all to Dr. Brockton

   d. Change *Consent* to *Yes*

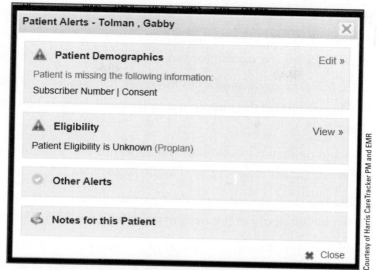

Figure 8-39   Pop-up Alert—Edit/Update Missing Information

e. Click on *Yes* in the *NPP* field

f. In the *Subscriber #*, enter the same information contained in the *Group #* in the *Insurance Plan(s)* section

g. Click *Save*

h. Once saved, the *Patient Alert* box will display "No missing patient information" in the *Patient Demographics* section. It is best practice to always update a patient's chart when needed and prompted.

4. Click the *Medical Record* module.

5. You see that Ms. Tolman's *Last Appt* displays as "03/20/17 New Patient CPE" (**Figure 8-40**).

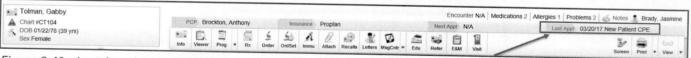

Figure 8-40   Last Appointment Displayed for Gabby Tolman

Courtesy of Harris CareTracker PM and EMR

6. In the *Clinical Toolbar*, click the *Recalls* icon.

7. If an encounter is in context, Harris CareTracker EMR displays the *Recalls* dialog box. If an encounter is not in context, Harris CareTracker EMR displays the *Select Encounter* dialog box. Select the encounter dated March 20, 2017.

8. Click + *New Recall* (**Figure 8-41**). Harris CareTracker EMR displays the *Add Patient Recall* dialog box.

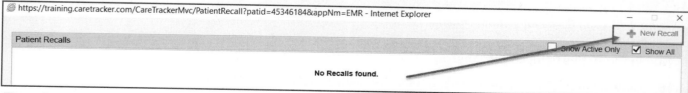

Figure 8-41   Add New Recall

Courtesy of Harris CareTracker PM and EMR

9. In the *Time Frame* list, click the time interval when the patient is expected to return to the office for a comprehensive physical exam (CPE). Select "2 Years."

10. In the *Appointment Type* list, click the reason for the patient recall. Select "Established Patient CPE."

11. In the *Resource* list, click the provider assigned to the recall (Dr. Brockton). This is the preferred provider the patient wants to see during the appointment. (**Note:** If there is no preference, select "Any Resource" from the list.)

12. In the *Location* list, click the preferred location for the appointment. If there is no preference, click "Any Location" from the list. Select "Napa Valley Family Associates."

    (**FYI**) In the *Case* list, click the case associated with the recall. If no case is associated with a recall, click "Default." A case list would apply in the case of workers' compensation. No case list applies.

    Note: If a recall is associated with a case, it is linked to the appointment when scheduled. For example, you can link workers' compensation and auto accident cases to an appointment.

13. By default, the *EMR Alert Status* is set to "No Alert." If required, add an alert to the recall by clicking either "Soft Alert" or "Pop-Up Alert." Select "Soft Alert."

> **TIP** The *pop-up alert* ⚠ displays when the patient's medical record is launched. The alert displays each time the patient's medical record is accessed and stops displaying when the alert is closed. You can also click the *Alert* icon next to the patient's chart number on the *Patient Detail* bar to view both soft and pop-up alerts.

14. In the *Recall Notes* box, enter additional comments for the recall. Enter "Schedule CPE and send Lab Order 30 days prior to appointment for complete panel." (**Figure 8-42**)

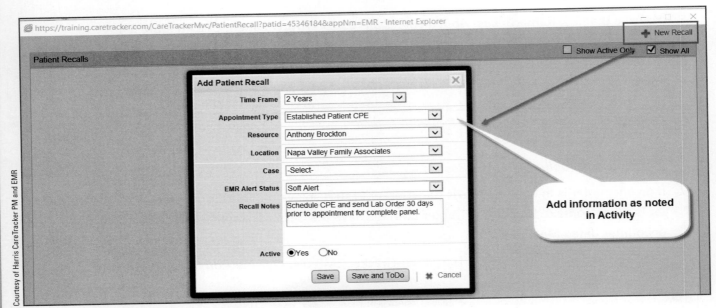

Figure 8-42   *Add Recall for Gabby Tolman*

Courtesy of Harris CareTracker PM and EMR

15. In the *Active* field, select "Yes."

16. Click *Save* to save the recall to the patient's record. (You could also click *Save and ToDo* to send a ToDo for the recall saved.) The *Recalls* dialog box displays with the recall just created (**Figure 8-43**).

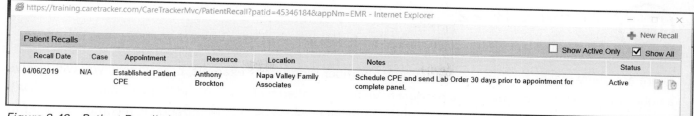

Figure 8-43   *Patient Recalls box*

Courtesy of Harris CareTracker PM and EMR

 Print a copy of the patient's recall. Label the recall summary "Activity 8-20," and place it in your assignment folder.

17. Close out of the *Patient Recalls* dialog box by clicking the "X" in the upper-right-hand corner.

Activity 8-21
Update Recall Details

The *Recall* application updates recall details recorded for the patient.

1. Pull patient Gabby Tolman into context.

2. Click on the *Medical Record* module.

3. In the *Clinical Toolbar,* click the *Recalls* 🖼️ icon.

4. If an encounter is in context, Harris CareTracker PM and EMR displays the *Recalls* dialog box. If an encounter is not in context, Harris CareTracker PM and EMR displays the *Select Encounter* dialog box. Select the encounter dated March 20, 2017.

5. Find the recall you want to update ("Established Patient CPE" you created in Activity 8-20).

6. Click on the *Edit* icon next to the recall and make the necessary changes to the available information. Dr. Brockton is having his non-Medicare patients see NP Torres for CPEs. Change the provider (*Resource*) to NP Torres.

7. Click *Save.* The existing recall for the patient is updated.

 Print a copy of the updated recall, label it "Activity 8-21," and place it in your assignment folder.

8. Close out of the *Patient Recalls* dialog box by clicking the "X" in the upper-right-hand corner.

> **TIP** To deactivate an open recall, click the *Edit* 🖊️ icon and change the *Active* field to "No." To activate a recall, click the *Edit* 🖊️ icon and change the *Active* field to "Yes."

RUNNING AN IMMUNIZATION LOT NUMBER REPORT

Learning Objective 5: Run an immunization report using the Clinical Export feature.

Activity 8-22

Run an Immunization Lot Number Report

There are many reasons to run immunization lot number reports. For example, occasionally you will receive a notice that certain lot numbers of a product have been recalled by the Food and Drug Administration (FDA). Lot numbers provide a source of comfort during a recall because each immunization is recorded in the EMR and various reports can be run to track that patients received the immunization. In addition, a practice can monitor inventory and expiration of immunizations on hand and also use the report for internal audit purposes.

1. With no patient in context, click on the *Reports* module and then click the *Reports* tab.

2. Under *Medical Reports*, click on the *Other Reports* link.

3. Click the *Report* drop-down menu and select "Global – Immunization by Lot Number" (**Figure 8-44**).

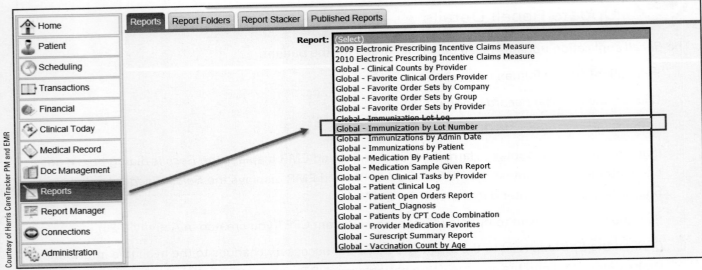

Figure 8-44   Select Global—Immunization by Lot Number

4. Enter the lot number you created in Activity 7-7 in the *Enter the Lot Number* box and also in the *Saved Report Name* box (see **Figure 8-45**). **Hint:** The lot number should be "Hep" followed by your operator number.

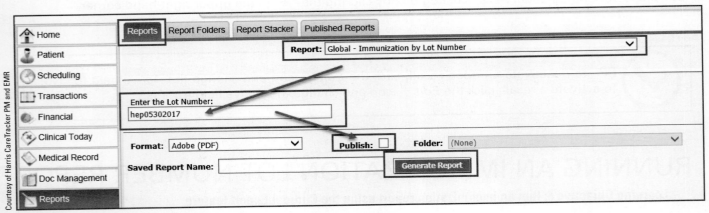

Figure 8-45   Enter the Lot Number

5. Uncheck "Publish."

6. Click *Generate Report*.

7. In the lower portion of your screen, you will see the report generated (**Figure 8-46**).

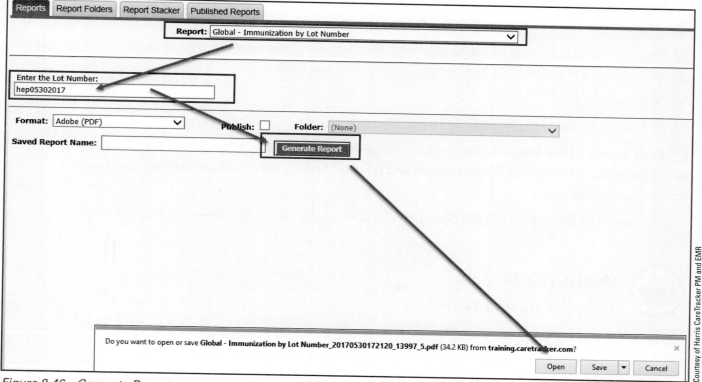

Figure 8-46   *Generate Report*

8. Click *Open* on the *PDF generated report* to view the report (**Figure 8-47**). **Note:** You also have the option to "Save," "Save as," or "Save and open" so you can store the file on your computer to print later (**Figure 8-48**). **Hint:** You might get a pop-up window asking if you want to *Open* or *Save* the PDF report. Select *Open* and the report will display.

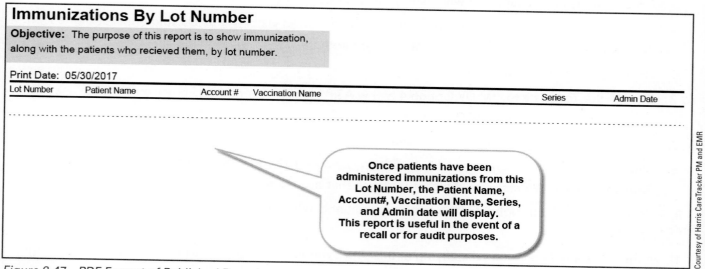

Figure 8-47   *PDF Format of Published Reports*

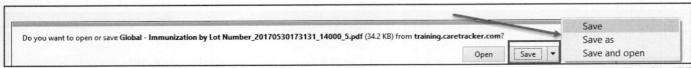

Figure 8-48   Alternative Methods to Save PDF Format of Published Reports

9. Click on the *Print* icon in the PDF to print the report.

10. Now repeat the activity, this time selecting the "Global – Immunizations by Admin Date" report using the begin date of 01/01/2013 and today's date as the end date.

11. Uncheck "Publish."

12. Generate and print the report.

 Print a copy of the Immunization by Lot Number report and label it "Activity 8-22a." Print a copy of the Immunizations by Admin Date report and label it "Activity 8-22b." Place both copies in your assignment folder.

13. Close out of the *Patient Recalls* dialog box by clicking the "X" in the upper-right-hand corner.

Activity 8-23
Sign Progress Notes

Before ending this chapter, be sure to sign the *Progress Notes* for patients with encounters that have visits captured. You may refer to the instructions in Activity 7-20 to complete this activity.

1. Click on the *Home* module > *Dashboard* tab > *Practice* tab > *Clinical* heading > *Open Encounters* link.

2. Select **All** providers and click on the refresh icon to the right of the *Provider* dropdown.

3. The screen will display any unsigned notes and whether or not the visit has been captured.

4. To determine if a visit has been captured, look at the *Description* column. A saved visit will display the *Visit Diags* codes. A visit that has not been captured will say "None" after "*Visit Diags*" as illustrated in **Figure 8-49**. In addition, a *Visit* that has not been captured displays the *Visit* icon. A *Visit* that has been captured will display the *Visit* icon with a checkmark.

5. Sign <u>all</u> of the progress notes for the patients with captured visits () by clicking on "Not Signed" in the *Note* column. Do <u>not</u> sign any *Notes* that are noted *as Missing (Required)*.

6. The progress note will display.

7. Change the *Template* to "IM OV Option 4 (v4) w/A&P" (except for patient Francisco Jimenez, leave the *Template* as "Pediatric OV Option 4 (v1)").

8. Click on the *Sign* icon in the *Progress Note*.

9. Click back on the *Open Encounters* link on the *Dashboard*, change *Provider* to *All*, and click the *Refresh* icon. The *Note*(s) with the captured visit that has been signed will disappear from the screen.

10. Continue steps 5 through 9 for the remaining patients with a completed *Visit* and a *Note* that is "Not Signed."

11. If there are any *Encounters* displaying at this time without *Visits*, do <u>not</u> sign the *Note*(s). Do <u>not</u> sign any *Note* noted *as Missing (Required)*.

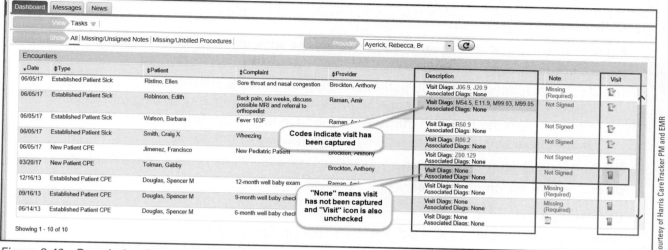

Figure 8-49   Description Column in Encounters

12. You will now be able to complete the *Billing* and *Collection* activities in Chapters 9 and 10.

🖫 **Print a screenshot of the *Open Encounters* screen after signing any unsigned notes with *Visit*s captured. Label it "Activity 8-23" and place it in your assignment folder.**

CRITICAL THINKING Having completed the activities in this chapter, reflect on your ability to integrate the patient relationship aspect and the clinical side of your duties. At the beginning of the chapter, you were encouraged to think about the patient's peace of mind as you receive and enter lab results, and the process of promptly notifying the provider. The other very important piece of processing and recording lab results is the integrity of the data entered. Referring back to Activity 8-11, what measures were taken to ensure data accuracy? Although the majority of lab results are sent electronically to the patient's EMR in a live practice, there are still some instances where the practice will receive lab result by paper and/or fax. Some practices scan the results to the patient's chart; some enter the data into the patient's electronic chart; some do both. Think about the complexity of lab results and how your duties as a medical assistant reply on your ability to accurately record laboratory results in the EMR. After completing the activities in this chapter, considering the likelihood that you will be entering multiple complex lab results in a live practice, what conclusions have you reached about your responsibilities? Would you advocate one method over another? Why or why not? Describe the "best practice" for entering lab results.

CASE STUDIES

Case Study 8-1

Patient: Adam Thompson

(**Note:** You must have completed Case Study 7-3 in order to complete Case Study 8-1.) Add an *Addendum* to Adam Thompson's progress note as follows: "Patient went to ED and was admitted to NVGH for treatment." Refer to Activity 8-7 for guidance if needed.

🖫 **Print a screenshot of the screens that illustrate you entered the addendum. Label them "Case Study 8-1" and place it in your assignment folder.**

Case Study 8-2

Patient: Alex Brady

a. Create an addendum for Alex Brady's encounter dated December 12, 2016 as follows: "Mother called on 12/18/2016 to inquire if any vaccinations are required for overseas travel. Sent the CDC recommendations for traveling to South America." Refer to Activity 8-7 for guidance if needed.

(continues)

CASE STUDIES (*continued*)

📼 **Print a screenshot that illustrates you entered the addendum. Label it "Case Study 8-2a" and place it in your assignment folder.**

b. Create an addendum for the patient's encounter dated March 10, 2017 as follows: "Mother called on 03/12/2017 at 4:50 pm to say Alex is refusing to eat solid foods; asked her to bring him into office for immediate follow-up. She will go to Urgent Care for after-hours visit." Refer to Activity 8-7 for guidance if needed.

📼 **Print a screenshot that illustrates you entered the addendum. Label it "Case Study 8-2b" and place it in your assignment folder.**

Case Study 8-3

Create *ToDos* as listed in **Table 8-2**. For each *ToDo* in **Table 8-2** use the *Category* "Interoffice," *Type* "EHR," and *Reason* "Phone Call (Patient)." Refer to Activity 8-13 for guidance if needed.

Table 8-2   New *ToDo* Messages

FROM	TO	SUBJECT	SEVERITY	NOTES (MESSAGE)	PATIENT
You	You *Though you have selected You for the To field, in the real world, you would be sending this to Dr. Raman.*	Medication Question	Medium	Patient wants to know if he can take a multivitamin while he is taking Coumadin. Please advise and I will return call to patient. Thank you.	Bradley Torez
You	You (see above comment)	Referral/ Authorization Status	Medium	Patient called and wants to know if her request for referral and authorization for MRI has been ordered. Please call patient at home phone between 3:00 p.m. and 5:00 p.m. OK to leave message on voicemail.	Kimberly Johnson

Courtesy of Harris CareTracker PM and EMR

📼 **Print a screenshot from the Messages tab that reflects the *ToDos* you created. Label it "Case Study 8-3" and place it in your assignment folder.**

Case Study 8-4

Create *Recalls* for the following patients, using each patient's PCP as provider. Refer to Activity 8-20 for guidance if needed.

a. Jane Morgan (recall for CPE due two years from today). Include a note to send lab (complete panel) and mammogram orders one month prior to CPE.

b. Harriet Oshea (recall for CPE due two years from today). Include a note to send lab (complete panel) and mammogram orders one month prior to CPE.

📼 **Print a screenshot that illustrates you entered the recalls. Label it "Case Study 8-4" and place it in your assignment folder.**

MODULE 4
Billing Skills

This module includes:

- Chapter 9: Billing
- Chapter 10: ClaimsManager and Collections

As a health care professional, you may use Harris CareTracker PM and EMR to manually enter and edit charges, and generate claims.Once claims are generated you will perform the steps to work claims, print patient statements, review overdue accounts, and perform collection actions. All the activities you will complete in this module mimic a real-world setting using the administrative and financial features of electronic health records.

QUICK START

In the patient workflow, billing tasks are performed after the patient has been seen by the provider. Because Harris CareTracker is a live EMR, you will need to complete several tasks to simulate a live clinic where patient accounts are ready for billing. The following activities are required in order to complete the activities in this module. **If you have been following along in this book from the beginning and have completed all the Required ⚑ activities as you've moved sequentially through the text, then you have already completed the activities below and can move forward. If you are beginning with this module, then you will need to complete the activities below before you can complete any other activities in this module.**

Be sure you are working in a supported browser (Internet Explorer 11 or Safari for iPad) before you begin. Other browsers (such as Chrome and Firefox) are not supported. Review Best Practices.

- ❑ Activity 1-1: Disable Toolbars
- ❑ Activity 1-2: Set Up Tabbed Browsing
- ❑ Activity 1-3: Turn Off Pop-Up Blocker
- ❑ Activity 1-4: Change Page Setup
- ❑ Activity 1-5: Add Harris CareTracker to Trusted Sites
- ❑ Activity 1-6: Clear Your Cache
  - *Note: Remember that you should clear your cache each time before you being working in CareTracker.*
- ❑ Activity 1-8: Disable Download Blocking
  - *Note: Once you have completed the system set-up requirements (Activities 1-1, 1-2, 1-3, 1-4, 1-5, and 1-8), you will not need to repeat these activities unless you change the device you are using or the settings automatically default back to prior settings.*
- ❑ Activity 1-9: Register Your Credentials and Create Your Harris CareTracker PM and EMR Training Company
  - *Note: It will take up to 24 hours for your CareTracker "Student Company" to be created. Plan accordingly.*

❑ Activity 2-1: Log in to Harris CareTracker PM and EMR
  • *Note: Be sure to write down your new password inside the front cover of your book for easy reference.*

❑ Activity 2-5: Open a New Fiscal Year
  • *Note: Every January 1, you will need to open a new fiscal year.*

❑ Activity 2-6: Open a Fiscal Period
  • *Note: Every first of the month, you will need to open a new fiscal period.*

❑ Activity 3-1: Searching for a Patient by Name
  • *Complete steps 1 and 2 only.*
  • *Note: You will search for patients throughout the text using the steps in Activity 3-1.*

❑ Activity 4-1: Book an Appointment
  • *Book an appointment for Jane Morgan, Ellen Ristino, Craig X. Smith, Adam Thompson, and Edith Robinson, but do **NOT** book an appointment for Francisco Powell Jimenez at this time.*
  • *The directions for this activity state to book the appointment for one week from today. Instead, book the appointment for today (the day you are working). If no appointments are available today, then book the appointment for a day within the past week.*
  • *Also book an "Established Patient Sick" appointment for today for Barbara Watson with Amir Raman. Her chief complaint is "Fever—103F."*

❑ Activity 4-12: Create a Batch
  • *Note: At various times throughout the activities, you will be directed to create batches.*

❑ Activity 4-13: Accept/Enter a Payment

❑ Activity 4-15: Accept/Enter a Payment
  • *Complete steps 1 through 12 only. You do not need to print receipts for this activity at this time.*

❑ Activity 4-17: Post a Batch
  • *Note: At various times throughout the activities, you will be directed to post batches.*

❑ Activity 7-18: Capture a Visit
  • *Also capture the visit for Jane Morgan. Enter the CPT codes 99213 and 90746 in the Procedures tab. Enter the ICD-10 codes N39.0, R30.0, and I10 in the Diagnosis tab. View the Visit Summary tab and save the information, making sure to receive the message "An error occurred connecting to Claims manager. Transaction saved" before moving on.*

❑ Activity 7-21(a–d): Capture a Visit
  • *Complete only parts A–D for Ellen Ristino, Craig X. Smith, Barbara Watson, and Edith Robinson at this time. You do NOT need to complete parts E, F, or G.*

Once you have completed these activities as part of this Quick Start, you will not need to complete them again if you come across the activities while working in Chapters 1–7.

PREREQUISITES FOR CASE STUDIES

In addition to the activities listed in the Quick Start, you will need to complete the following case study if you plan to complete case studies in this module:

❑ Case Study 7-3
  • *Complete part B only.*

Billing

Learning Objectives

1. Create a batch for financial transactions.
2. Manually enter a charge.
3. Edit an unposted charge.
4. Generate electronic and paper claims.
5. Perform activities related to electronic remittance including: posting payments and adjustments, and reconciling insurance payments.

Real-World Connection

Your challenge is to become familiar with the many different types of insurance plans and the effects on the practice when there is an issue regarding noncovered services. In order for the medical practice to be profitable, fees must be collected from patients for services rendered. The fees and copay can be collected at the time of the visit, or you can bill the patient after a claim has been submitted to the insurance company, depending on the type of insurance and the policy of the practice. It is NVFHA policy that copays must be collected from the patient at the office for each encounter. We only bill the copay when the patient does not have any form of payment available at the time of service. Upon receipt of payment from the insurance company and after any adjustment to the contracted rate is applied, the balance due will be billed to the patient.

Although it may be a delicate issue, you will be responsible for communicating the fees for services to patients. This discussion should take place prior to the patient's appointment with the physician to avoid an awkward situation, and again at any time there is a test ordered that will also include separate fees. With the ever-changing insurance environment and mandates from the Affordable Care Act (ACA), and the possible repeal and replacement of the ACA, you must verify the patient's insurance plan, deductibles, out-of-pocket amounts, and confirm that NVFHA is in fact contracted with the patient's insurance company before providing services. The deductibles with insurance plans available through the ACA and exchanges are extremely high (average for individuals is $6,500 per year or more and $10,000 or more per family). Consider how such a high deductible and out-of-pocket expenses will affect the patient's ability to pay and also the possibility that the patient may delay seeking health care due to the high insurance deductible.

If the patient's insurance is not contracted with NVFHA, the patient will be responsible for the entire fee. In some cases, patients will be forced to change providers to one that is contracted with their insurance; otherwise the costs would be unaffordable to the patient. Changing doctors is very stressful to many patients. Often they have developed relationships that span many years or decades. Therefore, it is important that you have an understanding of the various types of insurance and how to communicate effectively with patients in an articulate and compassionate manner. Even within the many types of insurance, copays and deductibles can vary widely. Some health plans have large deductibles and large copays. Other plans may require no copay at the time of visit, but the patient will pay a percentage of the contracted rate for the service.

When you register a new patient and collect patient demographic information over the phone, you will gather insurance information as well. This will help determine what type of fee or payment will be required of the patient, and confirm that our practice is contracted with the patient's insurance carrier. The office policy

Real-World Connection (continued)

must be clearly stated to the patients on the telephone, by written communication (on forms the patient must complete and sign), and by way of posted notices in the waiting room. Patients should be gently reminded in a very professional manner that payment will be expected at the time of service. Our automated answering system also conveys fee and payment options available.

Before you begin the activities in this chapter, refresh your memory on working with Harris CareTracker by referring back to the Best Practices list on page xiv of this workbook. Following best practices will help you complete work quickly and accurately.

CREATE A BATCH

Learning Objective 1: Create a batch for financial transactions.

Activity 9-1

Create a Batch for Billing and Charges

In order to perform any financial transactions, you must create a batch or have a batch open. Harris CareTracker PM will prompt you to create a batch unless you have already created a batch that has not yet been posted. You can view open batch(es) by clicking on the *Home* module > *Dashboard* tab > *Billing* header > *Open Batches* link **(Figure 9-1)**. You begin by setting the operator preferences as completed in Chapter 4, Activity 4-11. Create a *Batch* as instructed to begin your activities in this chapter.

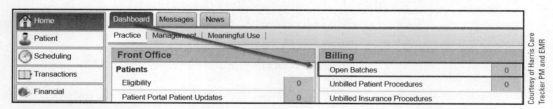

Figure 9-1   *Open Batches Link*

Because you will have been working in various activities in more than one fiscal period, always work in the "current" fiscal period unless otherwise instructed (e.g., if you begin an activity in September, complete all the related activities in that period. If you start a new activity unrelated to a previous period [e.g., in December], you would then use the new period [December]). Although you will be instructed to complete activities and post batches, *never* close a period.

1. Prior to creating a batch, you will need to open the fiscal period for which you will be entering activities. Go to the *Administration* module > *Practice* tab > *System Administration, Financial* headers > *Open/Close Period* link **(Figure 9-2)**.

2. Open the fiscal period for the activities you are posting. Since you will be posting financial information for patient Alex Brady whose visit was in September 2016, open the fiscal period (2016) and month (September). **Note:** You will first need to change the current *Fiscal Year* box field to 2016.

3. Click *Save* **(Figure 9-3)**.

4. Click the *Batch* ▌ icon on the *Name Bar* and the *Operator Encounter Batch Control* dialog box will display.

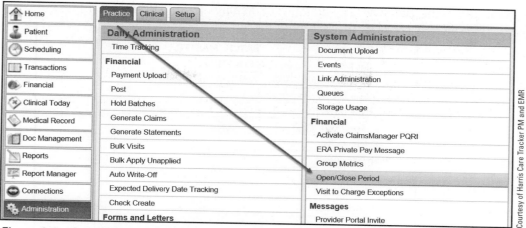

Figure 9-2   Open/Close Period Link

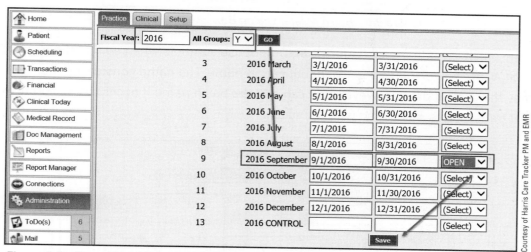

Figure 9-3   Open Fiscal Period for June 2016

5.   Then click *Edit.* **(Figure 9-4).**

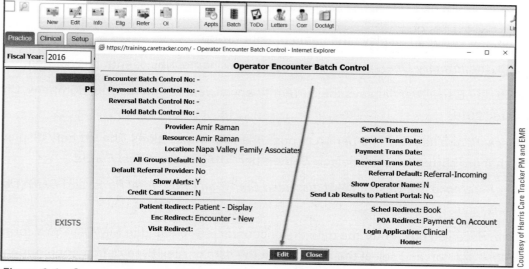

Figure 9-4   Operator Encounter Batch Control Dialog Box—Edit

6. Click *Create Batch.* The *Batch Master* dialog box displays **(Figure 9-5)**.

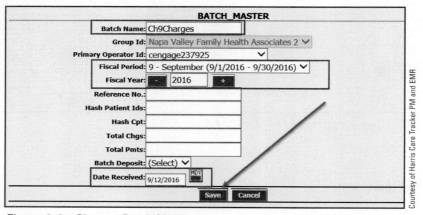

Figure 9-5   Batch Master Dialog Box

7. Name the batch "Ch9Charges" **(Figure 9-6)**. Do not use symbols when editing the name. By default, the *Batch Name* box displays a batch identification name. The name consists of your user name followed by the current date. However, you can edit the batch name if necessary to identify the types of financial transactions associated with the batch.

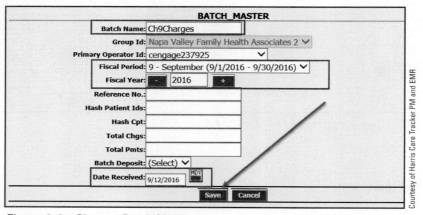

Figure 9-6   Change Batch Name

8. By default, the *Group Id* displays the name of your group.

9. By default, the *Primary Operator Id* displays your user name. This cannot be changed.

10. By default, the *Fiscal Year* displays the current financial year set up for your company. Change the year to "2016."

11. In the *Fiscal Period* list, click the period to post financial transactions. The list only displays fiscal periods that are currently open. Select "September 2016" as the *Fiscal Period*.

12. Leave the *Reference No; Hash Patient Ids; Hash Cpt; Total Chgs; Total Pmts;* and *Batch Deposit* fields blank.

13. In the *Date Received* box, enter the date the encounter was created in MM/DD/YYYY format or click the *calendar* icon and select the date. Select the date of Alex Brady's first appointment (September 12, 2016).

14. Click *Save*. If you have more than one period open, a pop-up warning **(Figure 9-7)** will appear asking you to confirm the fiscal period. Click *OK*.

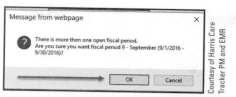

Figure 9-7   *Fiscal Period Pop-Up Warning*

15. Harris CareTracker PM and EMR displays the *Operator Encounter Batch Control* dialog box with the new batch information **(Figure 9-8)**.

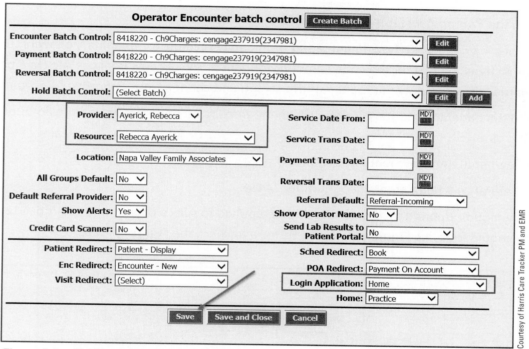

Figure 9-8   *Ch9Charges Batch Information*

16. Further *Edit* your batch using the drop-down arrow next to each field and updating the provider, resource, location, and so on, if needed.

   a. If not already selected, select "Rebecca Ayerick" as the *Provider* and *Resource*.

   b. Change your *Login Application* to *Home*.

   c. Leave the *Home* field as *Practice*.

17. Click *Save*.

18. Write down your "Encounter Batch Control No." for future reference (should include "Ch9Charges").

   _____.

📖 **Print the Operator Encounter Batch Control screen, label it "Activity 9-1," and place it in your assignment folder.**

19. Click the "X" in the upper-right corner to close the dialog box.

MANUALLY ENTER A CHARGE

Learning Objective 2: Manually enter a charge.

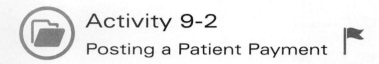

Activity 9-2
Posting a Patient Payment

Charges are financial transactions that require a batch to be created before entering and saving a charge. Having created your batch in Activity 9-1, complete this activity to post a patient payment.

1. Pull patient Alex Brady into context.

2. Open the *Transactions* module. The *Charge* application displays by default.

3. Click on the *Pmt on Acct* tab.

4. In Chapter 4, you learned how to enter and print copay receipts for patients. Following the instructions in Activity 4-15, enter the copay amount for patient Alex Brady. Because Alex is a pediatric patient, use the drop-down at the top of the screen and change from *Patient* to "*Responsibly Party.*"

5. Refer to the patient demographics or click on the *Info* icon to determine the amount of copay required ($10).

6. Enter Payment Type "Payment-Patient Check."

7. In the Reference # field, enter check number "4434."

8. Enter the appointment date (*Trans. Date*) to be applied to Alex's payment (September 12, 2016). Your screen should look like **Figure 9-9**. (**Note:** Be sure to check the "Copay?" box.)

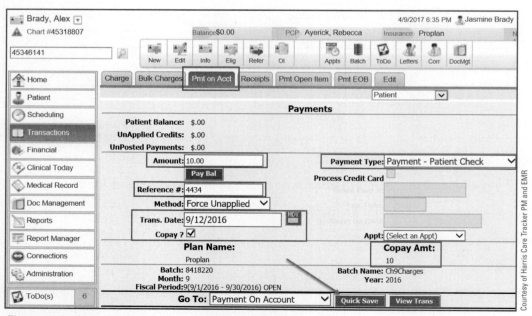

Figure 9-9   Alex Brady Payment on Account

9. Click *Quick Save*.

10. Click on the *Receipts* tab and print a receipt for Alex Brady.

Print the receipt, label it "Activity 9-2," and place it in your assignment folder.

You will <u>not</u> post the batch at this time because you will complete additional activities before running a journal and posting a batch.

 # Activity 9-3
Manually Enter a Charge for a Patient

Having entered the copay for Alex Brady in Activity 9-2, continue your billing activities by manually entering a charge for a patient not on the schedule.

1. Because you will be manually entering a charge in a different period, follow the steps in Activity 9-1 to create a new batch using today's current month and year. (**Note:** If the fiscal period and fiscal year are not already open, you will need to open them before creating the batch.) Set the batch parameters as follows:

   a. *Batch Name*: RobinsonSNF

   b. *Fiscal Year*: Use the current month

   c. *Fiscal Period*: Use the current year

   d. *Provider and Resource*: Raman, Amir

2. After the current fiscal period is open and you have the new batch created, pull patient Edith Robinson into context.

3. Open the *Transactions* module. The *Charge* application displays by default, displaying the charge screen.

 TIP You may get a pop-up stating "Please check Batch." If so, click *OK*. The *Operator Encounter Batch* screen will display. In the *Encounter Batch Control* field, you'll see that the "RobinsonSNF" batch you created is selected. Click "Save and Close."

4. Manually enter a "Skilled Nursing Facility" charge using the following charge-related information:

   a. Using the *Location* drop-down, select "NVSNF."

   b. Using the [Tab] key will automatically populate the *POS* with "SKILLED NURSING FACILITY."

   c. Enter *Ref Provider* "Dr. Raman."

5. If there have been previous ICD codes entered for this patient, you can place a check mark by the desired code to select it. Select codes E11.9, I10, M54.5, M99.03, and M99.05. If any of these codes are not listed, type the code (e.g., "I10") in the *Search Diagnosis* field and then click *Search*. Harris CareTracker PM will pull in the diagnosis code of I10 in the *Diag* field (**Figure 9-11**). Repeat code searches as necessary until you have all the five codes listed.

6. Click on *EncoderPro.com* to review the codes selected and determine if they are appropriate for the visit/charge. Click "X" to close the *EncoderPro* window.

FYI In the center of the screen, the *Visit* button will be grayed out **(Figure 9-10)**. In a live application, clicking the *Visit* button allows you to access the *Visit* window in which CPT and ICD-10 codes can be selected for the patient.

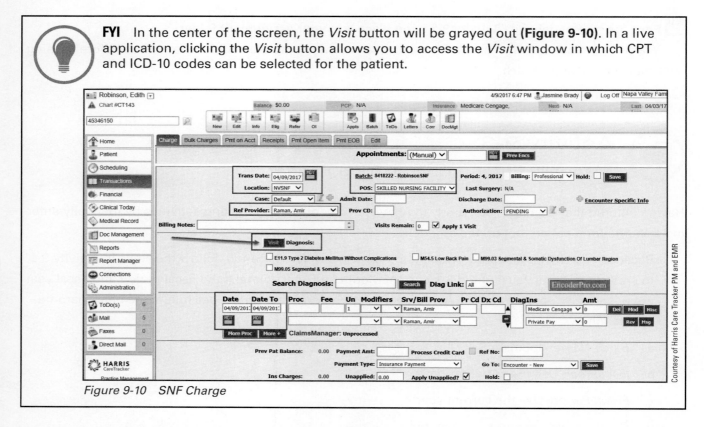

Figure 9-10   *SNF Charge*

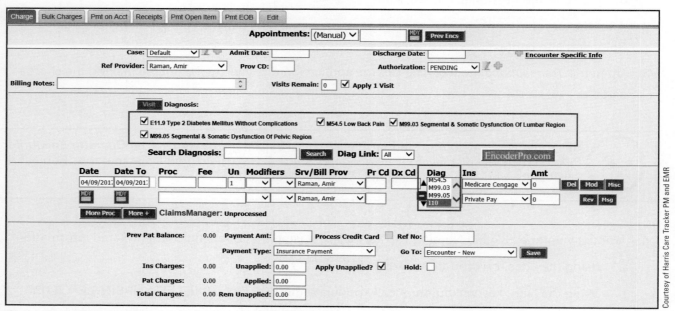

Figure 9-11   *Diagnosis Codes Selected—Charge Screen*

7. Enter today's date in the *Date* and *Date To* fields. A date can either be entered manually in MM/DD/YYYY format or can be selected from the *Calendar* 📅 function. The date must be within the open period in your current batch.

8. Enter the code "99212" in the *Proc* field, and hit the [Tab] key. The procedure description, fee, and the amount to be charged to the patient's insurance and to the patient will be populated, and the *Modifiers* will become the active field.

9. Click on the *More Proc* button, which brings up another billing line. Enter CPT® code "G0180" in the *Proc* field. Hit the [Tab] key and the *Procedure Search* pop-up box will appear **(Figure 9-12)**. Click on the code or description and the procedure will be pulled in to the charge box.

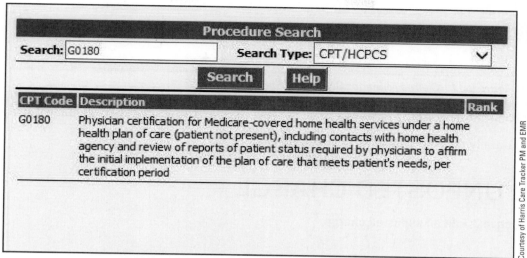

Figure 9-12   *Error Message When Saving a Charge*

10. Enter $100 in the *Fee* field because this CPT® code is not on the NVFHA fee schedule.

11. Select "Raman, Amir" from the *Srv/Bill Prov* drop-down list, if not already selected **(Figure 9-13)**.

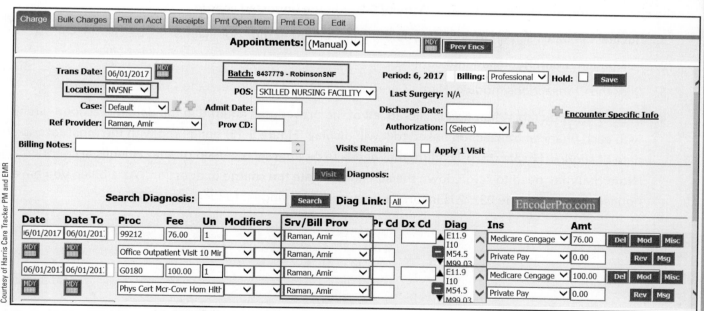

Figure 9-13   *SNF Procedure (CPT) Codes in Charge Screen*

🖳 **Print the Charge Screen, label it "Activity 9-3," and place it in your assignment folder.**

12. Click *Save.* You will receive an error message **(Figure 9-14)** because your student version is not connected to *ClaimsManager*. However, the transaction will be saved, and the patient is taken out of context. (**Note:** It may take a few moments for this task to save. You <u>must</u> wait until you receive the "error" message "Transaction Saved" before moving on.)

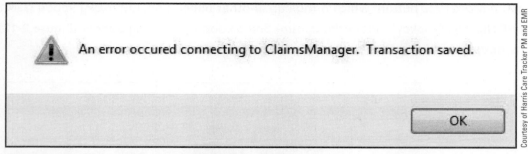

Figure 9-14   Claims Manager Screening Status

13. Click *OK* and the patient is removed from context and "Encounter Added" displays on your screen.

14. Your manually entered charge is now saved.

EDIT AN UNPOSTED CHARGE

Learning Objective 3: Edit an unposted charge.

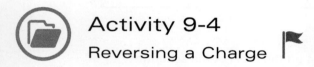

Activity 9-4
Reversing a Charge

Although it is not required to edit charges, there will be times when you will find it necessary to edit an unposted charge (e.g., a biller is reviewing a charge and sees that an incorrect CPT® code was assigned to the claim). Using the charge entered in Activity 9-3, edit the unposted charge.

1. Review the batch screen to confirm you are still working in the "RobinsonSNF" batch.

2. Pull patient Edith Robinson into context.

3. Click the *Transactions* module. Harris CareTracker PM and EMR opens the *Charge* application.

4. Click on the *Edit* tab. When *Edit* is clicked, all of the procedures entered in the patient's account along with each financial transaction linked to it will display (**Figure 9-15**) beginning with the most recent date of service. Locate the procedure that needs to be entirely reversed on the patient's account. (**Note:** You may need to scroll down the screen to locate the charge in question.) As a biller, you have noticed that CPT® code 99212 is incorrect, and want to change it to CPT® code 99214.

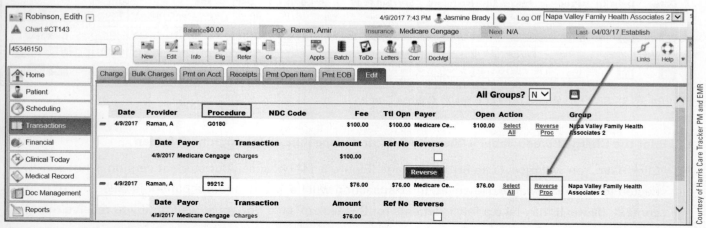

Figure 9-15   Edit Unposted Charge for Edith Robinson

5. Select the *Reverse Proc* link on the 99212 charge only (see **Figure 9-15**). (**Note**: If you click on the *Reverse* button, all of the selected transactions are reversed. Do <u>not</u> click on *Reverse*.)

6. You will receive a pop-up warning message (**Figure 9-16**) asking "Are you sure you want to reverse the selected Financial Transactions?" Click *OK*. The transaction will be reversed (see **Figure 9-17**). (**Note:** If you receive the error message "The Reversal Date must be within Period Start and End Dates: xx/xx/20xx and: xx/xx/20xx," it may be due to a "compatibility" issue with your browser. Refer to Best Practices regarding compatibility.)

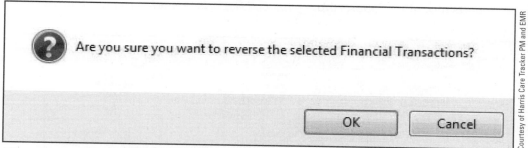

Figure 9-16   *Reverse Financial Transaction Warning*

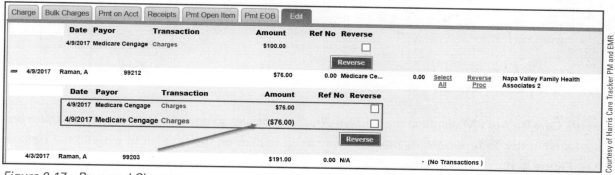

Figure 9-17   *Reversed Charge*

💾 **Print the Edit Unposted Charge screen, label it "Activity 9-4a," and place it in your assignment folder.**

7. Click back on the *Charge* tab in the *Transactions* module and complete the charge screen:

   a. *Location*: NVSNF

   b. *POS*: SKILLED NURSING FACILITY

   c. *Ref Provider*: Raman, Amir

   d. *Diagnosis*: E11.9, I10, M54.5, M99.03, M99.05

   e. *Date* and *Date To*: Use today's date

   f. Enter "99214" in the *Proc* field, and hit the [Tab] key. $245 should populate in the *Fee* field. If not, enter $245 into the *Fee* field.

💾 **Print the Charge screen, label it "Activity 9-4b," and place it in your assignment folder.**

8. Click on *Save* to save the charge. **Important!!** Be sure to wait for the message "An error occurred connecting to ClaimsManager. Transaction saved." before moving forward.

9. Click *OK*, and your transaction is saved.

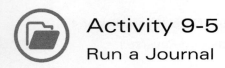

Activity 9-5
Run a Journal

Now that you have manually entered and edited unposted charges, the common workflow would be to complete the process by running a journal and posting your batch.

When you have finished entering data into your batch, you will run a journal to verify your batch and entry information. It is best practice to run a journal (as in Activity 4-16) prior to posting your batch to verify that you have entered all the financial transactions correctly in Harris CareTracker PM.

1. Go to the *Reports* module > *Reports* tab > *Financial Reports* header > *Todays Journals* link **(Figure 9-18)**.

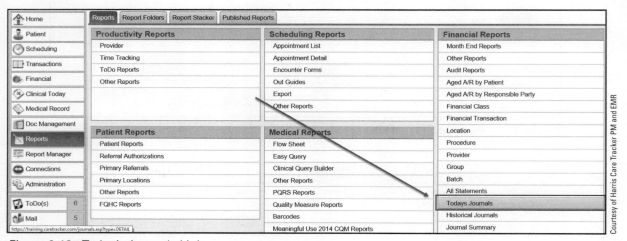

Figure 9-18 Today's Journals Link

2. Harris CareTracker PM displays the *Todays Journal Options* screen. All of your group's open batches are listed in the *Todays Batches* box. You may need to click on the [+] sign to expand the *Batches* field (see **Figure 9-19**).

3. Select a batch to include in the journal either by double-clicking on the batch name or by clicking on the batch and then clicking *Add >*. Harris CareTracker PM adds the selected batches to the box on the right. Select batches "Ch9Charges" and "RobinsonSNF."

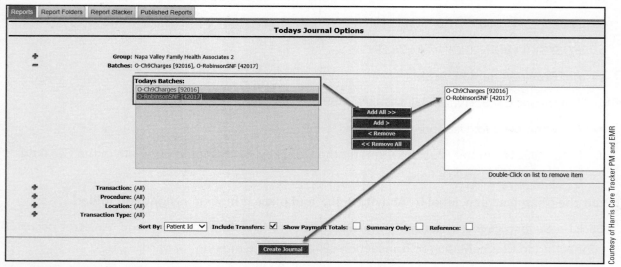

Figure 9-19 Expand Journal Batch Options

4. Scroll down to the bottom of the screen. From the *Sort By* drop-down list, select *"Entry Date"* **(Figure 9-20)**.

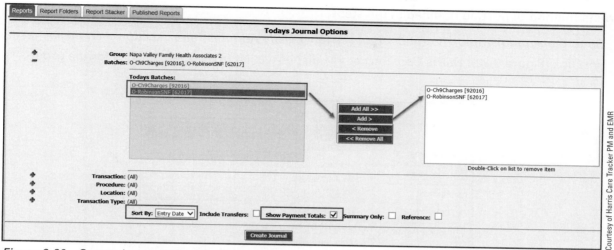

Figure 9-20   Create Journal—Sort By Entry Date

5. Select the *Show Payment Totals* checkbox (see Figure 9-20).

6. Click *Create Journal*. Harris CareTracker PM generates the journal **(Figure 9-21)**.

Financial Report
Journal
Print Date: Saturday, October 28, 2017 (10:58:49 AM)
Run By: Training Operator Cengage238039
Napa Valley Family Associates

Procedure: (All)
Location: (All)
Group: Napa Valley Family Health Associates 2
Transaction Type: (All)
Transaction Class: (All)

Patient	Serv Dt	Trans Dt	Transaction	Charges	Payments	Adjustments	Provider	Payer	CPT	MOD	Diag
Batch: Ch9Charges-8488221											
(45757117) Brady, Alex		9/12/2016	Payment - Patient C...		($10.00)			Unapplied			
Batch Totals:				**Batch Chg** $0.00	**Batch Pmts** ($10.00)	**Batch Adj** $0.00		**Batch Net** ($10.00)			
Batch: RobinsonSNF-8488222											
(45757126) Robinson, Edith	10/28/2017	10/28/2017	Charges	$76.00			Raman, Amir	Medicare Cengage	99212		(E11.9, M99.03, M99.05, I10)
(45757126) Robinson, Edith	10/28/2017	10/28/2017	Charges	$100.00			Raman, Amir	Medicare Cengage	G0180		(E11.9, M99.03, M99.05, I10)
(45757126) Robinson, Edith	10/28/2017	10/28/2017	Charges	-$76.00			Raman, Amir	Medicare Cengage	99212		(E11.9, M99.03, M99.05, I10)
(45757126) Robinson, Edith	10/28/2017	10/28/2017	Charges	$245.00			Raman, Amir	Medicare Cengage	99214		(E11.9, M99.03, I10, M99.05)
Batch Totals:				**Batch Chg** $345.00	**Batch Pmts** $0.00	**Batch Adj** $0.00		**Batch Net** $345.00			
Grand Totals:				**Tot Chg** $345.00	**Tot Pmts** ($10.00)	**Total Adj** $0.00		**Net Total** $335.00			

Payment Totals

Payment Description.	Payment Amount
Payment - Patient Check	($10.00)
Payment Grand Total	($10.00)

Figure 9-21   Journal—Financial Report

7. To print, right-click on the journal and select *Print* from the shortcut menu.

📇 **Print the journal, label it "Activity 9-5," and place it in your assignment folder.**

8. Close out of the *Journal* report.

Activity 9-6
Post a Batch

Having balanced the money in your journal, post an open batch as directed in this activity following the alternate method of posting outlined in the steps.

1. Go to the *Administration* module > *Practice* tab > *Daily Administration* section > *Financial* header > *Post* link **(Figure 9-22)**. Harris CareTracker PM displays a list of all open batches for the group.

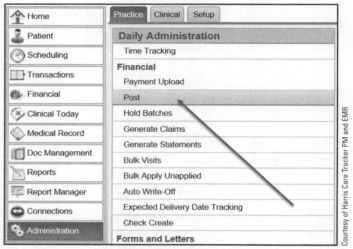

Figure 9-22   Post Link from Practice Tab

2. Check the box next to the batch(es) you want to post. Select <u>only</u> the batch "Ch9Charges" **(Figure 9-23)**. Do <u>not</u> select or post the "RobinsonSNF" batch at this time.

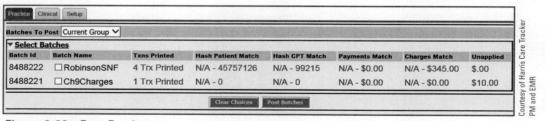

Batch Id	Batch Name	Txns Printed	Hash Patient Match	Hash CPT Match	Payments Match	Charges Match	Unapplied
8488222	☐ RobinsonSNF	4 Trx Printed	N/A - 45757126	N/A - 99215	N/A - $0.00	N/A - $345.00	$.00
8488221	☐ Ch9Charges	1 Trx Printed	N/A - 0	N/A - 0	N/A - $0.00	N/A - $0.00	$10.00

Figure 9-23   Post Batches

📧 **Print the Post Batches screen, label it "Activity 9-6," and place it in your assignment folder**

3. Then click *Post Batches*.

BUILD AND GENERATE CLAIMS

Learning Objective 4: Generate electronic and paper claims.

Activity 9-7
Workflow for Electronic Submission of Claims

Harris CareTracker PM transmits electronic claims directly to insurance companies and to clearinghouses.

Claims can only be generated after your batch has been posted. Most claims in a medical practice are transmitted electronically to a clearinghouse or directly to an insurance company; however, some claims will need to be printed out and mailed.

In a live environment, after completing the activities of posting payments, charges, running the journal, and posting the batch, Harris CareTracker PM will electronically submit the claims through *ClaimsManager*. You will simulate generating claims by following the steps in Activity 9-7. Because the *ClaimsManager* feature is not active in your student version of Harris CareTracker PM, the claim will not actually generate, but you will be able to complete the steps.

1. Go to the *Administration* module > *Practice* tab > *Daily Administration* section > *Financial* header > *Generate Claims* link **(Figure 9-24)**. Harris CareTracker PM launches the *Generate Claims* application.

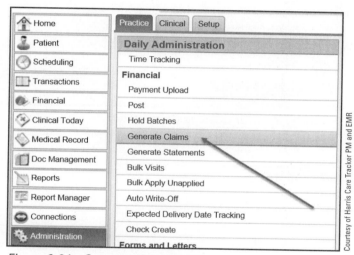

Figure 9-24   Generate Claims Link

2. Click *Generate Claims For This Group* **(Figure 9-25)**. You may receive an error message stating "Error Queuing Claims" **(Figure 9-26)** or a message saying "Claims are being Generated..." because the *ClaimsManager* feature of your student version is not active. In a live environment, your screen would look like **Figure 9-27**, which states "Claims are Queued for all Groups under this Parent Company."

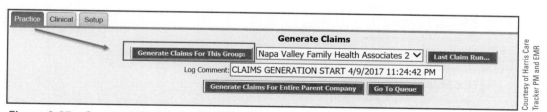

Figure 9-25   Generate Claims for This Group

3. Whether or not you have received an error message, click on *Go to Queue* and a report will generate **(Figure 9-28)**. **Figure 9-29** represents an example of the *Claims Queue* in a live environment, which displays the *Claims Worklist*. Since you are working in a student environment, all of your queues will be empty.

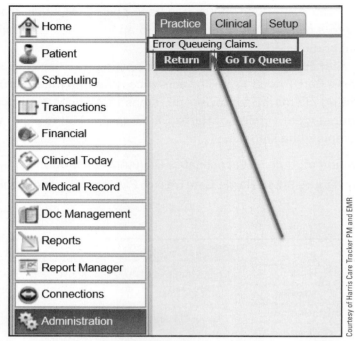

Figure 9-26   Error Queuing Claims (Your message might say "Claims are being Generated for Group [#]" instead.)

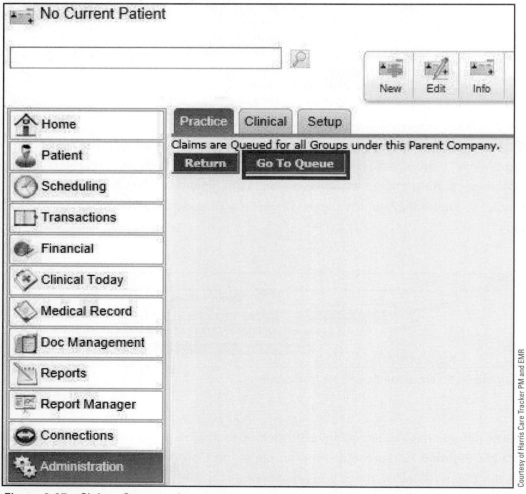

Figure 9-27   Claims Generated

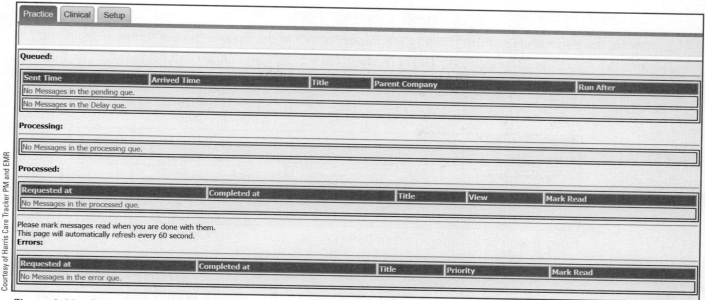

Figure 9-28   Claims Queue (The messages on your screen may differ.)

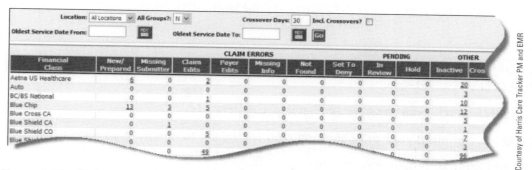

Figure 9-29   Claims Worklist

Print the Claims Queue window, label it "Activity 9-7," and place it in your assignment folder.

4. Click back on the *Administration* module to exit the claims queue. (**Note:** Claims wait in *Queue* to be processed at 5 P.M.)

Activity 9-8
Apply Settings to Print Paper Claims

Although paper claims are rare, there are occasions when you will need to submit one. In Harris CareTracker PM, paper claims are generated by way of the method outlined in Activity 9-9. To print paper claims, you must first apply print settings, as in Activity 9-8.

There are two ways to apply print settings in Harris CareTracker. For this activity, use the Harris CareTracker *Dashboard*.

1. Go to the *Home* module > *Dashboard* tab > *Billing* section > *Unprinted Paper Claim Batches* link. The application displays the *Print Options* window.

2. Click the *Print Options* button in the upper-right corner of the screen.

3. Locate the desired claim form ("1500 CMS Paper Form") in the list and then enter the margin size for the form in the corresponding *Offset Top* field (enter "10") and *Offset Left* field (enter "10") if not already populated **(Figure 9-30)**.

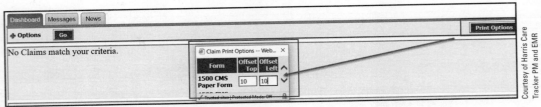

Figure 9-30   Apply Settings to Print Paper Claims

💾 **Print the Claim Print Options window, label it "Activity 9-8," and place it in your assignment folder.**

4. Scroll to the bottom of the dialog box and click *Update*. You must log out and then log back in to Harris CareTracker PM and EMR before the setting takes effect.

📁 # Activity 9-9
Build and Generate a Paper Claim 🚩

Now that you have entered your print settings, you will be set to generate paper claims.

1. Pull patient Edith Robinson into context.

2. Click the *Ol* ▊ tab in the *Name* bar.

3. Click on *Instant Claim* in the *First Clm* column **(Figure 9-31)** for Procedure code 99214. Harris CareTracker PM displays the *Claims Summary* in the lower frame of the screen.

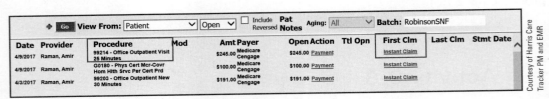

Figure 9-31   First Clm Column—Edith Robinson

4. Place a check mark in the rows for Procedure codes 99214 and G0180. Do **not** place a check mark in the row for Procedure code 99212.

5. Then click *Build Claim*. You will then note that the date you performed the activity is listed in the *First Clm* column.

6. Click on the date in the *First Clm* column for Procedure 99214. Harris CareTracker PM displays the *Claims Summary* in the lower frame of the screen.

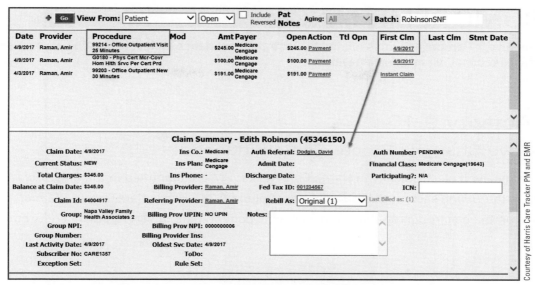

Figure 9-32   First Clm Column—Claim Summary; Edith Robinson

Print the Claims Summary window, label it "Activity 9-9," and place it in your assignment folder.

7. Scroll down and click the *Rebill To = = >* drop-down list at the bottom of the screen and select "*Paper 1500*." Click *Rebuild Paper* **(Figure 9-33)**. Because this is a simulated activity you will receive an error message (see Figure 9-33).

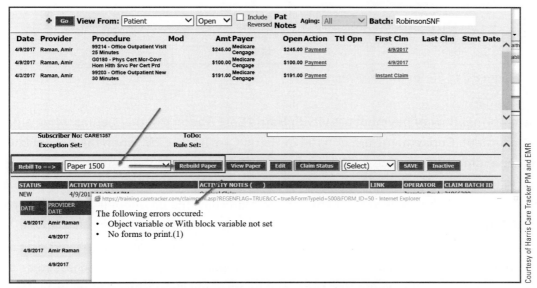

Figure 9-33   Select Rebuild Paper Claim—Paper Claim Error Message

8. Close out of the *Open Items* screen by clicking on "X."

ELECTRONIC REMITTANCE

Learning Objective 5: Perform activities related to electronic remittance including: posting payments and adjustments, and reconciling insurance payments.

Activity 9-10

Save Charges; Process a Remittance

Remittances received electronically in Harris CareTracker PM are identified in the *Electronic Remittances* application in the *Billing* section of the *Dashboard* **(Figure 9-34)**. Harris CareTracker PM matches the transactions on the electronic remittance to a specific patient, date of service, CPT® code, and charge amount.

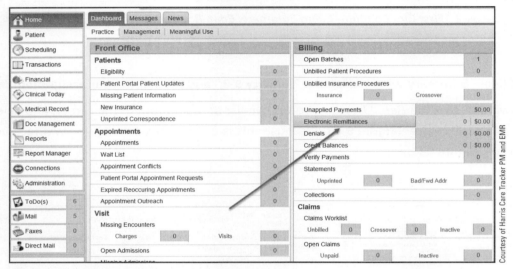

Figure 9-34   Electronic Remittances Link

There is a normal flow of payment activity in Harris CareTracker PM that begins when a patient pays his or her copayment. Copayments are entered in Harris CareTracker PM when the patient checks in or checks out (depending on the office workflow). Next, a claim is sent to the insurance company after the patient visit. In Harris CareTracker PM, most claims are transmitted electronically; however, paper forms are sometimes mailed. When bills are transmitted electronically, the payment is received electronically or on a paper EOB/RA.

Open Items is an application in the *Financial* module. There is an identical application accessed via the *Pmt Open Item* tab in the *Transactions* module, and this application can also be accessed as a window by clicking the *OI* button on the *Name Bar*. The *Open Items* application is used to view all dates of service and the associated procedures, financial transactions, and claims activity **(Figure 9-35)**. In this application, you can enter many different types of financial transactions including patient payments, insurance payments, third-party payments, transfer balances, refunds, and apply unapplied money. You can also view the procedure details of each procedure, enter denial descriptions, attach statement messages to appear on patient statements, view a claim history, potentially rebill a claim, view electronic responses received from insurance companies, and view EOB/RAs attached to payments.

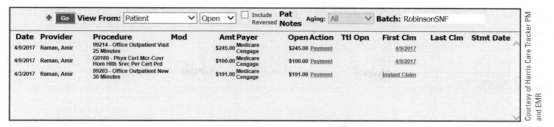

Figure 9-35   Open Items

TIP You can access *Open Items* in the following ways:

- Left-click on an appointment in the *Book* application and select *Open Items.*
- Click the *OI* button on the *Name Bar.*
- Click the *Pmt Open Item* tab in the *Transactions* module. If you receive an error message that the batch in not open, click on the *Batch* icon in the *Name Bar.* The "RobinsonSNF" batch will display. Click *Edit*, then click *Save*. Click back on the *Transactions* module and the *Pmt Open Item* tab, and the *Open Item*(s) will display.

The total number and sum of remittances received electronically into Harris CareTracker PM displays on the *Dashboard* and a list of the received remittances that need to be posted into the system is accessed by clicking on the *Electronic Remittances* link. Electronic remittances should only be posted after the check (or electronic payment) is received from the insurance company.

Before posting payments via *Electronic Remittances*, select one patient from the remittance, pull the patient into context, click the *OI* button on the *Name Bar,* and verify that the date of service is still open in Harris CareTracker PM **(Figure 9-36)**.

1. Before you begin this activity, pull Edith Robinson into context and refer back to Ms. Robinson's encounter from Activity 4-1. (**Hint**: refer to the *Scheduling* module, *History* tab to locate the appointment date.) Record the date of the encounter for this activity: _____

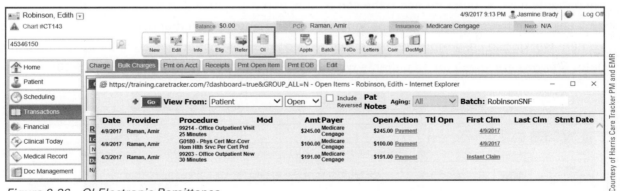

Figure 9-36   OI Electronic Remittance

2. Create a new batch and name it "9-10PostRAs." Use today's date for the *Fiscal Period* and *Fiscal Year*.

3. Update the *Provider* and *Resource* to Edith Robinson's provider and PCP.

4. Click *Save and Close* on the newly created batch. If you receive a message that the "Service Date From is before today. Are you sure you want to save?", click *OK.*

5. Go to the *Home* module > *Dashboard* tab > *Visit* header > *Missing Encounters* > *Charges* link **(Figure 9-37)**.

Courtesy of Harris Care Tracker PM and EMR

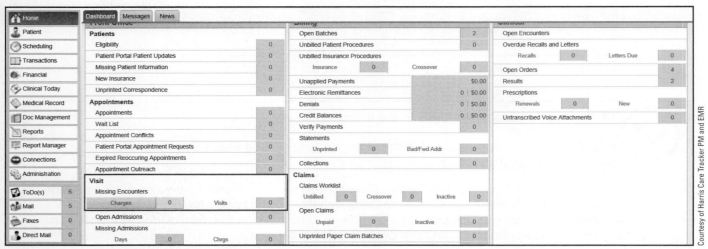

Figure 9-37 Missing Encounters/Charges Link

6. Set the fields as follows:
   - Change the beginning date to January 1, 20XX (current year) and change the ending date to today's date. (**Note**: By default, the ending date is yesterday and will not contain any entries made on the current date unless you change the ending date to today's date.) Be sure the dates include the date of the patient encounter from Activity 4-1.
   - Select *All providers*.
   - Select *All locations*.
   - Select *Visits Yes*.
   - Select *Charges No*.

7. Then click *Go* **(Figure 9-38)**. You will see the *Charges* that have not been saved **(Figure 9-39)**. If multiple patients have appointments on the same date, you will notice that the *Visits* and *Charges* buttons only appear in the row for the first patient with an appointment on that date. This is because when you are working in *OI*, if more than one charge (e.g., multiple patient visits) appears on the same date, *Charges* are saved for all patients with appointments on that date (see **Figure 9-40**).

Courtesy of Harris Care Tracker PM and EMR

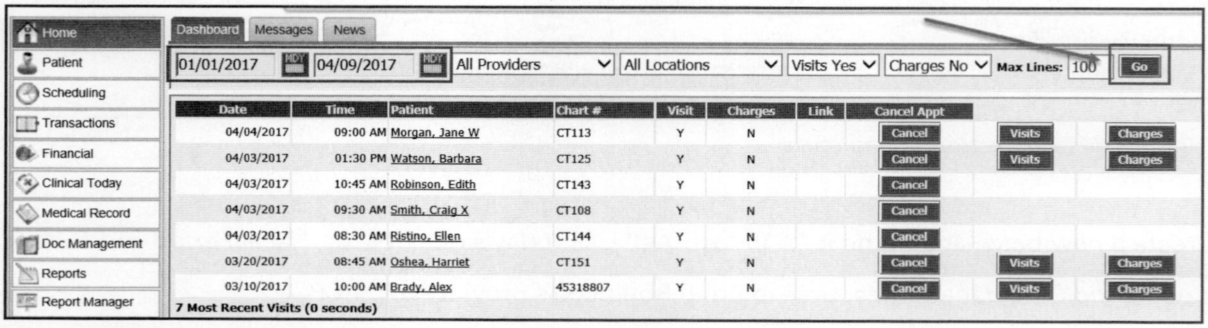

Figure 9-38 Charges Not Saved

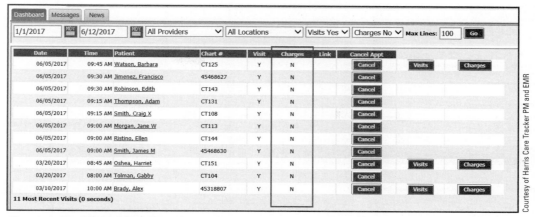

Figure 9-39   Visit(s) Not Saved

8. In the *Date* column, locate the visit date (Figure 9-40) for patient Edith Robinson's appointment from Activity 4-1. Then click on the *Charges* button on the right side of your screen for the date of service corresponding to her Activity 4-1 appointment. (Remember, the *Charges* button may not necessarily appear in Edith Robinson's row; it may appear in the row of a different patient who has the same date of service as her.)

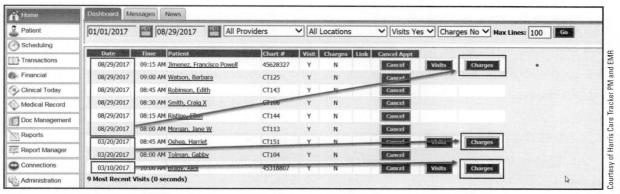

Figure 9-40   Visits and Charges Buttons

9. Now, click *Go* on the left side of your screen. The charges for all patient encounters on the Date of Service (DOS) display. **Note:** You may receive a popup message that says "Transaction Date must be within Period Start and End Dates: (of the date of your batch)." Click *OK* and the charges appear in the lower portion of your screen.

10. Since all the patients with charges display in the lower screen, you will need to scroll down to review the charges for patient Edith Robinson. We will assume here that the charges look okay.

11. Now, scroll down to the bottom of the lower screen, and click *Save* on the bottom left **(Figure 9-41)**. (**Note:** If more than one charge [e.g., multiple patient visits] appear on the date, the *Charges* will be saved for all patients).

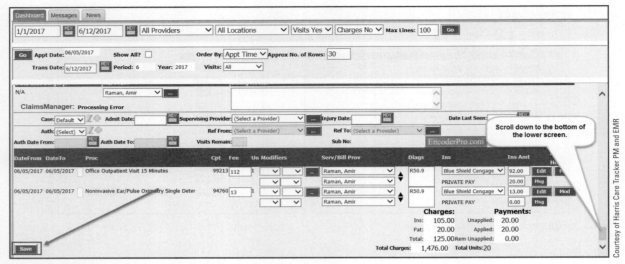

Figure 9-41   Save Visit—Jane Morgan

12. You must wait until the "Transaction Saved" message appears before moving on. Then click *OK*. You will receive another pop-up stating "Bulk Charges Saved." Click *OK*.

13. With patient Edith Robinson in context, click on the *OI* 🔲 button in the *Name Bar*. All captured charges for Ms. Robinson's Activity 4-1 appointment now display.

14. Click on *Instant Claim* in the *First Clm* column for Procedure 99203.

15. Place a checkmark next to the "99203" charge.

16. Click *Build Claim*. The *Open Items* dialog box will now display with a date in the *First Clm* column.

17. Click on the *Payment* link in the *Action* column next to Procedure 99203. Harris CareTracker PM displays the payment window in the lower frame of the screen **(Figure 9-42)**.

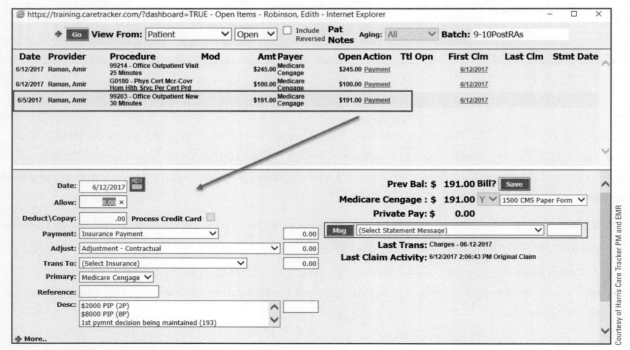

Figure 9-42   Payment Window in OI

18. In the payment window on the lower part of the screen, enter the information from Edith Robinson's EOB/RA (Source Document 9-1a, found at the end of this activity) for Procedure 99203 as instructed below. 92203 is a covered charge. A covered charge will have no amount listed in the "Not Covered (DENIAL)" column of the EOB/RA. You will also note that the EOB/RA also contains information for the SNF charge you entered in Activity 9-3 (Source Document 9-1b). **Important!!** Only enter the EOB/RA information for Procedure 99203. Your completed screen should look like **Figure 9-43**.

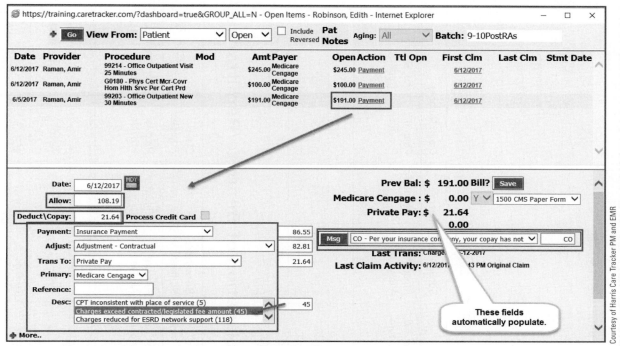

Figure 9-43   *Remittance Information in Payment Window*

a. *Date:* This should be today's date, the date you "received the EOB/RA" for the appointment you created in Activity 4-1.

b. *Allow:* Enter the information from the *Amount Allowed* column on the EOB/RA (Source Document 9-1a). Now hit the [Tab] button on your keyboard.

c. *Deduct/Copay:* Enter the information from the *Deduct/Coins/Copay* column on the EOB/RA (Source Document 9-1a). Now hit the [Tab] button and this will populate the amount in the *Adjust* and *Transfer* To fields based on the information entered in the *Demographics* screen.

d. *Payment:* Confirm that "*Insurance Payment*" is selected.

e. *Adjust:* Confirm that "*Adjustment – Contractual*" is selected.

f. *Trans To:* Confirm that "*Private Pay*" is selected.

g. *Primary:* Confirm that "*Medicare Cengage*" is selected.

h. *Reference:* Leave blank.

i. *Desc:* Enter "45" in the blank box to the right of the *Desc* field, and hit the [Tab] key.

j. *Msg:* Enter "CO" in the blank box to the right of the drop-down menu and hit the [Tab] key.

Source Document 9-1a: Explanation of Benefits/Remittance Advice

MEDICARE CENGAGE

Medicare Cengage
P.O. Box 234434
San Francisco, CA 94137

AMIR RAMAN, D.O.
Napa Valley Family Health Associates (NVFHA)
101 Vine Street
Napa, CA 94558

Date: MM/DD/YYYY (use today's date)
Payment Number: 12808957
Payment Amount: $ 145.01

Account Number	Patient Name					Subscriber Number		Claim Number			
Dates of Service	Description of Service	Amount Charged	Not Covered	Prov Adj Discount	Amount Allowed	Deduct/ Coins/ Copay	Paid to Provider	Adj Reason Code	Rmk Code	Patient Resp	
CARE1357	Robinson, Edith										
(Appt. date used in Activity 4-1)	99203	$191.00	$0.00	$82.81	$108.19	$21.64	$86.55	45*		$21.64	

Source Document 9-1b: Explanation of Benefits/Remittance Advice

Account Number	Patient Name					Subscriber Number		Claim Number			
Dates of Service	Description of Service	Amount Charged	Not Covered	Prov Adj Discount	Amount Allowed	Deduct/ Coins/ Copay	Paid to Provider	Adj Reason Code	Rmk Code	Patient Resp	
CARE1357	Robinson, Edith										
(SNF. date used in Activity 9-3)	99214	$245.00	$245.00		$0.00	$0.00	$0.00	96*		$245.00	
(SNF. date used in Activity 9-3)	G0180	$100.00		$26.93	$73.07	$14.61	$58.46			$14.61	

Print the Process Remittance (OI screen), label it "Activity 9-10a," and place it in your assignment folder.

19. Once you have entered the EOB/RA information, click *Save.* Your transaction will be saved and the claim disappears.

20. (FYI) If you were working multiple charges, you would enter the additional charge information (following steps 18 and 19 for guidance) for each of the charges listed on the EOB/RA. (**Note:** Do <u>not</u> enter the additional payments at this point.)

21. Close out of the *Open Items* window by clicking the "X" in the upper-right corner of the window.

22. Run a *Journal* for batch "9-10PostRAs."

Print the Journal, label it "Activity 9-10b," and place it in your assignment folder.

Activity 9-11

Enter a Denial and Remittance

Denials are claims that an insurance company has determined it will not pay, such as when a patient has not met his or her deductible. By working your denials separately from posting payments, you will improve the workflow and efficiency in your practice. Your student version of Harris CareTracker PM will not post *Denials* in your *Dashboard* because *ClaimsManager* is not active. The *Denials* screen can be accessed by going to the *Home* module > *Dashboard* tab > *Billing* header > *Denials* link **(Figure 9-44).**

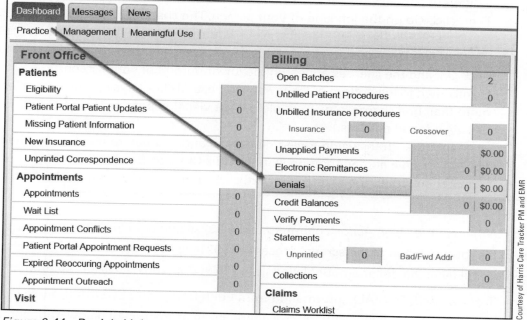

Figure 9-44   Denials Link

Using the same patient from Activity 9-10 (Edith Robinson), you will now post a denial and additional remittance to her account.

1. Before beginning this activity, click on *Batch* in the *Name Bar* and confirm you are still working in the "9-10PostRAs" batch.

2. With patient Edith Robinson in context, click on the *OI* button on the *Name Bar*.

3. You will see the charges for Ms. Robinson's *Open Items*. You are going to now work the SNF edited charges for Procedure codes 99214 and G0180.

TIP

1. **Important!!** Only if you do not see the edited SNF charges for Procedure codes 99214 and G0180, go to the *Home* module > *Dashboard* tab > *Visit* header > *Missing Encounters/Visit* link and you will see that the *Charge* has not been saved.
   To save the *Charges*, set the fields as follows:

   - Include the date of the patient encounter.
   - Select *All providers*.
   - Select *All locations*.
   - Select *Visits Yes*.
   - Select *Charges No*.
   - Click *Go*.

2. In the *Date* column, locate the visit date for patient Edith Robinson's SNF charges from Activity 9-3. Then click on the *Charges* button on the right side of your screen for the date of service corresponding to Edith's Activity 9-3 charges. (Remember, the *Charges* button may not necessarily appear in Edith Robinson's row; it may appear in the row of a different patient who has the same date of service as her.)

3. Then click *Go* on the left side of your screen. The charges for all patient encounters on the Date of Service (DOS) display. **Note:** You may receive a pop-up message that says "Transaction Date must be within Period Start and End Dates: (of the date of your batch)." Click *OK*, and the charges appear in the lower portion of your screen.

4. Scroll down to the bottom of the lower screen, and click *Save* on the bottom left. (**Note:** If more than one charge [e.g., multiple patient visits] appear on the date, the *Charges* will be saved for all patients.)

5. Wait until the "Transaction Saved" message appears before moving on. Then click *OK*. You will receive another pop-up stating "Bulk Charges Saved." Click *OK*.

6. With patient Edith Robinson in context, click on the *OI* button on the *Name Bar*.

---

4. Click on *Payment* in the *Open Action* column for code 99214 and the *Open Items* dialog box will display in the lower portion of the screen. Procedure 99214 is not a covered charge. A charge that is not covered will have the dollar amount listed in the "Not Covered (DENIAL)" column of the EOB/RA.

5. Enter the "Not Covered (DENIAL)" information from Edith Robinson's EOB/RA (Source Document 9-1b, found at the end of activity 9-10) for Procedure 99214 as instructed below. Your completed screen should look like **Figure 9-45**.

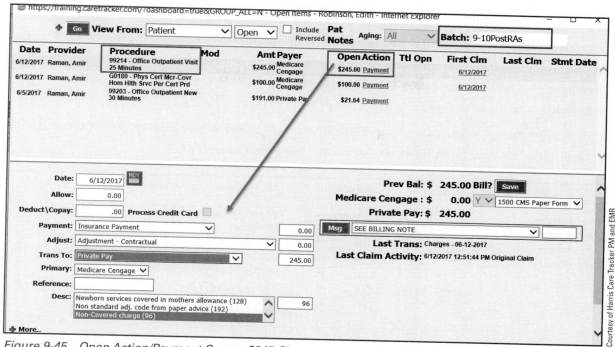

Figure 9-45   Open Action/Payment Screen $245 Charge

Note: Be sure to use the [Tab] key so that fields automatically populate.

a. *Date*: Enter today's date (within the *Fiscal Period Fiscal Year* set in your batch).

b. *Allow*: Leave blank. (0.00)

c. *Deduct/Copay*: Leave blank. (0.00)

d. *Payment*: Using the drop-down, select "Insurance Payment." **Note**: You may need to change the field first to (Select Payment Type) and then back to "Insurance Payment." Be sure you use the [Tab] key so that amounts will populate in the proper fields.

e. *Adjust*: Select "Adjustment – Contractual." Make sure this field is "0.00." If you need to enter "0.00," be sure you use the [Tab] key so that amounts will populate in the proper fields.

f. *Transfer To*: Use the drop-down and select "*Private Pay.*" This will automatically populate the amount field to the right of *Trans To*, as well as the *Prev Bal* and it *Private Pay* fields.

g. *Primary*: Leave blank (or it can remain "Medicare Cengage.")

h. *Reference*: Leave blank.

i. *Desc*: Type "96" in the blank box to the right of *Desc* and hit [Tab]. This will select "Non-Covered charge (96)."

j. In the *Msg* field, use the drop-down list and select "*SEE BILLING NOTE.*"

k. Your screen should reflect the same entries as noted in Source Document 9-1b for Procedure code 99214.

🖫 **Print the Not Covered (DENIAL) Charge screen, label it "Activity 9-11a," and place it in your assignment folder.**

l. Click *Save.* You will have to close out of the *OI* screen and re-open it before the claim disappears.

6. Click back on the *OI* button.

7. In the *Open Items* window, click the *Payment* link under the *Action* header for the G0180 Procedure code charge. G0180 is a covered charge. A covered charge will have <u>no</u> amount listed in the "Not Covered (DENIAL)" column of the EOB/RA. (If needed, refer back to Activity 9-10, step 18 for guidance on entering a covered charge.)

8. Enter the remittance information from Edith Robinson's EOB/RA (see Source Document 9-1b) for Procedure G0180. Your completed screen should look like **Figure 9-46**.

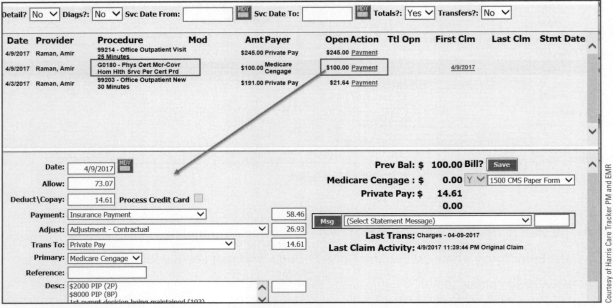

Figure 9-46   Open Action/Payment Screen $100 Charge

Print the Covered Charge screen, label it "Activity 9-11b," and place it in your assignment folder.

9. Click *Save*.

10. You have now saved all the information from the EOB/RA related to the SNF charge you created in Activities 9-3 and 9-4 for Edith Robinson (as noted in **Figure 9-47**). You will have to close out of the *OI* screen and re-open it before the claim disappears.

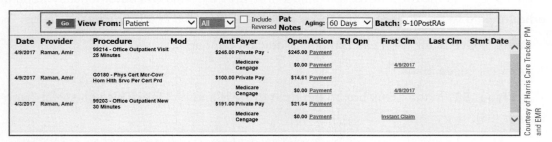

Figure 9-47   Denial and Remittance Information Saved-SNF Charge

11. Do **not** post the "9-10PostRAs" batch at this time. You will be instructed to post it later.

12. (FYI) Having entered the denial in Activity 9-11, the balance has now been transferred to private pay. **Note:** It is important to remember that it takes 24 hours for *Denials* to display in the *Dashboard* in a live environment. You can adjust your filters to set your display options. The *Dashboard* only shows *Denials* for the month.

PROFESSIONALISM CONNECTION

For many patients and staff members, discussing the subject of money owed is touchy and uncomfortable. You must always address the topic in a calm and non-judgmental way and comply with office policy, even if a patient requests special payment arrangements. Special requests should be documented and forwarded to the appropriate person or department, often the office manager, billing department, or managing provider. When asking for payment, use positive expressions. Practice your professionalism by role-playing with co-workers the following scenarios. Adjust the wording to your comfort level and to that of a service provider professional:

- When making an appointment by phone: "Copayment is expected at the time of service" or "Your office visit will be approximately $___. For your convenience we accept cash, checks, and credit card."
- For the patient checking in at the front desk: "Your copayment today will be $___."
- For patients checking out: "Your charges for today's office visit are $___. Would you like to pay by cash, check, or credit card?" or "I see your deductible has been met and your insurance pays 80%. Your portion of the bill comes to $___. Would you like to pay by cash, check, or credit card?"

My challenge to you is to demonstrate how you would approach collection of payment in a positive and professional manner.

Activity 9-12
Work Credit Balances

Working credit balances by batch should be done immediately after an electronic remittance has been posted in Harris CareTracker PM. Credit balances are created when either a patient or an insurance company pays more money for a specific procedure for a specific date of service than what was billed. Credit balances can be identified by the *Credit Balances* link under the *Billing* section of the *Dashboard* in the *Home* module for a specific batch or group **(Figure 9-48)**. After you post payments via electronic remittances, it is best practice to work credit balances for the batch you were working in before posting the batch.

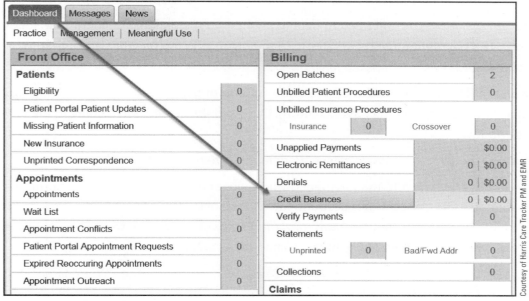

Figure 9-48   Credit Balances Link

There are two ways to work credit balances: *by Batch* or *for Refunds* (**Figure 9-49**). Once you post the batch, this will create a charge on the patient's account. You can then post a payment to create the credit balance.

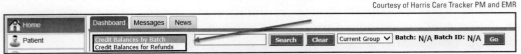

Figure 9-49   Work Credit Balances—By Batch or for Refunds

 TIP There is a big difference between a "Credit" and an "Unapplied Credit." A credit is an overpayment on an account, and an unapplied credit is only a patient payment (not insurance) that has not been attached to a DOS.

In order to work a *Credit Balance*, you must first have a credit in the patient's account.

1. Pull patient Edith Robinson into context.

2. Create a new batch and name it "9-12CreditBalance" using the following parameters:

   a. *Fiscal Period*: The fiscal period of Ms. Robinson's SNF charge created in Activity 9-3.

   b. *Fiscal Year*: The fiscal year of Ms. Robinson's SNF charge created in Activity 9-3.

   c. *Provider*: Select Ms. Robinson's PCP (Dr. Raman).

   d. *Resource*: Select Dr. Raman as *Resource.*

   e. *Location*: Napa Valley Family Associates.

   f. Leave *Service Date From*, *Service Trans Date*, and *Payment Trans Date* blank.

3. Click *Save and Close* on the batch screen.

4. Click on the *OI* button on the *Name Bar*. Harris CareTracker PM displays the *Open Items* application.

5. To see a credit balance, you will need to post a payment to the patient's account first, following these instructions. The payment must be greater than the balance in the patient's account in *OI* in the *Open Action* column:

   a. Click on the *Payment* line in the *Open Action* column of her G0180 *Procedure* (which should be listed as "Private Pay" in the *Payer* column). The *payment* screen will display in the lower portion of the window.

   b. Using the *Payment* drop-down, select "*Payment – Patient Cash (PATCSH).*"

   c. In the amount field next to the *Payment* drop-down, enter a payment in the amount of $50.00 more than the *OI* balance of her account. In this instance, her *OI* balance displays as $14.61, so you would add $50.00 to that amount for a total entry of $64.61. (**Note:** Do not enter the dollar sign.) You will see the *Private Pay* balance change to "$-50.00."

   d. In the *Msg* drop-down select (or leave as) "Select Statement Message." Your screen should look like **Figure 9-50**.

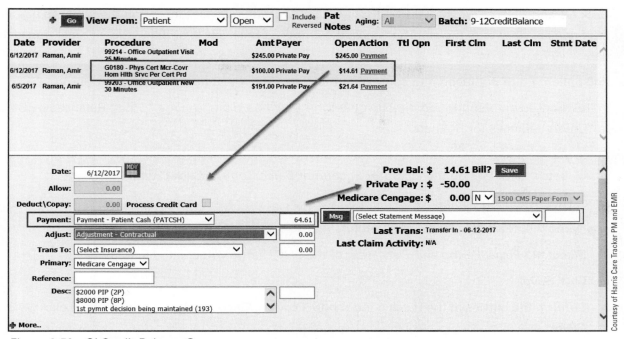

Figure 9-50   OI Credit Balance Screen

e. Click *Save*.

f. To close the *Open Items* screen, click "X."

g. Run a *Journal* for the "9-12CreditBalance" batch.

h. *Post* the "9-12CreditBalance" batch.

6. Go to the *Home* module > *Dashboard* tab > *Billing* header > *Credit Balances* link (see Figure 9-48).

7. Click on the *Search* button and Harris CareTracker PM displays a list of open batches in the *Search* dialog box.

   a. Because you have already posted your batch, it does not display in the *Search* box.

   b. Type in "9-12" and check the "Includes Closed Batches" and "All Groups" checkboxes **(Figure 9-51)**, and then click *Search*.

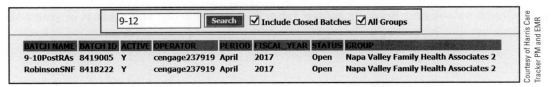

Figure 9-51   CreditBalance Search Criteria

8. Click on the "9-12CreditBalance" batch and it is pulled into context **(Figure 9-52)**.

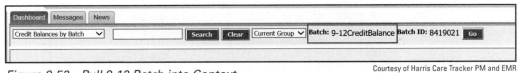

Figure 9-52   Pull 9-12 Batch into Context

9. Click *Go* and Harris CareTracker PM displays a list of credit balances including the patient's name, the financial class with the credit balance, the amount of the credit, and the patient's last transaction date.

10. Pull patient Edith Robinson into context on the *Name Bar* if you have not already done so.

11. In the drop-down menu found directly under the *Dashboard* tab, change "Credit Balances by Batch" to "Credit Balances for Refunds."

12. Since you posted the "CreditBalance" batch previously in this activity, you will be prompted to create a new batch. Click *Edit* on the *Operator Encounter Batch Control*. Click *Create Batch*.

13. Create a batch using the following parameters:

    a. Name the new batch "9-12CrBalRefunds."

    b. Select the *Fiscal Period* and *Fiscal Year* of the SNF charge you created in Activity 9-3.

    c. Click *Save*.

    d. Confirm the entries in the batch control box (Provider/Resource/Location) and then click *Save and Close*.

    e. Your new batch has now been created.

14. Confirm that the date for the charge is included in the *Date From* and *Date To* fields. **Hint**: Always change the *Date To* field to include today's date.

15. Click *Go* and Ms. Robinson's credit balance will pull in to the screen.

16. In the *Action* Column, use the drop-down and select "*Refund-Patient (P)*" **(Figure 9-53)**.

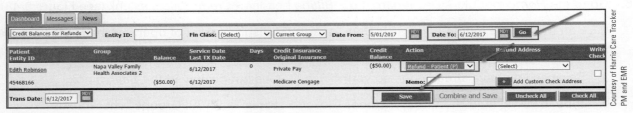

Figure 9-53   *Select Patient for Credit Balances for Refunds*

📇 **Print the Credit Balance for Refunds screen, label it "Activity 9-12," and place it in your assignment folder.**

17. Click *Save*.

18. The *Credit Balance Transfer* dialog box will display.

19. Click on *Write Transactions* **(Figure 9-54)**.

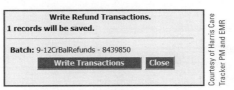

Figure 9-54   *Write Transactions*

20. The *Credit Balance Transfer* dialog box will confirm that the transaction has been saved **(Figure 9-55)**.

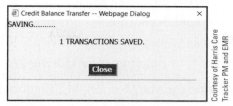

Figure 9-55   Credit Balance Transfer Dialog Box

21. Click *Close*, and the credit balance is removed from your screen.

Activity 9-13

Save Charges, Process Remittance, and Transfer to Private Pay

In order to continue with billing and collections activities, you must build and generate claims, save the charges, and process the EOB/RAs for the additional following patients.

In this activity, you will work with the following patients. Before you begin, refer back to the patient encounters and record the date of the encounters for this activity's patients:

      9-13a: Jane Morgan (Source Document 9-2): _____

      9-13b: Ellen Ristino (Source Document 9-3): _____

      9-13c: Craig X. Smith (Source Document 9-4): _____

      9-13d: Barbara Watson (Source Document 9-5): _____

1. Create a new batch and name it "9-13PostRAs" with the following parameters:

    a. Select the *Fiscal Period* and *Fiscal Year* for today's date.

    b. Click *Save*.

    c. Leave the *Provider/Resource/Location* as is.

    d. Click *Save and Close*.

2. Check that charges have been saved for each of the patients listed above. To do this, go to the *Home* module > *Dashboard* tab > *Visit* header > *Missing Encounters* > *Charges* link and set the fields as follows:

    • Change the beginning date to January 1, 20XX (current year) and change the ending date to today's date. Be sure the dates include the date of the patient's encounter.

    • Select *All providers*.

    • Select *All locations*.

    • Select *Visits Yes*.

    • Select *Charges No*.

3. Then click *Go*. You will see *Charges*(s) that have <u>not</u> been saved. You may or may not see the charges for these four patients here. That is because charges for the four patients in this activity would have

already been saved in Activity 9-10 if the patients had appointments on the same date as Edith Robinson. If an appointment was on a different date than Edith Robinson's, that appointment will appear here and the charges will need to be saved. If charges for any of these four patients are displaying, save the charges now. You can refer back to steps 8–12 of Activity 9-10 for assistance if needed. If no charges are displaying for any of these four patients, move forward to step 4.

4. Generate claims for all procedures listed for Ms. Morgan, Ms. Ristino, Mr. Smith, and Ms. Watson (refer to the steps noted below):

   - Pull patient into context.
   - Click the *OI* tab in the *Name* bar.
   - Click on *Instant Claim* in the *First Clm* column for one of the procedures. Harris CareTracker PM displays the *Claims Summary* in the lower frame of the screen.
   - Place a check mark next to each claim and then click *Build Claim.* You will then note that the date you performed the activity is listed in the *First Clm* column.

5. For each patient noted above, process the EOB/RAs from Source Documents 9-2 through 9-5 provided at the end of this activity. Refresher steps are provided as a "Tip." **Hint**: Denials should be entered as they were in Activity 9-11, step 5. A denial is when the *Amount Charged* and the *Not Covered* is the same amount, and when the *Amount Allowed* is 0.00 on the EOB/RA.

TIP   *Refresher:* **Process an EOB/RA**

1. If you are not already viewing the *Open Items* window, click on the *OI* button in the *Name Bar*.
2. Click on the *Payment* link in the *Action* column next to the Procedure(s).
3. Harris CareTracker PM displays the payment window in the lower frame of the screen (refer to Figure 9-42).
4. In the payment window on the lower part of the screen, enter the information from the patient's EOB/RA (see the Source Documents provided at the end of this activity) for the visit as follows. First determine if the charge is covered or not covered. To do this, look in the "Not Covered (DENIAL)" column of the EOB/RA. A covered charge will have no amount listed in the "Not Covered (DENIAL)" column. A not covered charge has an amount listed in the "Not Covered (DENIAL)" column. As described below, the process you follow for entering the charge will vary depending on if the charge is covered or not covered.

Covered Charges:
- *Date:* This should be today's date, the date you "received the EOB/RA" for the patient's visit.
- *Allow:* Enter the information from the *Amount Allowed* column on the EOB/RA. Now hit the [Tab] button on your keyboard.
- *Deduct/Copay:* Enter the information from the *Deduct/Coins/Copay* column on the EOB/RA. Now hit the [Tab] button and this will populate the amount in the *Adjust* and *TransferTo* fields based on the information entered in the *Demographics* screen.
- *Payment*: Confirm that "*Insurance Payment*" is selected.

- *Adjust*: Confirm that "*Adjustment – Contractual*" is selected.
- *Trans To:* Confirm that "*Private Pay*" is selected.
- *Primary:* Confirm that the patient's correct insurance is selected.
- *Reference:* Leave blank.
- *Desc:* Leave as is.
- *Msg:* Leave as is.

Not Covered Charges:

- *Date:* This should be today's date; the date you "received the EOB/RA" for the patient's visit.
- *Allow:* Enter the information from the *Amount Allowed* column on the EOB/RA. Now hit the [Tab] button on your keyboard.
- *Deduct/Copay:* Enter the information from the *Deduct/Coins/Copay* column on the EOB/RA. Now hit the [Tab] button and this will populate the amount in the *Adjust* and *Transfer To* fields based on the information entered in the *Demographics* screen.
- *Payment:* Confirm that "*Insurance Payment*" is selected and $0.00 is the amount in the field
- *Adjust:* Confirm that "*Adjustment – Contractual*" is selected. Delete the amount in the *Adjust* field, enter "0.00" and then hit the [Tab] button.
- *Trans To:* Confirm that "*Private Pay*" is selected. The *Trans To* field should then populate with "*Private Pay*" and the amount of the charge denied. (**Note**: If it does not populate, manually enter the amount to *Trans To* "*Private Pay*." The "*Private Pay*" amount would be the same as noted in the "Patient Resp" column on the EOB/RA.)
- *Primary:* Confirm that the patient's correct insurance is selected
- *Reference:* Leave blank
- *Desc:* Leave as is
- *Msg:* Leave as is

5. Once you have entered the EOB/RA information, click *Save*. Your transaction will be saved and the claim disappears. (You have now saved all the entries from the EOB/RA related to the charge you created. You have to close out of the *OI* screen and re-open it before the claim disappears.)
6. If you were working multiple charges, you would repeat the steps to enter each of the charges listed on the EOB/RA. Refer to Figure 9-43 for an example of what your completed screen should look like.
7. Close out of the *Open Items* window by clicking the "X" in the upper-right corner of the window.
8. Repeat the above steps for each patient.

6. Upon completion of *ALL* payment/denial entries, run a *Journal* (reference Activity 9-5 for assistance) and review for accuracy. Do **not** post the "9-13PostRAs" batch at this time.

Print the Journal after completing all the 9-13 activities, label it "Activity 9-13" and place in your assignment folder.

Source Document 9-2:   Explanation of Benefits/Remittance Advice

BLUE SHIELD CENGAGE

Blue Shield Cengage
P.O. Box 32245
Los Angeles, CA 90002

Date: MM/DD/YYYY (use today's date)
Payment Number: 5564856
Payment Amount: $0.00

AMIR RAMAN, D.O
Napa Valley Family Health Associates (NVFHA)
101 Vine Street
Napa, CA 94558

Account Number	Patient Name				Subscriber Number			Claim Number			
Dates of Service	Description of Service	Amount Charged	Not Covered (DENIAL)	Prov Adj Discount	Amount Allowed	Deduct/ Coins/ Copay	Paid to Provider	Adj Reason Code	Rmk Code	Patient Resp
BCBS97	**Morgan, Jane**									
(Appt. date used in Activity 4-1)	99213	$112.00		$36.00	$76.00	$76.00	$0.00			$56.00
(Appt. date used in Activity 4-1)	90746	$100.00		$23.00	$77.00	$77.00	$0.00			$77.00

Source Document 9-3: Explanation of Benefits

BLUE SHIELD CENGAGE

Blue Shield Cengage
P.O. Box 32245
Los Angeles, CA 90002

Date: MM/DD/YYYY (use today's date)
Payment Number: 5564854
Payment Amount: $81.64

ANTHONY BROCKTON, M.D.
Napa Valley Family Health Associates (NVFHA)
101 Vine Street
Napa, CA 94558

Account Number	Patient Name					Subscriber Number			Claim Number			
Dates of Service	Description of Service	Amount Charged	Not Covered (DENIAL)	Prov Adj Discount		Amount Allowed	Deduct/ Coins/ Copay		Paid to Provider	Adj Reason Code	Rmk Code	Patient Resp
BCBS97	**Ristino, Ellen**											
(Appt. date used in Activity 4-1)	99213	$112.00		$36.00		$76.00	$15.20		$60.80			$15.20
(Appt. date used in Activity 4-1)	86308	$45.00				$16.55	$3.31		$13.24			$3.31
(Appt. date used in Activity 4-1)	3210F	$24.00				$9.50	$1.90		$7.60			$1.90
(Appt. date used in Activity 4-1)	36415	$15.00	$15.00			$0.00						$15.00
(Appt. date used in Activity 4-1)	94760	$13.00	$13.00			$0.00						$13.00

Source Document 9-4:   Explanation of Benefits/Remittance Advice

MEDICAID CENGAGE

Medicaid Cengage
P.O. Box 221352
Fresno, CA 93701

Date: MM/DD/YYYY (use today's date)
Payment Number: 5644425
Payment Amount: $46.00

AMIR RAMAN, D.O.
Napa Valley Family Health Associates (NVFHA)
101 Vine Street
Napa, CA 94558

Account Number	Patient Name					Subscriber Number		Claim Number			
Dates of Service	Description of Service	Amount Charged	Not Covered (DENIAL)	Prov Adj Discount	Amount Allowed	Deduct/ Coins/ Copay	Paid to Provider	Adj Reason Code	Rmk Code	Patient Resp
CAID8002	**Smith, Craig X.**									
(Appt. date used in Activity 4-1)	99213	$112.00		$79.00	$33.00	$0.00	$33.00			$0.00
(Appt. date used in Activity 4-1)	J7650	$25.00		$18.00	$7.00	$0.00	$7.00			$0.00
(Appt. date used in Activity 4-1)	71020	$13.50		$7.50	$6.00	$0.00	$6.00			$0.00

Amount Allowed (45*) = Charges exceed your contracted/legislated fee arrangement
Amount Allowed (20*) = Not a covered code

Source Document 9-5:   Explanation of Benefits/Remittance Advice

BLUE SHIELD CENGAGE

Blue Shield Cengage
P.O. Box 32245
Los Angeles, CA 90002

Date: MM/DD/YYYY (use today's date)
Payment Number: 5564855
Payment Amount: $0.00

AMIR RAMAN, D.O
Napa Valley Family Health Associates (NVFHA)
101 Vine Street
Napa, CA 94558

Account Number	Patient Name				Subscriber Number		Claim Number			
Dates of Service	Description of Service	Amount Charged	Not Covered (DENIAL)	Prov Adj Discount	Amount Allowed	Deduct/ Coins/ Copay	Paid to Provider	Adj Reason Code	Rmk Code	Patient Resp
BCBS97	**Watson, Barbara**									
(Appt. date used in Activity 4-2)	99213	$112.00		$36.00	$76.00	$76.00	$0.00			$56.00
(Appt. date used in Activity 4-2)	94760	$13.00		$11.00	$2.00	$2.00	$0.00			$2.00

CRITICAL THINKING There was a lot to cover in this chapter! Describe your understanding of the many different types of insurance plans and the effects on the practice when there is an issue regarding noncovered services.

If you are tasked with communicating the fees for services to patients, collecting copays, or billing/collections on overdue accounts, describe what communication skills you would use. How would you incorporate empathy toward the patient while performing your financial responsibilities? How would using an electronic health record help with your duties? Write out some scenarios and practice on a family member, classmate, or friend.

CASE STUDIES
Case Study 9-1

1. Before beginning Case Study 9-1, create a new batch and name it "Ch9CS-Remit" with the following parameters:

   a. *Fiscal Period* and *Fiscal Year*. Select the current month and year for *Fiscal Period* and *Fiscal Year*. Click *Save*.

   b. Change *Provider* and *Resource* to Dr. Rebecca Ayerick.

   c. Location: Napa Valley Family Associates.

   d. Click *Save and Close*.

2. Pull patient Kevin Johnson into context.

3. Manually enter a charge for Kevin Johnson. Refer to Activity 9-3 and the following steps for help.

4. Select *Location* of "NVFA."

5. Select *POS*: Office

6. Search for and select ICD-10 code N41.0 in the *Dx Cd* field. (**Note:** This is a non-covered charge by Mr. Johnson's insurance.)

7. Using the following information, manually enter a charge for an "Online Service" for patient Kevin Johnson using today's date.

   a. Enter CPT code 99444 in the *Proc* field, and the *Fee* of $45.00.

8. Click *Save* and wait for the error message that the transaction has been saved.

9. Then click *OK*.

10. Upon completion, run a *Journal* (refer to Activity 9-5) and review. Do <u>not</u> post the "Ch9CS-Remit" batch at this time.

11. Enter a denial of the charge and transfer to private pay following instructions in Activity 9-11 and as noted on Mr. Johnson's EOB/RA (Source Document 9-6, located at the end of the Chapter 9 Case Studies). (**Hint:** First *Build the Claim* by clicking on *Instant Claim* in the *First Clm* column.)

12. Run the *Journal* again.

📧 Print the Journal after completing the 9-1 case study, label it "Case Study 9-1," and place in your assignment folder.

13. Now *Post* the batch "Ch9CS-Remit."

Source Document 9-6:   Explanation of Benefits/Remittance Advice

BLUE SHIELD CENGAGE

Blue Shield Cengage
P.O. Box 32245
Los Angeles. CA 90002

Date: MM/DD/YYYY (use today's date)
Payment Number: 2322144
Payment Amount: $0.00

REBECCA AVERICK, M.D.
Napa Valley Family Health Associates (NVFHA)
101 Vine Street
Napa, CA 94558

Account Number	Patient Name					Subscriber Number			Claim Number			
Dates of Service	Description of Service	Amount Charged	Not Covered (DENIAL)	Prov Adj Discount	Amount Allowed	Deduct/ Coins/ Copay	Paid to Provider	Adj Reason Code	Rmk Code	Patient Resp
9706416	Johnson, Kevin									
(Date of Case Study 9-1 manual charge)	99444	$45.00	$45.00	$0.00	$0.00	$45.00	$0.00			$45.00

Case Study 9-2

In order to complete Case Study 9-2, you must have completed the prior chapter Case Studies for patient Adam Thompson. Having captured the visit for Adam Thompson (in Case Study 7-3), you will now build the claim, and then enter the EOB/RA.

1. Create a new batch and name it "Ch9CS-RA" with the following parameters:

   a. *Fiscal Period* and *Fiscal Year*: Select the *Fiscal Period* and *Fiscal Year* of the encounter/visit you created for Adam Thompson in Activity 4-1. Click *Save*.

   b. Change *Provider* and *Resource* to Dr. Anthony Brockton.

   c. Location: Napa Valley Family Associates.

   d. Click *Save and Close*.

2. Pull patient Adam Thompson into context.

3. Click on the *OI* button in the *Name Bar* and Mr. Thompson's charges will appear. **Hint**: If Mr. Thompson's charges aren't appearing in *OI*, you will need to first save the charges. To save the charges for Mr. Thompson's visit, refer back to Activity 9-13.

4. Click on *Instant Claim* in the *First Clm* column.

5. All of Mr. Thompson's charges appear in the lower screen.

6. Place a check mark next to each charge and then click *Build Claim*.

7. Now click on the *Payment* link in the *Open Action* column (repeat for each Procedure listed in the claim).

8. Referring to Source Document 9-7 located at the end of this case study, enter the EOB/RA amounts. Refer to Activities 9-9 and 9-10 for help.

9. Run a *Journal*.

🖫 **Print the screen after completing the 9-2 case study, label it "Case Study 9-2," and place in your assignment folder.**

10. Now *Post* the batch "Ch9CS-RA" (refer to Activity 9-6 for help).

Source Document 9-7:   Explanation of Benefits/Remittance Advice

MEDICARE CENGAGE

Medicare Cengage
P.O. Box 234434
San Francisco, CA 94137

Date: MM/DD/YYYY (use today's date)
Payment Number: 11235784
Payment Amount: $81.12

ANTHONY BROCKTON, M.D.
Napa Valley Family Health Associates (NVFHA)
101 Vine Street
Napa, CA 94558

Account Number	Patient Name				Subscriber Number			Claim Number			
Dates of Service	Description of Service	Amount Charged	Not Covered (DENIAL)	Prov Adj Discount	Amount Allowed	Deduct/ Coins/ Copay	Paid to Provider	Adj Reason Code	Rmk Code	Patient Resp	
CARE1357	**Thompson, Adam**										
(Appt. date from Activity 4-1)	94760	$13.00		$10.36	$2.64	$0.53	$2.11			$0.53	
(Appt. date from Activity 4-1)	99213	$112.00		$53.11	$58.89	$11.78	$47.11			$11.78	
(Appt. date from Activity 4-1)	71020	$13.50		$3.50	$10.00	$2.00	$8.00			$2.00	
(Appt. date from Activity 4-1)	93000	$46.50		$16.50	$30.00	$6.00	$24.00			$6.00	

ClaimsManager
and Collections

Learning Objectives

1. Use the features of ClaimsManager in Harris CareTracker PM and EMR.
2. Check status and work unpaid/inactive claims.
3. Generate patient statements.
4. Review collection status and transfer private pay balances.
5. Create collection letters.
6. Generate collection letters.

Real-World Connection

It cannot be overstated that all personnel, including office staff or collections agents, must act with the utmost professionalism during the collection process. Not only do numerous laws and regulations apply to the collection process, but also the sensitive nature of the relationship between provider and patient must be protected. Credit information of the patient is considered confidential and may not be released without the patient's expressed permission. Financial information regarding the patient is also confidential and must be protected according to the law. Both in-person and telephone discussions should be conducted in an area that is out of view and hearing of other patients.

Credit arrangements and interest charges must be disclosed in writing. Enforcing the credit policy can be uncomfortable for both patients and staff. You must overcome any inhibitions regarding discussion of fees and payments. The success of the practice relies heavily on the medical assistant's ability to politely yet firmly ask for payment from patients. The first step in the collection process is to advise patients of the office policy regarding payment when they call to schedule an appointment. It is important that you remain calm, compassionate, and empathetic to patients. If you encounter a difficult patient, follow these steps to diffuse and resolve the matter:

1. Let the patient vent.
2. Express empathy to the patient. The tone of your voice goes a long way. Use a genuinely warm and caring tone to enhance the meaning of empathetic phrases.
3. Begin problem-solving. Ask the patient questions to help clarify the situation and cause of the problem and double-check the facts.
4. Mutually agree on the solution. Be careful not to make a promise you cannot keep.
5. Follow up. You will score big points by following up with your patient to resolve the problem. This is sometimes referred to as service recovery.

You must demonstrate professionalism with every contact and treat each patient with the utmost respect. Your collection activities should be client-oriented and demonstrate the proper attitude and temperament with close attention given to protecting the goodwill established with your patient. Let me challenge you to role-play with your co-workers various collection scenarios that you might encounter. This will help with preparedness, conveying empathy, and noting the tone and inflection in your voice.

> Before you begin the activities in this chapter, refresh your memory on working with Harris CareTracker by referring back to the Best Practices list on page xiv of this workbook. Following best practices will help you complete work quickly and accurately.

CLAIMSMANAGER

Learning Objective 1: Use the features of ClaimsManager in Harris CareTracker PM and EMR.

The *ClaimsManager* application in Harris CareTracker PM electronically screens a claim and the associated CPT®, ICD, and HCPCS codes and modifiers at the time the claim is created.

Activity 10-1
Work the Claims Worklist

Most claims are sent electronically in Harris CareTracker PM. Any claims identified with a problem that would prevent them from being paid will show up on a *Claims Worklist* to be resolved. The *Claims Worklist* identifies the following:

- Newly prepared claims that will be transmitted during your next claim run
- Claims that cannot be transmitted electronically due to a missing submitter number
- Claims that cannot be transmitted from Harris CareTracker PM because of missing information
- Claims that are not transmitted because of errors identified by *ClaimsManager*
- Claims that will not be accepted by a payer because of missing information
- Claims that you manually flagged as missing information or in review
- Claims that a payer does not have on file and claims with a denial status

Any claims flagged in any of the *Claims Worklist* columns, except *New/Prepared*, need to be followed up on, which typically requires you to add and/or edit information and rebill the claim. Harris CareTracker PM performs an electronic claim status check and, based on its status, moves the claim to one of the *Claims Worklist* categories. You can also manually flag a claim to move it to a *Claims Worklist* category.

The *Claims Worklist* is grouped into four main categories: *New/Prepared*, *Claim Errors*, *Pending*, and *Other* (**Figure 10-1**).

			CLAIM ERRORS					PENDING		OTHER	
Financial Class	New/ Prepared	Missing Submitter	Claim Edits	Payer Edits	Missing Info	Not Found	Set To Deny	In Review	Hold	Inactive	Crossovers
Commercial Insurance	1	0	0	0	0	0	0	0	0	1	0
Medicare Cengage	2	0	0	1	0	0	0	0	0	0	0
Total:	3	0	0	1	0	0	0	0	0	1	0

Figure 10-1   Claims Worklist Categories

Courtesy of Harris CareTracker PM and EMR

The *Claim Summary* screen (**Figure 10-2**) displays when an individual claim line is clicked. In this screen, actions can be performed on the selected claim only.

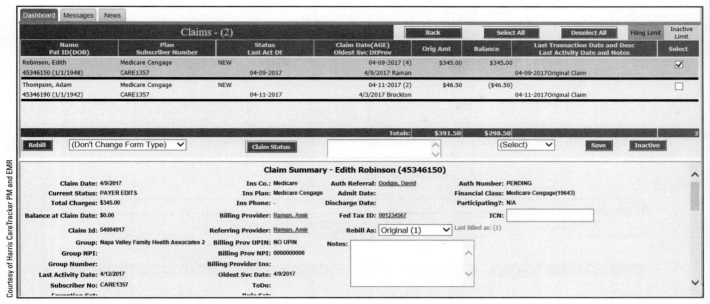

Figure 10-2   Claims Summary Screen

To Work the Claims Worklist

1. Go to the *Home* module > *Dashboard* tab > *Billing* section > *Claims Worklist* link. There are three options: *Unbilled, Crossover,* and *Inactive* (**Figure 10-3**). Select *Unbilled.* This will take you to the *Claims Worklist* screen.

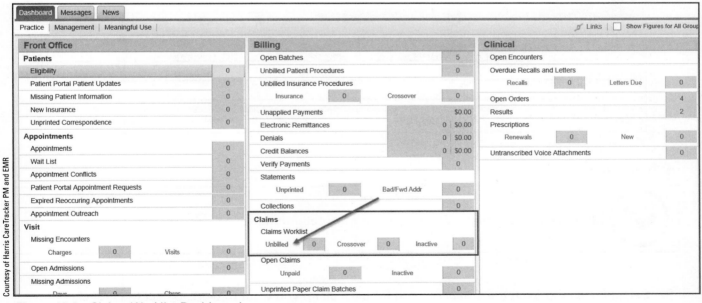

Figure 10-3   Claims Worklist Dashboard

2. The *Location* list defaults to "All Locations." You have the option to select a specific location if needed. Leave as is.

3. The *All Groups* list defaults to "N" for No. Select "Y" for Yes if you want to include claims for all groups. Select "Y."

4. Enter "180" in the *Crossover Days* field.

5. Select the *Incl. Crossovers?* checkbox to include crossover claims.

6. Leave the *Oldest Service Date From/To* as is. If you wanted to view claims from a specific time period, you would enter a date range here.

7. Click *Go.* The application displays a list of all claims broken down by financial class (**Figure 10-4**).

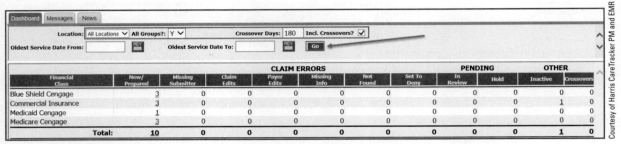

Figure 10-4   Claims by Financial Class

8. Click on a number in the *New/Prepared* column for the corresponding financial class you need to work (select the column for "Medicare Cengage"). The *New/Prepared Claims* screen will display (**Figure 10-5**).

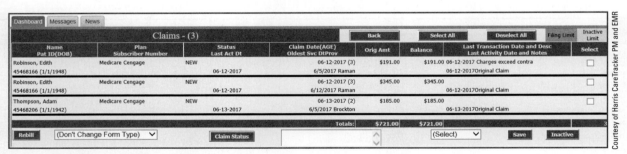

Figure 10-5   New/Prepared Claims Screen

 TIP Click the column headings to re-sort the column data.

9. Select the checkbox in the *Select* column for each claim you want to work. Select the first claim for Edith Robinson and click the *Claim Status* button. (**Note:** You can select all of the claims by clicking *Select All.*) You will receive a pop-up (**Figure 10-6**) advising you of the claim's status (which displays "Processing. . . . "). **Do NOT** click the *Close* button in the pop-up as this will remove the claim from the *Unbilled Claims* screen. Rather, click on the "X" in the upper-right-hand corner to close out of the window.

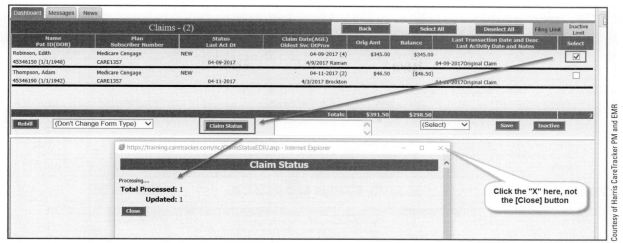

Figure 10-6   Claim Status Pop-Up

10. Click directly in the claim summary line containing Edith Robinson's first visit. The claim line now appears in yellow and the application displays the *Claim Summary* in the lower frame of the screen (see Figure 10-2). This allows you to review, edit, check claim status, or rebill an individual claim.

11. Scroll down and look under the *Activity Notes* column to determine the inaccurate or missing claim information that, triggered by *ClaimsManager*, prevented the claim from being transmitted from Harris CareTracker PM, that prevented the claim from being accepted by a payer, or that caused the claim to be denied by the payer (**Figure 10-7**).

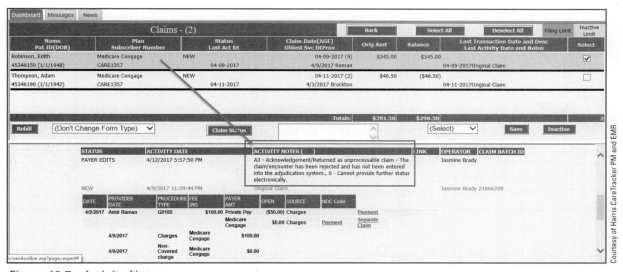

Figure 10-7   Activity Notes

12. Perform the desired action on the claim(s):

Confirm that *Billing Provider* and *Referring Provider* displays Dr. Raman. If not, scroll down and click *Edit* on the *Claim Summary* screen (**Figure 10-8**). The *Claim Transaction Summary* window displays the location, place of service, encounter-specific claim information, referring provider, diagnosis code, and modifiers. Click *Save*. You may briefly receive the "error" message noted in **Figure 10-9**. Click *OK*. Your *Claim Summary* will now reflect the change to *Referring Provider*.

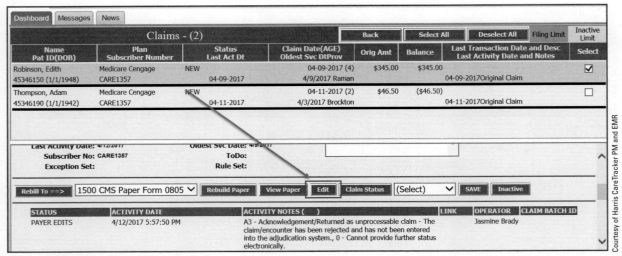

Figure 10-8   Edit Claim Summary

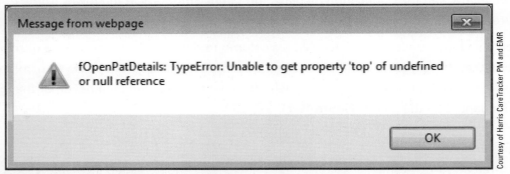

Figure 10-9   Update Claim Message

TIP

- When the billing provider, dates of service, procedure codes, fee, units, servicing provider, or insurance need to be changed, the charge must be reversed from Harris CareTracker PM via the *Edit* application in the *Transactions* module. The charge will then need to be put back into the system.
- When rebilling claims, the form type is not typically changed.

13. Now select the same claim by clicking in the claim summary line (which will turn yellow) and checking the *Select* box even if there were no edits. The only "edit" noted in step 12 was to confirm or change the *Billing Provider* and *Referring Provider* to Dr. Amir Raman.

14. Now, scroll down and click *Rebill To ==>*. Harris CareTracker PM places the claim in the *New/Pending* category of the *Claims Worklist* and the claim will be transmitted during the next claim run.

15. Scroll down the screen and in the *Activity Notes* column, you will now see the activities completed (**Figure 10-10**).

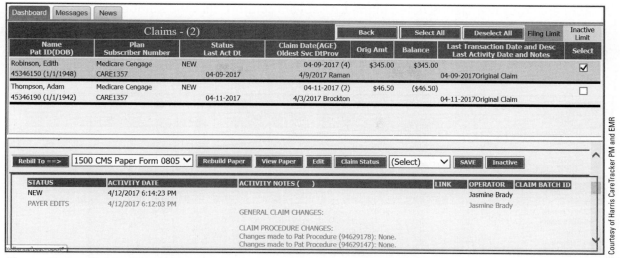

Figure 10-10   Claims Status Activity Note

Print the Claim Status Activity screen, label it "Activity 10-1," and place it in your assignment folder.

Activity 10-2
Search Crossover Claims

A crossover claim is a claim that is automatically forwarded from Medicare to a secondary insurer after Medicare has paid its portion of a service.

1. Go to the *Home* module > *Dashboard* tab > *Billing* section > *Claims Worklist* link. Select *Crossover* from the three options. Harris CareTracker PM opens the *Claims Worklist* application.

2. The *Location* list defaults to "All Locations." Leave as is.

3. The *All Groups* list defaults to "N" for No. Select "Y" for Yes to include claims for all groups.

4. Adjust the crossover days to 180.

5. Select the *Incl. Crossovers?* checkbox.

6. Leave the *Oldest Service Date From/To* as is. If you wanted to view claims from a specific time period, you would enter a date range here.

7. Click *Go*. Harris CareTracker PM displays a list of all claims organized by financial class (**Figure 10-11**).

Financial Class	New/ Prepared	CLAIM ERRORS						PENDING			OTHER	
		Missing Submitter	Claim Edits	Payer Edits	Missing Info	Not Found	Set To Deny	In Review	Hold	Inactive	Crossovers	
Blue Shield Cengage	4	0	0	0	0	0	0	0	0	0	0	
Commercial Insurance	2	0	0	0	0	0	0	0	0	1	0	
Medicaid Cengage	1	0	0	0	0	0	0	0	0	0	0	
Medicare Cengage	1	0	0	0	0	0	0	0	0	0	0	
Total:	**8**	**0**	**0**	**0**	**0**	**0**	**0**	**0**	**0**	**1**	**0**	

Figure 10-11   Crossover Claims

Print the Crossovers search screen, label it "Activity 10-2," and place it in your assignment folder.

8. If there are crossover claims noted in the *Crossovers* column, click the number that corresponds to the financial class in which you want to work. Harris CareTracker PM displays a list of crossover claims (**Figure 10-12**). **Hint:** There are no *Crossover Claims* for you to work here.

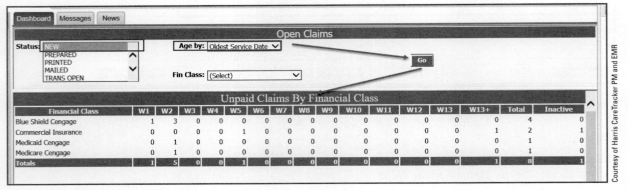

Figure 10-12   *Crossover Claims Displayed*

FYI   In a live environment, you would do the following:

a. In the *Bill?* column, select the checkbox next to each claim you want to bill to secondary insurance. Alternatively, click *Check All* to bill all claims as crossover claims.

b. Click *Set to Bill*. All crossover claims are saved as Secondary 1500 Forms under the *Unprinted Paper Claims* link for printing in the next bill run.

WORK UNPAID CLAIMS

Learning Objective 2: Check status and work unpaid/inactive claims.

Activity 10-3
Individually Check Claim Status Electronically

Harris CareTracker PM automatically checks the status of unpaid claims every evening with specific payers and will check the status of all claims with an outstanding balance. When a status check is complete, the claim's status is updated, attached to the claims, and if necessary will also be flagged in *Claims Worklist* if a status of "Not Found," "Set to Deny," or "In Review" is returned.

Claim status is automatically checked every evening for every claim that has an outstanding balance. Typically, a manual claim status check is not necessary. However, if you need to manually check claim status, you do so individually or in a batch. Claim status for individual claims can be checked from any application in Harris CareTracker PM where the *Claim Summary* screen displays.

1. Go to the *Home* module > *Dashboard* tab > *Billing* section > *Open Claims/Unpaid* link. Harris CareTracker PM displays the *Open Claims* application.

2. Select the desired filter options, as outlined (**Figure 10-13**):
   - *Status*: NEW
   - *Age By*: Oldest Service Date
   - *Financial Class*: Leave as is

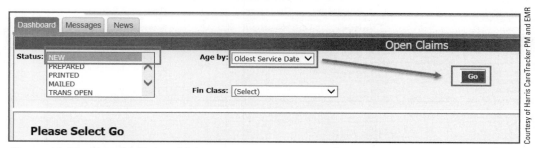

Figure 10-13   Unpaid Claims Link

3. Click *Go*. Harris CareTracker PM displays the *Unpaid/Inactive* claims, broken down by financial class and by week. The total inactive claims for a financial class displays in the *Inactive* column. Totals for all unpaid claims for a financial class displays in the *Total* column, and for each week, the total number of unpaid claims displays in the *Totals* row (**Figure 10-14**).

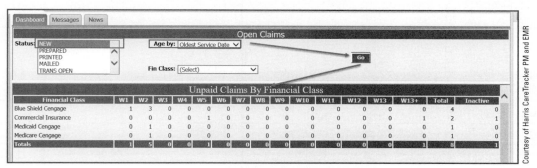

Figure 10-14   Open Claims

4. To work the "Blue Shield Cengage *Financial Class*" line, click on the corresponding number in the *Total* column. Harris CareTracker PM displays a claim line for all corresponding *Unpaid/Inactive* claims with the patient's name, ID number, date of birth, subscriber number, the insurance plan for which the claim was transmitted, the claim status, last activity date on the claim, claim date, claim age, oldest service date on the claim, the provider on the claim, the original amount, balance remaining, and the last activity notes saved for the claim.

5. Place a check mark in Ellen Ristino's *Select* column.

6. Then click directly on the patient's claim line. The line turns yellow and Harris CareTracker PM displays the *Claim Summary* in the lower frame of the screen.

7. You may need to scroll down the screen to be able to view the claim history (**Figure 10-15**). Click *Claim Status*.

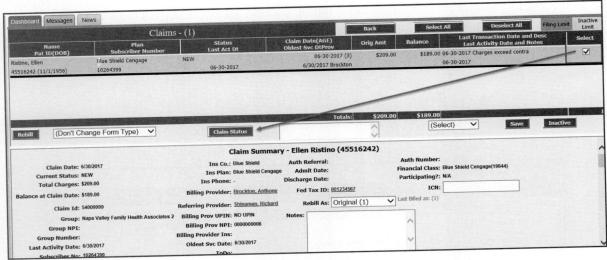

Figure 10-15 Claim History

8. When the *Claim Status* window has finished processing, close out of it by clicking only the "X" in the upper-right corner (**do <u>not</u>** click on the *Close* button).

9. Re-select the claim by directly clicking on the patient's claim line.

10. You must scroll down and click the *Claim Status* button just above *Activity Notes* (**Figure 10-16**).

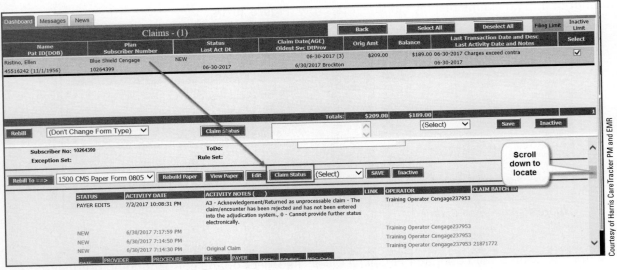

Figure 10-16 Select Claim Status Button

11. Click on the *Claims Status* button. Harris CareTracker PM displays the *Claim Status History* window (**Figure 10-17**), which includes all previous status checks that have occurred, including the date of the status check, the operator who performed the check, the claim status category, and the *Claim Status* code. (**Note**: If the message says no history, close the box and click it again.)

12. Click on the *Claim Status* button on the top right corner of the *Claim Status History* window to perform another claim status check. When the claim status check is complete, the status of the current claim is automatically updated. Click on the "X" in the upper-right corner of the *Claim Status* window to close it (**do <u>not</u>** click on *Close*).

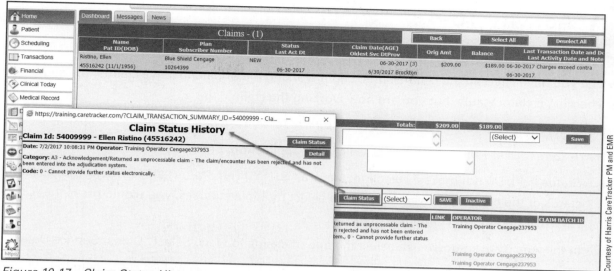

Figure 10-17   Claim Status History

✓ TIP   When a claim's status has been returned, except for "Set to Pay," the claim will be moved to the corresponding column on the *Claims Worklist* screen.

---

13. To view the details of the check, click on the *Detail* button in the *Claim Status History* box, and the *Claim Status Detail* dialog box displays (**Figure 10-18**). (**Note:** The *Claim Status Detail* displayed will not match your patient, provider, and insurance. That is because this is an educational environment.)

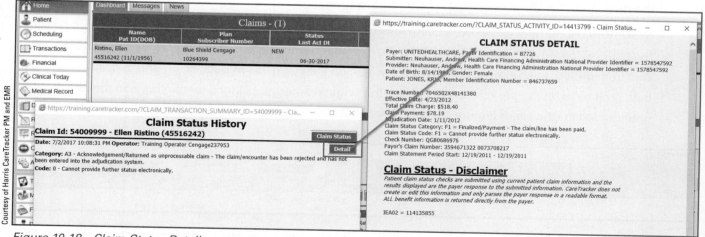

Figure 10-18   Claim Status Detail

🖶 **Print the Claim Status Detail screen, label it "Activity 10-3," and place it in your assignment folder.**

14. Click "X" in the top right corner of the *Claim Status Detail* and the *Claim Status History* windows to close out of them.

Activity 10-4
Work Unpaid/Inactive Claims

Now that you have checked the claim status, begin working the unpaid/inactive claims. The steps are similar to checking a claim status, but you are now working the claim.

1. Go to the *Home* module > *Dashboard* tab > *Billing* section > *Open Claims/Unpaid* link.

2. Harris CareTracker PM displays the *Open Claims* application. Enter the following:

   a. *Status* field: Do not make a selection; leave as is. (**FYI**) The *Status* field is where you select the status of the claims you want to view. To select multiple statuses, you would press the *[Ctrl]* key while clicking to select multiple statuses.

   b. In the *Age by* drop-down list, select the age of claims to view. Select "Oldest Service Date."

   c. (Optional) From the *Fin Class* drop-down list, select the financial class containing the claims you want to view. Leave as "(Select)."

   d. Click *Go*. Harris CareTracker PM displays the unpaid/inactive claims by financial class and by week.

TIP Unpaid Claims by Financial Class:
- The *Inactive* column displays the total inactive claims for a financial class.
- The *Total* column displays the total unpaid claims for a financial class.
- The *Totals* row displays the total unpaid claims for each week.

---

3. Locate the claims you want to work. Select the number in the *Total* column for "Medicare Cengage," and click on the corresponding number. Harris CareTracker PM displays a claim line for each unpaid/inactive claim. (**Note:** You cannot click on a zero total.)

   (**Note:** When a number is clicked, a claim line for all corresponding *Unpaid/Inactive Claims* displays with the patient's name, ID number, date of birth, subscriber number, the insurance plan for which the claim was transmitted, the claim status, last activity date on the claim, claim date, claim age, oldest service date on the claim, the provider on the claim, the original amount, balance remaining, and the last activity notes saved for the claim (**Figure 10-19**). Claims that have reached their *Filing Limit* will display in red.)

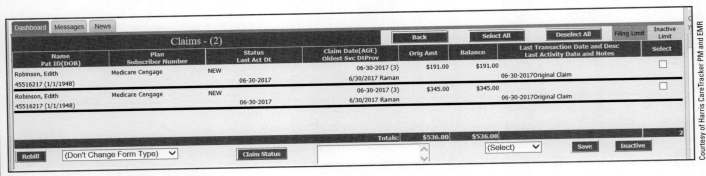

Figure 10-19 Unpaid/Inactive Claims

4. To work claims in a batch:

   a. To review or work an individual claim, click directly on the claim line (select Edith Robinson's first claim). The claim line will turn yellow. Harris CareTracker PM displays the *Claim Summary* in the lower frame of the screen.

   b. You will need to scroll down on both the upper and lower screens to view all the claims and the *Claim Summary* information for the claim selected.

   c. Scroll down and click *Edit* on the *Claim Summary* screen (**Figure 10-20**) to change the location, place of service, encounter-specific claim information, referring provider, diagnosis code, and modifiers. The *Claim Transaction Summary* window displays (**Figure 10-21**), where you can make changes. **Note:** Dates of service, procedure codes, fees, the insurance company, and the amount of the claim may not be edited from this window.

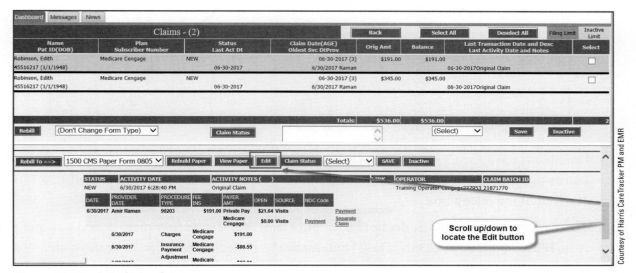

Figure 10-20   Edit Claim Summary

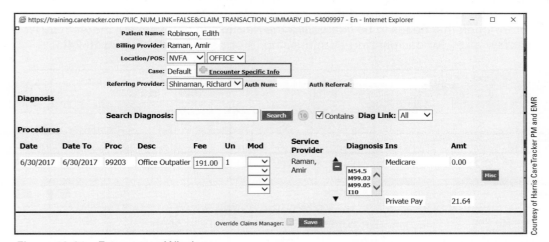

Figure 10-21   Encounters Window

   d. Click on the [+] icon next to *Encounter Specific Info* and a pop-up *Preferred Patient Case* dialog box will appear.

   e. In the *Claim Information* tab, use the drop-down arrow and select "Dr. Raman" as both the *Supervising* and *Ordering Provider* (**Figure 10-22**).

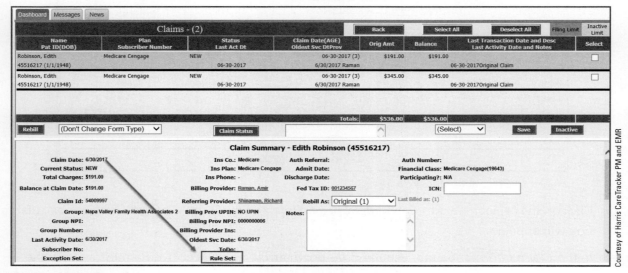

Figure 10-22   Preferred Patient Case Dialog Box

f. If you see a *Save For Charge* button, click on it, and the dialog box disappears and the screen returns to the *Encounters* dialog box. If no *Save For Charge* button is displaying, click "X" to close out of the dialog box.

g. Then click the *Save* button at the bottom of the *Claim Transaction Summary* dialog box and it will close. **Hint:** If the box does not "close" automatically, click on the "X" to close the dialog box.

TIP If there is a number in *Rule Set*, click the number link next to *Rule Set* (**Figure 10-23**) to view descriptions of the rules for the insurance company. This can be helpful when determining the information that needs to be fixed. Click the *Key* link (in blue) next to the *Activity Notes* heading to view a key for deciphering each missing information code (**Figure 10-24**).

Figure 10-23   Rule Set

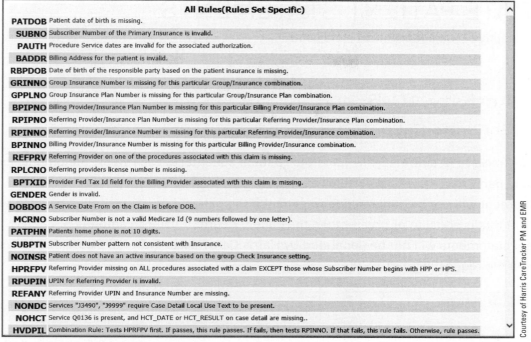

Figure 10-24   Claims Rules Set Key

5. Scroll down and click *Rebill To ==>*. Harris CareTracker PM will place the claim in the *New/Pending* category of the *Claims Worklist* screen and will transmit the claim during the next bill run (**Figure 10-25**). When rebilling claims, the form type typically is not changed.

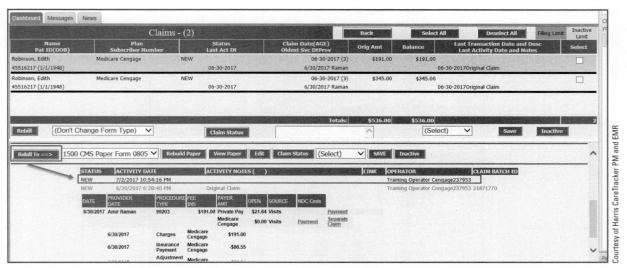

Figure 10-25   Last Transaction Update

Print the Unpaid/Inactive screen, label it "Activity 10-4," and place it in your assignment folder.

GENERATE PATIENT STATEMENTS

Learning Objective 3: Generate patient statements.

Activity 10-5
Generate Patient Statements

Harris CareTracker PM automatically generates patient statements each week. Statements are sent to responsible parties who owe a private pay balance.

A statement will not be generated for a patient if the patient has an unapplied balance saved on his or her account that is equal to or greater than the patient's current balance amount.

Patient statements will not be generated by Harris CareTracker PM until 5 p.m., regardless of when you submit the request (**Figure 10-26**)

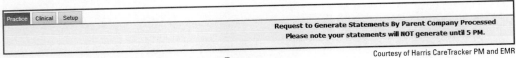

Request to Generate Statements By Parent Company Processed
Please note your statements will NOT generate until 5 PM.

Courtesy of Harris CareTracker PM and EMR

Figure 10-26   Statements Generate at 5 p.m.

1. Before beginning this activity, post the following batches: "9-12CrBalRefunds," "9-10PostRAs," and "RobinsonSNF."

2. With patient Edith Robinson in context, go to the *Administration* module > *Practice* tab > *Daily Administration* section > *Financial* header > *Generate Statements* link (**Figure 10-27**). If a patient is in context, the application displays the option to generate statements for the parent company or the responsible party. You can generate statements for only the parent company when no patient is in context.

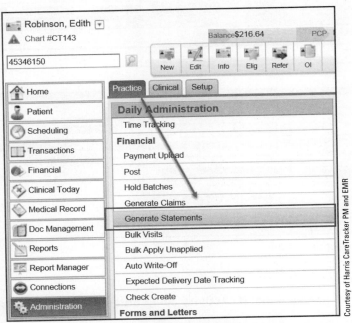

Figure 10-27   Generate Statements Link

3. In the *Generate Statements for Responsible Party* field, select the responsible party for whom you want to generate statements (select patient Edith Robinson) and then click *Go!* (**Figure 10-28**).

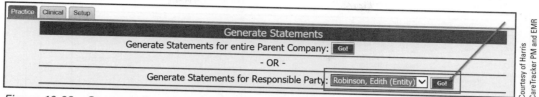

Figure 10-28   *Generate Statements for Responsible Party—Edith Robinson*

4. The application schedules the statements to be printed. Your screen will look like **Figure 10-29**.

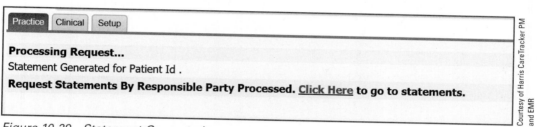

Figure 10-29   *Statement Generated*

SPOTLIGHT   If no statements are displaying, recheck after 24 hours (or after 5 p.m. on the date the activity is performed). Continue with your activities, and repeat Activity 10-5 in 24 hours.

5. Click on the blue "Click Here" prompt (see **Figure 10-29**) to go to the statements. **Note:** You may need to click on *Generate* and *Click Here* (in blue) again for the statement(s) to appear. If you receive an error message, click out of the *Administration* module and repeat the activity steps. Your screen will now look like **Figure 10-30**. (**Note:** If no results are showing, change the *Date Range* to "All Dates.")

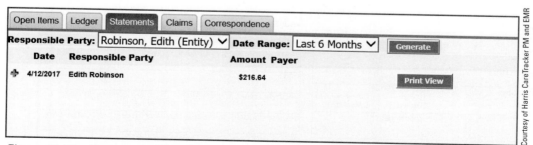

Figure 10-30   *Statements Display*

6. Click on the *Print View* button. The patient's statement will display in a new window (**Figure 10-31**).

Napa Valley Family Associates

RESP PARTY ACCT #	101616-45346150	STMT DATE	4/12/2017
LAST PMT	$64.61	STMT TOTAL	$216.64

Statement - Page 1

DATE OF SERVICE	PATIENT	DESCRIPTION OF SERVICES	PROCEDURE CODE	SERVICING PROVIDER	AMOUNT	PATIENT AMT DUE
4/3/2017	Robinson, Edith (45346150)	Office Outpatient New 30 Minutes	99203	Raman, Amir	-$86.55	$21.64
		Per Your Insurance Company, Your Copay Has Not Been Paid In Full. The Balance Is Your Responsibility. Thank You.				
		Transaction 04/03/2017, Adjustment - Contractual			-$82.81	
		Transaction 04/03/2017, Charges			$191.00	
4/9/2017	Robinson, Edith (45346150)	Phys Cert Mcr-Covr Hom Hlth Srvc Per Cert Prd	G0180	Raman, Amir	$100.00	-$50.00
		Transaction 04/09/2017, Insurance Payment			-$58.46	
		Transaction 04/09/2017, Payment - Patient Cash			-$64.61	
		Transaction 04/09/2017, Adjustment - Contractual			-$26.93	
		Transaction 04/09/2017, Non-Covered charge				
4/9/2017	Robinson, Edith (45346150)	Office Outpatient Visit 25 Minutes	99214	Raman, Amir	$245.00	$245.00
		See Billing Note				
		Transaction 04/09/2017, Non-Covered charge				

PLEASE PAY THIS AMOUNT	$216.64

MAKE CHECKS PAYABLE TO: Napa Valley Family Associates

TO ENSURE PROPER CREDIT, PLEASE DETACH AND RETURN BOTTOM PORTION WITH YOUR PAYMENT

Napa Valley Family Associates
101 Vine Street
Napa, CA 94558

707- 555-1212 Ext:

RESP PARTY ACCT #	101616-45346150	STMT DATE	4/12/2017
AMT ENCLOSED $		STMT TOTAL	$216.64

PATIENT ID# 45346150

☐ CHECK BOX AND ENTER ADDRESS OR INSURANCE CORRECTIONS ON THE REVERSE SIDE

☐ IF PAYING BY CREDIT CARD, FILL OUT THE INFORMATION ON THE REVERSE SIDE

ADDRESSEE:
EDITH ROBINSON
3072 SACRAMENTO ST
SONOMA, CA 95476

REMIT TO:
NAPA VALLEY FAMILY ASSOCIATES
101 VINE STREET
NAPA, CA 94558

Statement - Page 2

IF ANY OF THE INFORMATION HAS BEEN CHANGED SINCE YOUR LAST STATEMENT, PLEASE INDICATE...

ABOUT YOU:

YOUR NAME (Last, First, Middle Initial)

ADDRESS

CITY   STATE   ZIP

TELEPHONE	MARITAL STATUS
( )	☐ Single ☐ Divorced ☐ Married ☐ Widowed

EMPLOYER'S NAME   TELEPHONE
( )

EMPLOYER'S ADDRESS   CITY   STATE   ZIP

IF PAYING BY CREDIT CARD, FILL OUT BELOW

☐ AMERICAN EXPRESS   ☐ MASTERCARD ☐ VISA
CARD NUMBER   CSV

CHARGE THIS AMOUNT   EXPIRATION DATE

SIGNATURE   CARDHOLDER NAME

ABOUT YOUR INSURANCE:

YOUR PRIMARY INSURANCE COMPANY'S NAME   EFFECTIVE DATE

PRIMARY INSURANCE COMPANY'S ADDRESS   PHONE

CITY   STATE   ZIP

POLICYHOLDER'S ID NUMBER   GROUP PLAN NUMBER

YOUR SECONDARY INSURANCE COMPANY'S NAME   EFFECTIVE DATE

SECONDARY INSURANCE COMPANY'S ADDRESS   PHONE

CITY   STATE   ZIP

POLICYHOLDER'S ID NUMBER   GROUP PLAN NUMBER

Figure 10-31 Patient Statement

7. Print the statement by right-clicking on the screen and selecting *Print* from the drop-down menu.

💾 **Print the patient statement, label it "Activity 10-5," and place it in your assignment folder.**

8. Close out of the *Statement* by clicking on the "X" in the upper-right-hand corner.

Activity 10-6
View and Reprint a Patient Statement Using the Financial Module

The *Statements* application in the *Financial* module (**Figure 10-32**) allows you to view and reprint statements that have been generated for the patient in context. A statement can be reprinted by clicking on the *Print View* button next to the appropriate statement line. When *Print View* is clicked, the patient's statement displays in a new window, and by right-clicking on top of it, the statement can be printed.

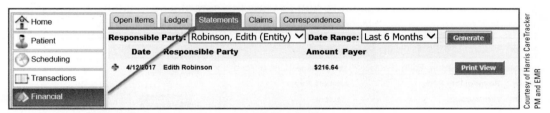

Figure 10-32   *Statements Application in Financial Module*

1. Pull patient Edith Robinson into context.

2. Click the *Financial* module. Click *Go.* The *Open Items* for the patient display (**Figure 10-33**). (**Note:** You can also access the open items by clicking the *OI* icon on the *Name Bar.*)

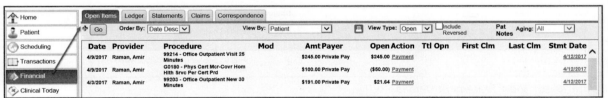

Figure 10-33   *Financial Open Items*

3. Click the *Statements* tab. Harris CareTracker PM opens the *Statements* application (see **Figure 10-34**).

    a. The *Responsible Party* list defaults to the responsible party set in the patient's demographic. Leave as is. (**Note:** You can select a different responsible party or "(All)" responsible parties, if applicable.)

    b. The *Date Range* list defaults to "Last 6 Months." Use the drop-down next to *Date Range* and select "All Dates."

4. Click *Generate.* Harris CareTracker PM generates a list of the patient's statements and displays a processing message in the lower frame of the screen.

5. Select the *Click Here* link in blue. The application displays the list of statements.

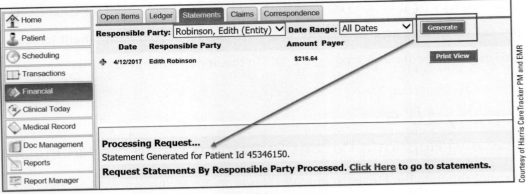

Figure 10-34   Financial Module/Statements Tab

TIP Click on a statement line to view the statement details in the lower frame of the screen. Click the *plus sign* [+] next to a statement line to view the procedure details included in the statement. Click on a procedure line to view the complete procedure details (**Figure 10-35**).

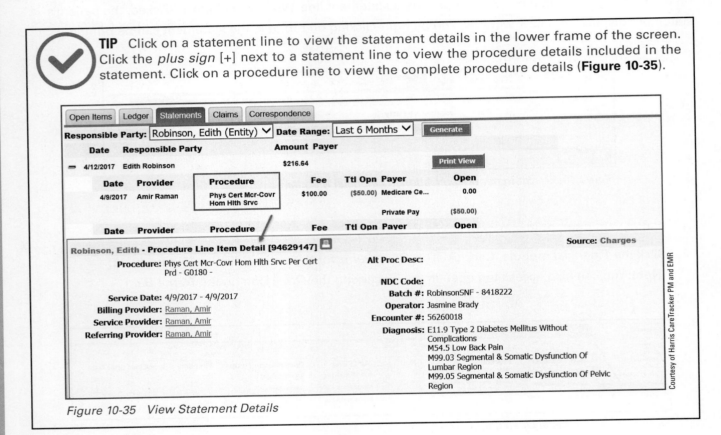

Figure 10-35   View Statement Details

6. Click *Print View* next to the statement you want to print. Select the most recent statement. The application displays the statement in a new window. **Note:** It may take a few moments to display.

7. Right-click on the statement and then select *Print* from the shortcut menu.

💾 **Print the statement, label it "Activity 10-6," and place it in your assignment folder.**

8. Close the statement window when the statement has printed.

PATIENT COLLECTIONS

Learning Objective 4: Review collection status and transfer private pay balances.

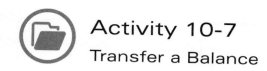

Activity 10-7
Transfer a Balance

The *Collections* application in Harris CareTracker PM allows you to focus collection efforts on patients with balances at least 30 days overdue. You can determine whether patients are identified by the collections system immediately or after their balance is 30, 60, 90, or 120 days overdue.

A patient balance will automatically appear in *Collections* when the balance ages past the days set in *Days Overdue* and one additional statement has generated. When "Immediate" is selected, the system will send a patient directly to the *Collections* module after his or her first statement is generated. The collections' setting applies to all groups in the company.

All new patients added to the *Collections* application will have a collection status of "New" and should be reviewed weekly to determine if they should be removed from *Collections* or if some type of collection action should be taken. However, when the patient balance reaches zero, Harris CareTracker PM automatically removes the patient from the *Collections* list.

In addition to managing the balance transfers, when you send a patient's balance to a collection agency, you should change his or her patient status to *Collections*. This can be done in the *Demographics* application by selecting "Collections" from the *Category* drop-down list. This status will always display next to the patient's name in Harris CareTracker PM so all staff will know that this patient has been transferred to the collection agency. For the *Collections* notice to appear, you will have to take the patient out of context and then bring back into context before *Collections* status appears.

The *Collections* application is accessed from the *Home* module > *Dashboard* tab > *Billing* section > *Collections* link (**Figure 10-36**). There are seven collection statuses in Harris CareTracker PM: New, Open Collections, Review, Collections Actual, Collections Pending, Collections Pending – NS, and Hold (**Figure 10-37**).

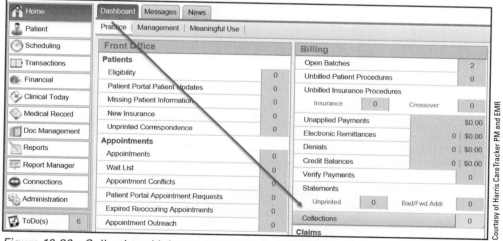

Figure 10-36   Collections Link

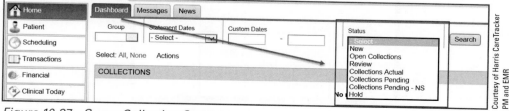

Figure 10-37   Seven Collection Statuses

TIP You must have a batch open to transfer any balances from private pay to *Collect Pend Statement.*

Harris CareTracker PM automatically moves patients into *Collections* when their overdue balance reaches the aging level assigned in the group settings and automatically removes patients from *Collections* when their overdue balance is paid. Operators can also move patients in and out of *Collections* manually. In *Open Items*, you can add a patient to *Collections* by clicking the *Add Responsible Party* link in the *Collections* work area or by transferring a balance to *Collections*.

Patients manually added to *Collections* are flagged with an asterisk (*) next to their name in the work area. Patients manually added to *Collections* must be removed from *Collections* manually as well. When manually adding a patient to *Collections*, Harris CareTracker PM pulls the patient into context and filters the *Collections* list to show the responsible party for that patient.

1. Go to the *Home* module > *Dashboard* tab > *Billing* section > *Collections* link. Harris CareTracker PM displays a list of collection statuses and the number of patients in each status.

2. If there is no patient listed, click the *Add Responsible Party* link in the upper-right corner of the screen.

3. In the *Add Manual Collection* window, click the *Search* icon and enter the name of the patient you are searching for (select patient Edith Robinson). Click on the patient name in the *Results* window. The patient name now populates in the *Add Manual Collection* window.

4. Click *Save*.

5. Click the *Edit* icon next to the balance you want to transfer to a new financial class. Harris CareTracker PM displays the *Edit* window (**Figure 10-38**).

   a. *Insurance*: Leave blank (-Select-).

   b. *Overdue*: Leave blank (-Select-).

   c. *Letter*: Leave blank (-Select-).

   d. *Change Status*: Select "Open Collections."

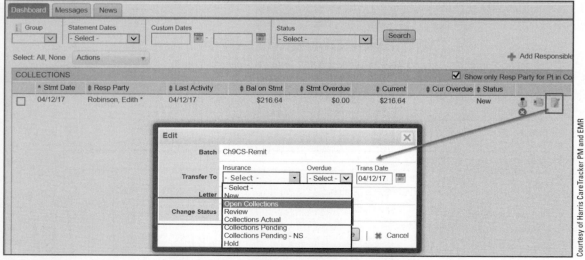

Figure 10-38   Edit Collections Dialog Box

6. Click *Save*.

7. In the *Updates Processed* window that appears, click *Close*. Harris CareTracker PM updates the patient's status in the *Collections* application, transfers the outstanding balance to the selected financial class, and adds the selected "TransferTo" financial class to the patient's *Demographics* record.

 Print the BalanceTransfer screen, label it "Activity 10-7," and place it in your assignment folder.

You can add the *Collections Pending Statement, Collections Pending No Statement, Collections Actual* financial classes, or your collection agency name to the *Insurance Plans* "quick pick" list in the *Quick Picks* application in the *Administration* module.

COLLECTION LETTERS

Learning Objective 5: Create collection letters.

PROFESSIONALISM CONNECTION

Collection letters should do two things: retain customer good will and help you get paid. One way to know if the letter is working is based on the response received. A good letter will generate multiple responses (phone calls and/or payments). If you send a batch of letters and there is no response, it may be time to revise your collection letters and/or procedure. Any correspondence from the medical office is a reflection of the practice, so keep it professional.

Your letter is intended to persuade someone to send you money; therefore, the wording and tone are critical, especially if this is a patient you want to continue to do business with. Enclosing an envelope for payment is always a good idea. If you can include postage on the payment envelope, that is even better. The easier you make it for the customer to make the payment, the better your chances are of getting paid. If you cannot include a pre-paid return envelope (due to high cost), propose an alternative form of payment (i.e., credit/debit card). Always remember to close the letter with an appropriate salutation.

Review the "Global Collection Letters" available in the templates provided and see if they fit with the "message" you want to send to the patient along with the appropriate "image" of the practice. How would you feel if you received one of the generic "collections" letter? How could you customize the language to accomplish the goal of collecting money due, yet keeping the relationship with the patient intact?

 # Activity 10-8

Create a Custom Collection Letter

The *Global Collection Letters* application contains the following letters, which are available to all users in Harris CareTracker PM.

- "Collections 1": Explains that the account is overdue and lists the overdue balance.
- "Past Due": Explains that the overdue balance or a portion of the balance is more than 60 days past due.
- "Delinquent": Explains that the overdue balance or a portion of the balance is more than 90 days past due.

- "Final Notice": Tells the patient that her overdue balance or a portion of her balance is more than 120 days past due. This is the final written notice the patient will receive, and, if payment is not received, the account will be sent to *Collections*.

- "75 Collection": States that if the overdue balance is not paid in full, the billing office will continue with its collection policy, which may include using a collection agency.

- "Collection Payment Plan": Informs the patient that she can set up a weekly or monthly payment plan to pay off the overdue balance. On a "Collection Payment Plan" letter, the patient can also indicate if she has insurance that covered the services for which she has an overdue balance. When a patient indicates that he or she has insurance to cover the services, the patient must also complete the insurance section on the back of a statement.

You can also create custom collection letters in the *Letter Editor* application in the *Administration* module. When you create a group-specific collection letter, the top portion of the letter by default includes patient information, such as name, address, and so on. The only portion of the letter you need to build in the *Letter Editor* is the text you want to appear in the letter.

Group-specific collection letters are built in the *Practice Letter Editor* in the *Administration* module. After creating a custom collection letter, you must add the letter to your *Form Letters Quick Picks* via the *Quick Picks* application in the *Administration* module. This will allow you to access the letter in the *Collections* module.

1. Go to the *Administration* module > *Practice* tab > *Forms and Letters* section > *Practice Letter Editor* link (**Figure 10-39**).

2. From the *Letters* drop-down list, select "Create New Letter" (**Figure 10-40**). The application displays the *New Letter* window (**Figure 10-41**).

3. Enter a descriptive name for the form letter in the *Letter Name* field. Enter "Missed Appointment Fee."

4. In the *Letter Type* field, select the radio button next to the type of form letter you are creating (select "Appointment").

5. Then click *Save* (see **Figure 10-41**). The application closes the *New Letter* window and pulls the new letter name and type into the *Letters* field (**Figure 10-42**). **Note:** It may take a few moments for the screen to refresh.

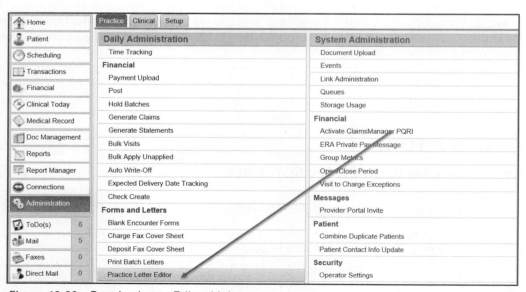

Figure 10-39   Practice Letter Editor Link

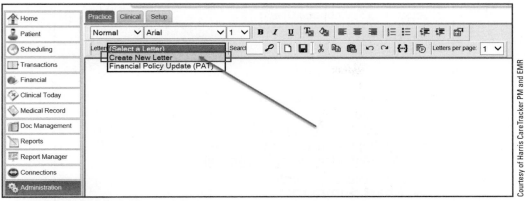

Figure 10-40   Create New Letter

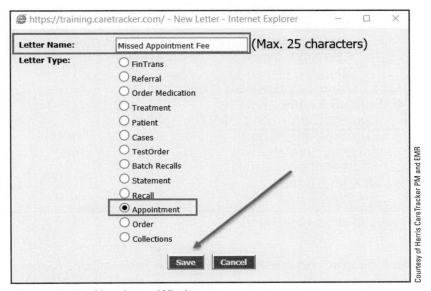

Figure 10-41   New Letter Window

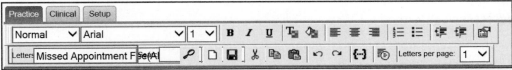

Figure 10-42   Letters Field

6. Enter the text to appear in the form letter and Insert data fields where necessary using the *Select Field* {··}
    icon. Select data fields from the drop-down list in the *Select Field* list (**Figure 10-43**) to complete your letter.
    (For example, for the first line of the letter, select "Current Date – Long" from the *Special Fields* section in the
    Select Field list.) As a best practice, you should click *Save* 🖫 icon periodically while building your letter. Be
    sure to format the letter as you would like it to appear, following the instructions below:

    a. Click on the *Select Field* icon, and scroll down to the *Special Fields* section and select "Current Date –
        Long," then click [enter] to move the line. Recall that the *Letter Editor* is preset to double space when
        you hit the [Enter] key to enter a new line of text. For single spacing, hold the [Shift] key down as you
        press the [Enter] key.

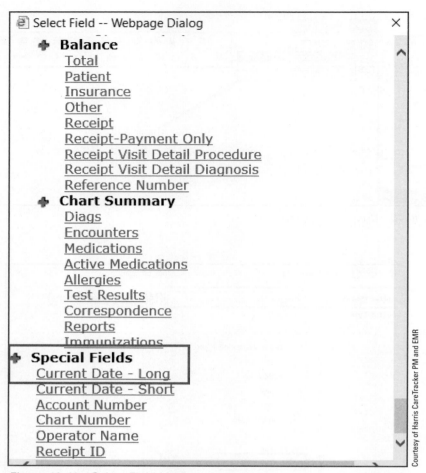

Figure 10-43   Select Field List

b. Click on the *Select Field* icon, and scroll down and in the *Patient Fields (General)* select "First Name."

c. Staying on the same line, click on the *Select Field* icon, and scroll down and in the *Patient Fields (General)* select "Last Name."

d. Staying on the same line, click on the *Select Field* icon, and scroll down and in the *Patient Fields (Billing Address)* select "Address 1."

e. Staying on the same line, click on the *Select Field* icon, and scroll down and in the *Patient Fields (Billing Address)* select "City."

f. Staying on the same line, click on the *Select Field* icon, and scroll down and in the *Patient Fields (Billing Address)* select "State Code."

g. Staying on the same line, click on the *Select Field* icon, and scroll down and in the *Patient Fields (Billing Address)* select "Zip Code."

h. Hit [Enter] to move to the next line.

i. Type "Dear" then a space.

j. Then staying on the same line, click on the *Select Field* icon, and scroll down and in the *Patient Fields (General)* select "Title."

k. Staying on the same line, click on the *Select Field* icon, and scroll down and in the *Patient Fields (General)* select "Last Name."

l. Click [Enter] to move to the next line.

m. Type in the following message:

"You missed your last scheduled appointment with Dr. _____ (click on the *Select Field* icon, and scroll down and in the *Primary Care Provider (PCP)* field select "Last Name") on _____ (click on the *Select Field* icon, scroll down, and in the *Appointment* field select "Date Only"). We are concerned about your health and would like to reschedule the appointment at your earliest convenience. There is a $35 charge for appointments that are canceled with less than 8-business hours' notice. Please remit to our billing office.

Please call the office to schedule or select an appointment via the Patient Portal.

If you have any questions, please don't hesitate to call.

Sincerely,

Jasmine Brady, MA, Office Manager"

n. Your screen should look like **Figure 10-44**.

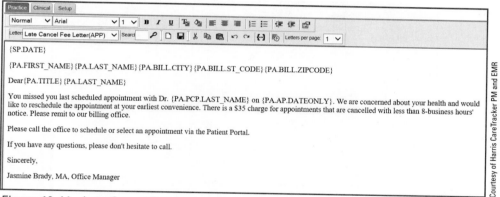

Figure 10-44   Late Cancel Fee Letter

7. Click the *Save File* 💾 icon when you are finished with your form letter.

💾 **Print the screen that displays the Custom Collection Letter, label it "Activity 10-8," and place it in your assignment folder.**

Activity 10-9
Add a Form Letter to Quick Picks

After creating a new form letter, you must add it to your *Quick Picks* to make it available for use in Harris CareTracker PM and EMR.

1. Go to the *Administration* module > *Setup* tab > *Financial* section > *Quick Picks* link.

2. From the *Screen Type* drop-down list, select "Form Letters" (**Figure 10-45**).

3. In the *Search* field, enter part of the name of the new form letter you created in Activity 10-8 (enter "Missed") and then click the *Search* 🔍 icon. The application displays a pop-up of all of the letters that match the search criteria (**Figure 10-46**).

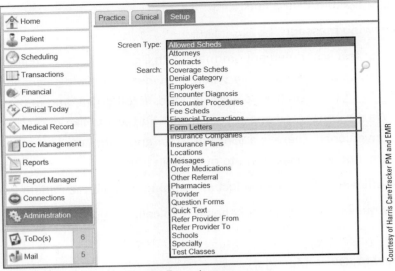

Figure 10-46   Screen Type—Form Letters

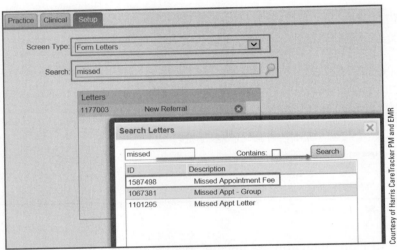

Figure 10-46   Search Letters Window

4. Click on the form letter you want to add to your *Quick Pick* list (select "Missed Appointment Fee"). You will receive a pop-up *Success* box stating "Quick Pick information has been updated." Click *Close* on the *Success* box (**Figure 10-47**).

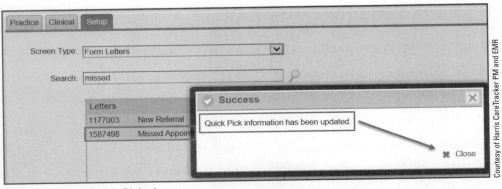

Figure 10-47   Quick Picks Letters

5. The application adds the letter to the *Quick Picks* list where it will be available to generate for patients.

🖫 **Print the Quick Pick list screen with the Form Letter added, label it "Activity 10-9," and place it in your assignment folder.**

GENERATE COLLECTION LETTERS

Learning Objective 6: Generate collection letters.

Activity 10-10

Generate Collection Letters

To generate collection letters, use one of two options: Harris CareTracker PM and EMR's global collection letters, or build a custom collection letter specific to your practice. After collection letters have been generated, they must be printed from the *Print Batch Letters* application in the *Administration* module. Generated collection letters are saved in the patients' record in the *Correspondence* application of the *Financial* module.

1. Go to the *Home* module > *Dashboard* tab > *Billing* section > *Collections* link. Harris CareTracker PM displays a list of collection statements (**Figure 10-48**).

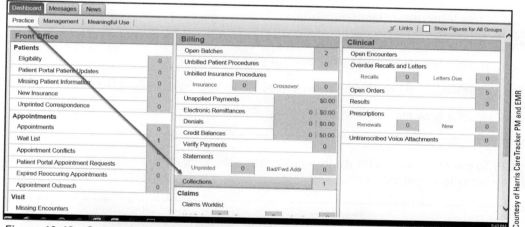

Figure 10-48   Search Collections Fields

2. (FYI) To search *Collections*, select an option from one or more of the following search fields and then click *Search* (**Figure 10-49**) to practice the options.

    *   *Group*—This field is only available when statements for the company are set up by group.
    *   *Statement Dates*—This allows you to view a week's worth of statements.
    *   *Custom Dates*—Enter a custom date range in the fields provided.
    *   *Status*—Select the status of the collection statements you want to view.

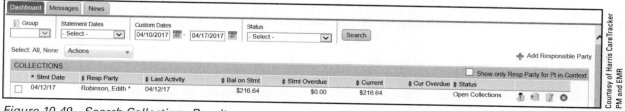

Figure 10-49   Search Collections Results

3. Use the filters at the top of the page to view statements by *Group, Status,* or date range. For this activity, in the drop-down list in the *Status* field, leave as (-Select-).

4. Double-click the name "Edith Robinson" in the line of the *Responsible Party* column to view the *Statement Details* (**Figure 10-50**). It is helpful to review this information when determining a status change and/or deciding what action to take on a patient's balance. Close the *Statement Detail* dialog box.

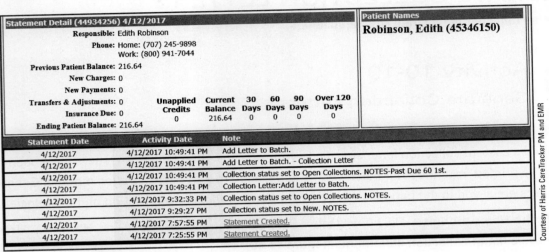

Statement Detail (44934256) 4/12/2017		Patient Names
Responsible: Edith Robinson		**Robinson, Edith (45346150)**
Phone: Home: (707) 245-9898 Work: (800) 941-7044		

	Unapplied Credits	Current Balance	30 Days	60 Days	90 Days	Over 120 Days
Previous Patient Balance: 216.64						
New Charges: 0						
New Payments: 0						
Transfers & Adjustments: 0	0	216.64	0	0	0	0
Insurance Due: 0						
Ending Patient Balance: 216.64						

Statement Date	Activity Date	Note
4/12/2017	4/12/2017 10:49:41 PM	Add Letter to Batch.
4/12/2017	4/12/2017 10:49:41 PM	Add Letter to Batch. - Collection Letter
4/12/2017	4/12/2017 10:49:41 PM	Collection status set to Open Collections. NOTES-Past Due 60 1st.
4/12/2017	4/12/2017 10:49:41 PM	Collection Letter:Add Letter to Batch.
4/12/2017	4/12/2017 9:32:33 PM	Collection status set to Open Collections. NOTES.
4/12/2017	4/12/2017 9:29:27 PM	Collection status set to New. NOTES.
4/12/2017	4/12/2017 7:57:55 PM	Statement Created.
4/12/2017	4/12/2017 7:25:55 PM	Statement Created.

Figure 10-50 Statement Details

5. Close out of the *Statement Detail* dialog box.

6. Click the *Edit* icon next to the statement line for which you want to generate a collection letter (Edith Robinson). Harris CareTracker PM displays the *Edit* box.

7. From the *Letter* list, select the letter you want to generate. Select "Past Due 60 1st" (**Figure 10-51**)

8. If needed, select a new status from the *Change Status* list. (Leave blank: "-Select-".)

TIP To generate letters for multiple patients, select the checkbox next to each patient for whom you want to generate a letter and then click *Actions > Edit*.

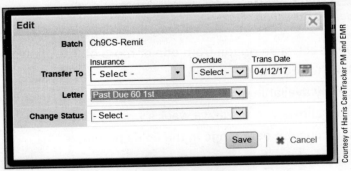

Edit			
Batch	Ch9CS-Remit		
	Insurance	Overdue	Trans Date
Transfer To	- Select -	- Select -	04/12/17
Letter	Past Due 60 1st		
Change Status	- Select -		

Save | ✖ Cancel

Figure 10-51 Generate Past Due 60 1st Letter

 Print the Edit window, label it "Activity 10-10," and place it in your assignment folder.

9. Click *Save.*

10. Then close out of the *Updates Processed* window. Generated collection letters can be printed from the *Print Batch Letters* application in the *Administration* module (**Figure 10-52**). You will receive an error message because you are not able to print batch letters in your student version of Harris CareTracker.

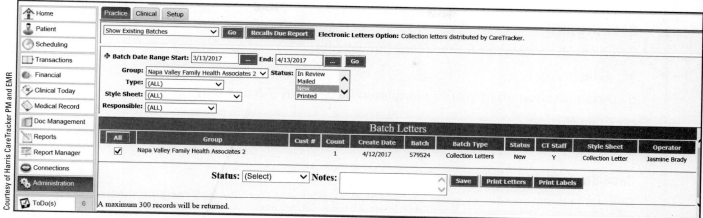

Figure 10-52 Print Batch Letters Application

 TIP If you do not print the collection letters, Harris CareTracker PM and EMR will automatically print the letters to send out to the patient the next day.

 ## Activity 10-11

Run a Journal and Post All Remaining Batches

1. Go to the *Reports* module > *Todays Journals* link.

2. Click on *Add All>>*.

3. Scroll down and place a check mark in the *Includes Transfers* checkbox.

4. Click *Create Journal*.

🖥 **Print the Journal, label it "Activity 10-11a," and place it in your assignment folder.**

5. Go to the *Home* module > *Dashboard* tab > *Billing* section > *Open Batches* link. Harris CareTracker PM displays a list of open batches.

6. Place a checkmark in the *Batch Name* column by each unposted batch.

🖥 **Print the Batches to Post screen, label it "Activity 10-11b," and place it in your assignment folder.**

7. Click *Post Batches*.

 CRITICAL THINKING Billing and collections activities require the utmost professionalism. Having completed your studies and activities in this chapter, do you feel more (or less) comfortable working collections? How would you apply professionalism skills to the situation where a patient desperately needs medical care and medication, but cannot afford either? How would you deal with an angry patient when you need to discuss finances? Can you think of ways to avoid difficult situations with patients and billing and collections? Consider also how the practice is affected by your ability to collect fees due.

If you have had the opportunity to role-play with your fellow students or a family member with various collection scenarios, did that help with preparedness, conveying empathy, and noting the tone and inflection in your voice? Share your experiences with your instructor and classmates.

CASE STUDIES

Complete all case studies for the following patients

a. Jane Morgan

b. Adam Thompson (if you've completed Case Study 7-3 and 9-2)

c. Ellen Ristino

d. Barbara Watson

Case Study 10-1

Generate statements for all patients (a–d above). (Refer to Activity 10-5 for guidance.)

(**Note**: If statements are not displaying after you complete the steps or you receive an error message, click back on the *Administration* module, *Generate Statements* link and repeat the steps.)

Print the Generated Statements, label them Case Study 10-1a through 10-1d, and place them in your assignment folder.

Case Study 10-2

Transfer any remaining balance to *Open Collections* for Jane Morgan, Adam Thompson, Ellen Ristino, and Barbara Watson. See Activity 10-7 for guidance. Note that you will need to click *Add Responsible Party* and add each of these four patients in order for them to appear in the *Add Manual Collection* window.

Once all balances have been transferred, print the screen showing all Transferred Balances, label it "Case Study 10-2" and place them in your assignment folder. Hint: If "Show only Resp Party for Pt in Context" is not checked, then you can take one screenshot that shows all of the patients.

Case Study 10-3

Generate collection letters (Past Due 60 1st) for all patients (a–d above). See Activity 10-10 for guidance. Once all patients (a–d above) have had the collections letter generated, click on the *Correspondence* icon after *Status* "Open Collections" of each patient. The *Patient Correspondence* dialog box displays. Print the *Correspondence Log* for each patient.

Print the Edit screens showing the Collection Letters generated for each patient, label them "Case Study 10-3a through 10-3d, and place them in your assignment folder.

MODULE 5
Apply Your Skills

QUICK START

This module includes:

- Chapter 11: Applied Learning for the Paperless Medical Office

This chapter is the finale of the text and should be completed only after you have completed all of the other modules (Get Started, Administrative Skills, Clinical Skills, and Billing Skills).

This chapter follows a typical patient workflow in a medical clinic. You will apply the skills learned throughout this textbook by completing case studies that test your comprehension of the material presented throughout the text without providing step-by-step instructions. You will build both competence and confidence from performing activities in this chapter.

Be sure you are working in a supported browser (Internet Explorer 11 or Safari for iPad) before you begin. Other browsers (such as Chrome and Firefox) are not supported. Review Best Practices.

Applied Learning for the Paperless Medical Office

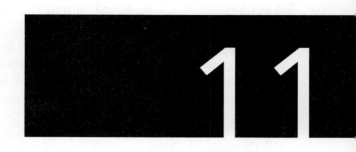

Learning Objectives

1. Perform EMR tasks related to registering and scheduling a patient, completing the visit, billing the appointment, and collecting payment

INTRODUCTION

Congratulations on completing the activities in Chapters 1 through 10! You will now apply what you learned to the case studies in this chapter. Completing these case studies will help you increase your proficiency in a real-world electronic health record.

 If you need help completing these case studies, a guide has been posted to the student companion website. This guide references activities within this book that you can review for assistance.

Before you begin the activities in this chapter, refresh your memory on working with Harris CareTracker by referring back to the Best Practices list on page xiv of this workbook. Following best practices will help you complete work quickly and accurately.

CASE STUDY 11-1: DELORES SIMPSON

Delores Simpson is an established patient of the practice who calls the office this morning to schedule an appointment with Dr. Raman, her primary care provider. She tells you she has not been feeling well and complains of chest discomfort. She has taken her blood pressure at home several times this morning and says it is normal. Just to be on the safe side, you encourage the patient to call the EMS so that she can be evaluated. The patient refuses to call and insists on coming into the office. Due to her age and the severity of her complaint, you message Dr. Raman and he replies to have her come in to the office this morning. If there are no appointments open, double-book the first available appointment for her to be seen. Delores has not been in to see Dr. Raman since the office converted to electronic records, but she is registered in the database.

Step 1: Search the Database and Schedule an Appointment

1. Search the database for patient Delores Simpson. Update her demographics to include Dr. Raman as her PCP, update her insurance *Subscriber Number* to that of her *Group #*, and change her *Consent* and *NPP* to "Yes."

2. Schedule an appointment for Delores with Dr. Raman, using the first available morning slot, or by double-booking the 11:00 a.m. slot. (**Note**: If you are entering data on a weekend, or a day when there is no availability in the schedule, select an appointment day on the first prior date available. This will ensure that you can complete activities by not working in a "future date." This applies to all of the case studies in Chapter 11.)

- *Appointment Type:* Follow Up
- *Complaint:* Chest pain (resolved, normal BP readings)
- *Location:* NVFA

Step 2: Check In Patient

3. When Delores arrives for her appointment, view her *At-A-Glance* patient information to confirm that she is still insured with Medicare and has no copay.

4. Check Delores in for her visit with Dr. Raman.

Step 3: Patient Work-Up

To begin EMR activities, create a new *Batch* titled "SimpsonCS" and edit your operator preferences for clinical workflows with Dr. Raman as the provider.

📧 **When you have completed Step 3: Patient Work-Up, print the patient's Chart Summary, and label it "Case Study 11-1a."**

Background Information about Delores Simpson

Delores is a kind, older patient who rarely complains. This morning she has been experiencing some chest discomfort. Upon her arrival, you immediately escort Delores to the cardiac bay. This room has equipment that can be used during a cardiac event. Normally, you would update the patient's medical history information, but the provider tells you just to get the patient's medication and allergy information to expedite the process.

1. *Transfer* Delores to the cardiac bay. (**Hint**: You would have added the Cardiac Bay as a Room in Activity 5-7. If it is not displaying, add the room first.)

2. Referring to **Table 11-1**, enter Delores's medical information into her patient record.

Table 11-1 Medical Information for Delores Simpson	
Medications	Levothyroxine Sodium Oral Tablet, 100 mcg tab, 1 per day Lisinopril, 20 mg tab, 1 per day
Allergies	Codeine (*Reaction*: Hives and Rash; *Start Date*: 02/15/1999; *Alert Status*: Popup Alert)

3. Take Delores's vital signs and record them in her patient chart. Refer to **Table 11-2** for Delores's vital sign information.

Table 11-2 Vital Signs for Delores Simpson					
Height	5' 2"	**Pulse Rate**	68 bpm	**Pulse Oximetry**	96%
Weight	143	**Temperature**	97.4°F	**Pain Level**	0/10
Blood Pressure	122/68	**Respiratory Rate**	14		

4. Because Delores is now ready to see Dr. Raman, create a *Progress Note* for her. Select progress note template "Cardio Option 3 (v4)." Refer to **Table 11-3** while completing the progress note. (**Note:** You will be acting as a scribe for the provider in this case study, meaning you will free text much of the medical record information in the *Progress Note*.)

Table 11-3   Progress Note for Delores Simpson

TAB	ITEM	ENTRY
CC/HPI	*Reason for Visit*	Click on the *REASON FOR VISIT* tab and check "Chest pain." In the *Other* box free text: "Chest pain (resolved)."
	HPI	Free text in the *HPI* box: Patient complains of early morning chest pain that lasted approximately 15 minutes and then subsided. No current chest pain. Patient described the pain as midsternal "tight, squeezing pressure radiating slightly to the left side of sternum." Pain rating at its worst around a "6." Patient denies any radiation of pain to other parts of the body, shortness of breath, or diaphoresis. There was no change in pain intensity upon movement. Patient took her blood pressure at least three times during the event but stated that each time her blood pressure was normal ("Around 110/68"). Patient denies any gastrointestinal or neurologic symptoms. Patient states that she has been under a great deal of stress lately because her daughter just moved to Boston. She feels that the pain may be related to stress. Patient does not recall any history of chest pain prior to this morning's event.
ROS		Select "N" for all categories in the *Cardiovascular ROS* sections, except select "Y" for chest pain. In the "other cardiovascular symptoms" box enter "Chest pain this morning, resolved."
		Do not mark any of the boxes in the *Review of Systems* section.
	Other Review of Systems box	Free-text the following entries: Denies fatigue, fever, weight changes, or pain (other than the chest discomfort she experienced this morning).
		HEENT: Denies headache, dizziness, or voice changes.
		CHEST: As stated in the HPI, patient denies any current chest pain or shortness of breath.
		CV: Refer to HPI.
		GI: Patient denies any nausea or vomiting, abdominal pain, or reflux. Has had some constipation lately but nothing out of the "ordinary."
		GU: Denies any frequency, dysuria, or changes in voiding habits.
		MUSC: Denies any muscular or joint pain or any joint swelling.
		NEURO: Denies vertigo, headache, ataxia, or syncope.
		PV: No changes in temperature or any swelling in extremities.

(continues)

Table 11-3 *(continued)*

TAB	ITEM	ENTRY
		PSYCH: As stated in the HPI, patient feels anxious over daughter moving to Boston. Feels like she will never see her daughter now that she is so far away.
PE		Select "N" for all applicable categories in the *Cardio PE* section. Click in the box beside *regular rate and rhythm*.
		Do not click on any of the responses in the *Physical Examination* box.
	Other Physical Findings box	Free-text the following: *General*: Patient appears alert and well.
		HEENT: Head, normocephalic, no pharyngeal exudate or erythema, uvula midline.
		NECK: Supple, no palpable masses or nodules, thyroid normal in size, trachea midline.
		CHEST: Thorax without distortion. Respiration regular and unlabored, no cough. Lung fields normal. Negative rales or rhonchi. Breath sounds clear.
		HEART (CARDIOVASCULAR): EKG findings—12 lead with NSR without ST elevation or depression.
		ABDOMEN: Round and soft. No tenderness, rash, or palpable mass. Nail beds pink with less than 2-second capillary refill. Pedal pulse 2 + 1.
		NEURO: Patient alert and oriented. No speech problems. Patient able to move all extremities and appears coherent. Other than being a little anxious regarding daughter's move, patient appears in good overall spirits.
EKG TESTS		Free text: EKG findings—12 lead with NSR without ST elevation or depression.
A&P	*Today's Selected Diagnosis*	Using the drop-down, scroll down and select "Chest pain, unspecified type (R07.9)"; search for and select "Anxiety (F41.9)." **Note**: You would need to click *Save* before the updates to all the fields display, including diagnosis updates.
	Assessment	In the *OTHER DIAGNOSES/CONDITIONS* of the A&P box, free-text the following: "R/O angina pectoris and MI. Chest discomfort may be related to the stress of her daughter's move."
	Other Plan Items box	1. 12-Lead EKG 2. Patient information sheet "Your Body's Response to Anxiety" 3. F/U in one week with Dr. Raman 4. Give patient a prescription for Xanax Oral Tablet MG (CIV) PRN (as needed), not to exceed 1 tablet in 24 hours, # 10, 0 refills; refill/reprint prescription for levothyroxine tabs, 100 mcg, Sig 1 tab daily, #30, 3 refills. 5. Order *Stat* lab test "Troponin I. cardiac [Mass/volume] in Serum or Plasma by Detection limit—0.01 ng/mL" for patient to have drawn at the lab tomorrow morning.

Step 4: Review the *Plan* Section of the *Progress Note* and Complete the Tasks Noted in the *Plan*

Delores's visit is now over with Dr. Raman. It is your responsibility to complete orders as indicated in the *A&P* section of the progress note.

1. Create and print the new prescription for Xanax.

💾 **Label the printed prescription "Case Study 11-1b."**

2. In the *Procedures* tab within the progress note, type the following: "Performed 12-Lead EKG per Dr. Raman."

3. Provide Delores with a copy of the Patient Information sheet(s) ordered in the *Plan* section of the progress note.

💾 **Print the Patient Information sheet and label it "Case Study 11-1c."**

Step 5: Capture the Visit and Sign the Note

Having completed all of the orders as indicated in the *Progress Note*, now capture the *Visit* and sign the progress note.

1. Capture the *Visit* by entering:

   a. *CPT® code(s):* 99213 and 93000
   Source: Current Procedural Terminology © 2013 American Medical Association.

   b. *ICD-10 code(s):* R07.9 and F41.9

2. Sign the progress note.

💾 **Print the signed progress note and label it "Case Study 11-1d."**

3. Before Delores leaves schedule her follow-up appointment noted in the *Plan* section of the progress note.

Step 6: Process Remittance (EOB/RA) and Transfer to Private Pay

1. Save the charges for the visit for Ms. Simpson. (**Hint:** Check your batch and make sure you are working in the batch "SimpsonCS." If not, edit the batch and use the drop-downs to select the parameters as set in the original batch.)

2. Build all claims for Delores's visit.

3. Refer to Delores's EOB/RA (Source Document 11-1 at the end of this case study) and process the remittance.

4. Run a journal to verify charges.

💾 **Print the journal and label it "Case Study 11-1e."**

Step 7: Work Claims and Generate Patient Statement

1. Work the *Claims Worklist*.

2. Post all open batches.

3. Generate a statement for Delores.

💾 **Print the statement and label it "Case Study 11-1f."**

Source Document 11-1: Explanation of Benefits/Remittance Advice

MEDICARE CENGAGE

Medicare Cengage
P.O. Box 234434
San Francisco, CA 94137

AMIR RAMAN, D.O.
Napa Valley Family Health Associates (NVFHA)
101 Vine Street
Napa, CA 94558

Date: MM/DD/YYYY (use today's date)
Payment Number: 1280977
Payment Amount: $126.80

Account Number	Patient Name				Subscriber Number			Claim Number		
Dates of Service	Description of Service	Amount Charged	Not Covered (DENIAL)	Prov Adj Discount	Amount Allowed	Deduct/ Coins/ Copay	Paid to Provider	Adj Reason Code	Rmk Code	Patient Resp
42399647	Simpson, Delores									
99213		$112.00								
(Appt. date used in Case Study 11-1)					$112.00	$22.40	$89.60			$21.64

Account Number	Patient Name				Subscriber Number			Claim Number		
Dates of Service	Description of Service	Amount Charged	Not Covered (DENIAL)	Prov Adj Discount	Amount Allowed	Deduct/ Coins/ Copay	Paid to Provider	Adj Reason Code	Rmk Code	Patient Resp
CARE1357	Simpson, Delores									
93000		$46.50								
(Appt. date used in Case Study 11-1)					$46.50	$9.30	$37.20			$9.30

CASE STUDY 11-2: CRAIG X. SMITH

Craig is an established patient who was last seen in the office for wheezing. He is returning today for a recheck from his prior visit.

Step 1: Search the Database and Schedule an Appointment

1. Search the database for patient Craig X. Smith.

2. Schedule an appointment for Craig with Dr. Raman, using the first available morning slot today. (**Note:** If you are entering data on a weekend, or day when there is no availability in the schedule, select an appointment day on the first prior date available. This will ensure you can complete activities by not working in a "future date." This applies to all of the case studies in Chapter 11.)

   - *Appointment Type:* Follow Up

     Chief Complaint: Follow Up

   - *Location:* NVFA

Step 2: Enter Payment and Check In Patient

1. When Craig arrives for his appointment, view his *At-A-Glance* patient information and confirm that he is still insured with Medicaid and has no copay.

2. Check Craig in for his visit with Dr. Raman.

Step 3: Patient Work-Up

To begin EMR activities, create a new *Batch* titled "CXSmithCS" and edit your operator preferences for clinical workflows with Dr. Raman as the provider.

Background Information about Craig X. Smith

Craig was seen two weeks ago for a fever and wheezing. His mother was unable to keep his follow-up appointment last week so she is following up today. Craig's symptoms have completely resolved. Fever has subsided and wheezing is gone.

1. *Transfer* Craig to Exam Room #1.

2. Now review the patient's medical history with his mother. Mom reports that there is no change since the last visit. (**Note:** This medical history was completed in Proficiency Builders 6-2a and 6-3a. If you did not complete that Proficiency Builder, you can skip this step without entering the medical history.) **Hint:** Be sure to access through *Clinical Today.*

3. Next, take Craig's vital signs and record them in his chart. Refer to **Table 11-4** for Craig's vital sign information.

Table 11-4 Vital Signs for Craig X. Smith

CATEGORY	ENTRY
Height	42 inches
Weight	49 lb 8 oz
Body Mass Index	Automatically populates after entering height and weight
LMP	N/A
Blood Pressure	94/60
Pulse Rate	96 bpm
Temperature	98.6°F
Respiratory Rate	20
Pulse Oximetry	98%
Pain Level	N/A
Head Circumference	N/A
Length	N/A

4. Because Craig is now ready to see Dr. Raman, create a *Progress Note* for him. Select a template of "Pediatric OV Option 4 (v1)." Refer to **Table 11-5** while completing the progress note.

💾 **When you have completed Step 3: Patient Work-Up, print the patient's Chart Summary, and label it "Case Study 11-2a."**

Table 11-5 Progress Note for Craig X. Smith

SECTION OF OV TAB	ENTRY
CC	Free text: Follow-up from last visit.
History of Present Illness	Free text: Patient's mother states that patient is doing much better. His symptoms have completely subsided and he is once again a happy and active boy.
Past Medical/Social/Family History	Free text: No changes since last visit.

SECTION OF OV TAB	ENTRY
Review of Systems	Free text the following: *General:* No acute distress at this time. *Ears, Nose, and Throat:* Symptoms have dissipated from previous exam. *Respiratory:* No wheezing or coughing at this time.
Physical Examination	Free text the following: *General:* Awake, well developed. *Ears, Nose, and Throat:* Normal oropharyngeal discharge, ears and nose clear. *Respiratory:* All lung fields clear, SaO$_2$ reading is 98% today. *Cardiovascular:* Normal rate and peripheral pulses are normal.
Tests	Leave blank.
Procedure Note	Leave blank.
Assessment	Free text: No active problems today.
Plan	Free text: Mother to call if symptoms return.

Step 4: Capture the Visit and Sign the Note

Having completed all the orders as indicated in the *Progress Note*, now capture the *Visit* and sign the progress note.

1. Capture the *Visit* by entering:
   a. *CPT® code(s):* 99392
      Source: Current Procedural Terminology © 2017 American Medical Association.
   b. *ICD-10 code(s):* R06.2 (**Note:** Although the symptoms have resolved, Craig is still being seen for a follow-up of this diagnosis.)
2. Sign the progress note.

📾 **Print the signed progress note and label it "Case Study 11-2b."**

Step 5: Process Remittance (EOB/RA) and Transfer to Private Pay

1. Save the charges for the visit.
2. Build all claims for Craigs's visit.
3. Refer to Craig's EOB/RA (Source Document 11-2 at the end of this case study) and process the remittance.
4. Run a journal to verify charges.

📾 **Print the journal and label it "Case Study 11-2c."**

Source Document 11-2:   Explanation of Benefits/Remittance Advice

MEDICAID CENGAGE

Medicaid Cengage
P.O. Box 221352
Fresno, CA 93701

Date: MM/DD/YYYY (Appt. date used in Case Study 11-2)
Payment Number: 2321442
Payment Amount: $30.00

AMIR RAMAN, D.O.
Napa Valley Family Health Associates (NVFHA)
101 Vine Street
Napa, CA 94558

Account Number	Patient Name				Subscriber Number		Claim Number			
Dates of Service	Description of Service	Amount Charged	Not Covered (DENIAL)	Prov Adj Discount	Amount Allowed	Deduct/ Coins/ Copay	Paid to Provider	Adj Reason Code	Rmk Code	Patient Resp
42399649	SMITH, CRAIG X.									
(Appt. date used in Case Study 11-2)	99392	$195.00		$165.00	$30.00	$0.00	$30.00			$0.00

Step 6: Work Claims and Generate Patient Statement

1. Work the *Claims Worklist.*

2. Post all open batches.

3. Craig does not have an outstanding balance, so you do not need to generate a patient statement.

CASE STUDY 11-3: TRANSFER TO COLLECTIONS

Scenario: It has now been more than 60 days since you generated a statement for Delores. Her final payment has not been received.

1. Manually transfer her account to *Collections.*

2. Generate a collection letter appropriate to the office policy for accounts older than 60 days.

🖳 **Print a screenshot of the Collections screen listing this outstanding account and label it "Case Study 11-3."**

CASE STUDY 11-4: OPERATOR AUDIT LOG

Having completed the activities in this textbook and the applied learning case studies, run an operator audit log to review the entries (refer to Activity 2-4).

🖳 **To print the log, click "Print Operator Audit Log", or right-click your mouse on the log and then select Print from the shortcut menu. Label the Operator Audit Log "Case Study 11-4."**

PROFESSIONALISM CONNECTION

Dear Student:

Congratulations on completing the Harris CareTracker PM and EMR Workbook activities, your first step toward becoming a "super-user" of electronic health records! As manager, I screen applicants for open positions within the practice. Once a job opening is posted and applications and résumés are received, I will begin the screening process. The following qualifications and characteristics are some of the ways applicants will be evaluated:

- Education (certification or degree from an accredited program)

- Experience (total length of each place of employment related to job opening)

- Quality of application and résumé (grammar, spelling, and punctuation)

- References (verify with former employers)
    - Length of employment
    - Eligible (or not) for re-hire
    - What would provider say about the applicant? (best and worst qualities)
    - What would co-workers say about the applicant? (best and worst qualities)
    - Attendance and punctuality
    - Attention to detail
    - Teamwork behavior
    - Work ethic and habits

(continues)

PROFESSIONALISM CONNECTION *(continued)*

Often a practice will provide placement for externs from local schools completing the clinical portion of their training. This affords the externs a good opportunity to observe the needed quality of clinical and administrative skills as well as work ethics and habits. Many times an externship position can lead to employment within the practice.

How would you rate your qualifications and characteristics? How will the information you learned from this workbook enhance your capabilities to obtain the desired position you are seeking? Have you created your résumé and portfolio yet? If not, it would be good practice to begin documenting your achievements. It has been our pleasure to have you as a "Student MA" here at NVFHA. Congratulations and best wishes on a successful career!

Sincerely,
Takari Miata, Office Manager
Napa Valley Family Health Associates

Resources

ABC News.com. (2009, July 16). *President Obama continues questionable "You Can Keep Your Health Care" promise.* Retrieved from http://abcnews.go.com/blogs/politics/2009/07/president-obama- continues-questionable-you-can-keep-your-health-care-promise/

American Academy of Family Physicians. (2003). The HIPAA privacy rules: three key forms. Retrieved from http://www.aafp.org/fpm/2003/0200/p29.html

American Association of Professional Coders (AAPC). https://www.aapc.com/

American Medical Association (AMA). https://www.ama-assn.org

Bureau of Labor Statistics, U.S. Department of Labor. (2014). *Occupational Outlook Handbook.* Medical Records and Health Information Technicians. Retrieved from http://www.bls.gov/ooh/healthcare/medical-records-and-health-information-technicians.htm

Centers for Medicare and Medicaid Services. (n.d.). Retrieved from http://www.cms.gov/Regulations-and-Guidance/HIPAA-Administrative-Simplification/Versions5010andD0/index.html

Centers for Medicare and Medicaid Services. (n.d.). Delivery system reform, medicare payment reform. Retrieved from https://www.cms.gov/Medicare/Quality-Initiatives-Patient-Assessment-Instruments/Value-Based-Programs/MACRA-MIPS-and-APMs/MACRA-MIPS-and-APMs.html

Centers for Medicare and Medicaid Services (CMS). (n.d.). Glossary. Retrieved from the CMS website http://www.medicare.gov/glossary/f.html

Centers for Medicare and Medicaid Services. (n.d.). *Meaningful use.* Retrieved from http://www.cms.gov/Regulations-and-Guidance/Legislation/EHRIncentivePrograms/Meaningful_Use.html

CertMedAssistants.com. (n.d.). Retrieved from http://www.certmedassistant.com/

Coding classification standards. (n.d.). Retrieved from www.ahima.org

Department of Health and Human Services (DHHS), *Centers for Medicare and Medicaid Services (CMS).* (2003, June 6). Medicare hospital manual. Retrieved from http://www.cms.gov/Regulations-and-Guidance/Guidance/Transmittals/downloads/R804HO.pdf

Department of Health and Human Services (DHHS), Centers for Medicare and Medicaid (CMS). (n.d.). Remittance advice information: an overview. Fact sheet. Retrieved from https://www.cms.gov/Outreach-and-Education/Medicare-Learning-Network-MLN/MLNProducts/Downloads/Remit-Advice-Overview-Fact-Sheet-ICN908325.pdf

Duke Clinical Research Institute. (n.d.). Beers criteria medication list. Retrieved from https://www.dcri.org/beers-criteria-medication-list/

General information: Nurse practitioner practice. (2011, April 13). Retrieved from http://www.rn.ca.gov/pdfs/regulations/npr-b-23.pdf

Health Information and Management Systems Society. (2008, August). *Real time adjudication of healthcare claims* (HIMSS Financial Systems Financial Transactions Toolkit Task Force White Paper). Retrieved from http://himss.files.cms-plus.com/HIMSSorg/content/files/Line%2027%20-%20Real%20Time%20Adjudication%20of%20Healthcare%20Claims.pdf

Health Information Technology for Economic and Clinical Health (HITECH). (2013, November 27). HITECH Act Enforcement Interim Final Rule.

HealthIT.gov. (n.d.). *EHR incentives and certification.* Retrieved from https://www.healthit.gov/providers-professionals/ehr-incentive-payment-timeline

HealthIT.gov. (n.d.). Meaningful use definitions and objectives. Retrieved from https://www.healthit.gov/providers-professionals/meaningful-use-definition-objectives

HealthIT.gov. (n.d.). What does "interoperability" mean and why is it important. Retrieved from https://www.healthit.gov/providers-professionals/faqs/what-does-interoperability-mean-and-why-it-important

HealthIT.gov. (n.d.). What is meaningful use? Retrieved from http://www.healthit.gov/policy-researchers-implementers/meaningful-use

HealthIT.gov. (2013, January). Are there penalties for providers who don't switch to electronic health records (EHR)? Retrieved from https://www.healthit.gov/providers-professionals/faqs/are-there-penalties-providers-who-don%E2%80%99t-switch-electronic-health-record

Health Resources and Services Administration (of the HHS). (n.d.). Retrieved from http://www.hrsa.gov/index.html

Indian Health Service. (n.d.). Medicare and Medicaid incentives for EPs. Retrieved from https://www.ihs.gov/meaningfuluse/incentivesoverview/incentivesep/

Institute for Healthcare Improvement. (n.d.). The five rights of medication administration. Retrieved from http://www.ihi.org/resources/pages/improvementstories/fiverightsofmedicationadministration.aspx

Institute of Medicine of the National Academies. (2003, July 31). *Key capabilities of an electronic health record system.* Retrieved from http://www.iom.edu/Reports/2003/Key-Capabilities-of-an-Electronic-Health-Record-System.aspx

Internal Revenue Service. (2016, November). Questions and Answers about Reporting Social Security Numbers to Your Health Insurance Company. Retrieved from https://www.irs.gov/affordable-care-act/questions-and-answers-about-reporting-social-security-numbers-to-your-health-insurance-company.

Kaiser Family Foundation. (2016, September). Key facts about the uninsured population. Retrieved from http://kff.org/uninsured/fact-sheet/key-facts-about-the-uninsured-population/

Lowes, Robert. (2015, August). e-Prescribing controlled substances now legal nationwide. Retrieved from http://www.medscape.com/viewarticle/850268

"Meaningful Use." *Centers for Medicare and Medicaid Services.* (2014, February 8). Retrieved from http://www.cms.gov/Regulations-and-Guidance/Legislation/EHRIncentivePrograms/Meaningful_Use.html.

Medicare.gov. (n.d.). Your medicare coverage. Is my test, item, or service covered? Retrieved from https://www.medicare.gov/coverage/cervical-vaginal-cancer-screenings.html

Menachemi, N., & Collum, T. H. (2011). Benefits and drawbacks of electronic health record systems. *Risk Management and Healthcare Policy*, 4, 47–55. Retrieved from http://www .ncbi.nlm.nih.gov/pmc/articles/PMC3270933/

National Healthcareer Association. (n.d.). *Certified electronic health records specialist (CEHRS™).* Retrieved from http://www.nhanow.com/health-record.aspx

New Health Advisor. (2016). 10 rights of medication administration. http://www.newhealthadvisor.com/10-Rights-of-Medication-Administration.html

Rowley, R. (2011). *Ambulatory vs. hospital EHRs.* Retrieved from http://www.practicefusion.com/ehrbloggers/2011/07/ambulatory-vs-hospital-ehrs.html

SNOMED Overview: Clinical Terms and SNOMED Terminology Solutions. (2008, July 3). Retrieved from /files/HIMSSorg/content/files/snomed_101overview.pdf

The American Health Quality Association, Quality Update. (2003, August 22). Retrieved from www.ahqa.org

The Fiscal Times. (2016, May). Even with obamacare, 29 million people are uninsured; here's why. Retrieved from http://www.thefiscaltimes.com/2016/05/10/Even-Obamacare-29-Million-People-Are-Uninsured-Here-s-Why

U.S. Department of Commerce, U.S. Census Bureau, American National Standards Institute. (2013). Retrieved from http://www.census.gov/geo/www/ansi/ansi.html

U.S. Department of Health and Human Services. (n.d.). *HIPAA for Individuals.* Retrieved from http://www.hhs.gov/hipaa/for-individuals/index.html.

U.S. Department of Health and Human Services. (n.d.). *Summary of the HIPAA privacy rules.* Retrieved from http://www.hhs.gov/ocr/privacy/hipaa/understanding/summary/

U.S. Department of Health and Human Services. (2013, February 11). *Construction of LMS Parameters for the Centers for Disease Control and Prevention 2000 Growth Charts,* by Katherine M. Flegal, Ph.D., Office of the Director, National Center for Health Statistics; and Tim J. Cole, Ph.D., MRC Centre of Epidemiology for Child Health, Institute of Child Health, University College London, UK. National Health Statistics Report (No. 63). Retrieved from http://www.cdc.gov/nchs/data/nhsr/nhsr063.pdf

U.S. Department of Health and Human Services, National Institutes of Health. (n.d.). *What health information is protected by the privacy rule?* Retrieved from http://privacyruleandresearch.nih.gov/pr_07.asp

U.S. Drug Enforcement Administration. (n.d.). Retrieved from www.dea.gov

U.S. Food and Drug Administration. (2013, April 1). *CFR - Code of Federal Regulations Title 21.* Retrieved from http://www.accessdata.fda.gov/scripts/cdrh/cfdocs/cfCFR/CFRSearch.cfm?fr=155.3